I0036767

Teenage Reproductive Health: Pregnancy, Contraception, Unsafe Abortion, Fertility

Teenage Reproductive Health: Pregnancy, Contraception, Unsafe Abortion, Fertility

Special Issue Editor

Jon Øyvind Odland

MDPI • Basel • Beijing • Wuhan • Barcelona • Belgrade

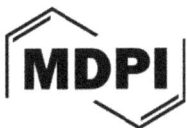

MDPI

Special Issue Editor
Jon Øyvind Odland
The Norwegian University for
Science and Technology
Norway

Editorial Office
MDPI
St. Alban-Anlage 66
Basel, Switzerland

This is a reprint of articles from the Special Issue published online in the open access journal *International Journal of Environmental Research and Public Health* (ISSN 1660-4601) from 2017 to 2018 (available at: http://www.mdpi.com/journal/ijerph/special_issues/teenage_reproductive_health)

For citation purposes, cite each article independently as indicated on the article page online and as indicated below:

LastName, A.A.; LastName, B.B.; LastName, C.C. Article Title. *Journal Name* **Year**, *Article Number*, Page Range.

ISBN 978-3-03897-061-3 (Pbk)
ISBN 978-3-03897-062-0 (PDF)

Articles in this volume are Open Access and distributed under the Creative Commons Attribution (CC BY) license, which allows users to download, copy and build upon published articles even for commercial purposes, as long as the author and publisher are properly credited, which ensures maximum dissemination and a wider impact of our publications. The book taken as a whole is © 2018 MDPI, Basel, Switzerland, distributed under the terms and conditions of the Creative Commons license CC BY-NC-ND (http://creativecommons.org/licenses/by-nc-nd/4.0/).

Contents

About the Special Issue Editor

Jon Øyvind Odland, Professor of Global Health. NTNU (the Norwegian University of Science and Technology). MD, PhD, Specialist Obstetrics, and Gynecology. Visiting Professor, Department of Public Health, University of Pretoria, South Africa (2013–); Visiting Professor, OB/GYN Department, College of Medicine, University of Malawi (2013–); Key National Expert, Sustainable Development Working Group, Arctic Council (2010–); President of the Norwegian Forum for Global Health Research (2009–2011); and Chair of AMAP Human Health Assessment Group (2009–). President, International Union of Circumpolar Health (2012–2015). Teacher and supervisor in Health Education, Obstetrics and Gynecology, and Public Health at Bachelor, Master, and PhD level in Norway, Russia, Denmark, Greenland, Faroe Island, Iceland, Canada, Malawi, South Africa, Zimbabwe, Ghana, Australia, Argentina, and Vietnam. Appr. 200 peer-reviewed publications in international journals.

Preface to "Teenage Reproductive Health: Pregnancy, Contraception, Unsafe Abortion, Fertility"

We are proud to present 14 papers that focus on teenager health in this Special Issue entitled "Teenage Reproductive Health: Pregnancy, Contraception, Unsafe Abortion, and Fertility".

Maternal mortality is still globally high, and reducing it is a top priority. Teenage pregnancies have more complications and are also unwanted in many cases. This contributes to high maternal mortality with both obstetric complications and the burden of unsafe abortion. Additionally, many teenagers live in areas with heavy pollution that affect the mother and the unborn child. Global public health is a very important issue that aims to prevent disease, prolong life, and promote physical, mental, and social well-being. Teenagers are the future, and maternal death is a disaster that should be prevented. Hence, research should aim to improve teenage reproductive health and influence policy makers. There are a variety of topics on this issue, with some conclusions and ways forward as described in different papers.

This book is meant to facilitate young scientists to develop studies and methodologies with the aim of improving teenage health, especially reproductive health on a global level. Young research, done by young people, for young people!

Jon Øyvind Odland
Special Issue Editor

International Journal of
*Environmental Research
and Public Health*

MDPI

Editorial

Teenage Reproductive Health: Pregnancy, Contraception, Unsafe Abortion, Fertility

Jon Øyvind Odland

Department of Public Health and Nursing, Faculty of Health Sciences, Norwegian University of Science and Technology (NTNU), 7491 Trondheim, Norway; jon.o.odland@ntnu.no

Received: 4 June 2018; Accepted: 4 June 2018; Published: 5 June 2018

We are proud to present 14 papers with focus on teenager health in this Special Issue entitled "Teenage Reproductive Health: Pregnancy, Contraception, Unsafe Abortion, Fertility".

Maternal mortality is still globally high and reducing it is a top priority. Teenage pregnancies have more complications and are also unwanted in many cases. This contributes to the high maternal mortality with both obstetric complications and burden of unsafe abortion. Additionally, many teenagers live in areas with heavy pollution that affects the mother and the unborn child. Global public health is a very important issue that aims to prevent disease, prolong life, and promote physical, mental and social well-being. Teenagers are the future, and maternal death is a disaster that should be prevented. Hence, research should aim to improve teenage reproductive health and influence policy makers. There are a variety of topics in this issue, with some conclusions and ways forward as described in different papers.

Oppong-Darko et al. [1] describe the dilemma between religious beliefs and traditions and the conflict with reproductive health and abortion laws in Ghana, which is a typical low-income country (LMIC). They conclude that the midwives make it clear that unsafe abortions are common, stigmatizing and contributing to maternal mortality, which are issues that must be addressed. They introduce various suggestions to reduce this preventable tragedy.

Grossman et al. [2] have a very interesting paper about parents' conversations with their teenagers about reproductive health and risks in sexual behavior. It seems like once teens entered high school, more parents described feelings comfortable with their conversations. However, parents also more often reported that their teens responded more negatively to the communication in high school than they had in middle school. These findings may help parents to anticipate their own as well as their teens' responses to family conversations about sex at different developmental time points and to strategize how to effectively talk with their teens about sex and relationships to improve their teens' overall reproductive health.

von Rosen et al. [3] describe how sexually transmitted infections (STIs) pose a significant threat to individual and public health. They disproportionately affect adolescents and young adults. In a cross-sectional study, they assessed self-rated and factual STI knowledge in a sample of 9th graders in 13 secondary schools in Berlin, Germany. Differences by age, gender, migrant background and school type were quantified. Knowledge of human immunodeficiency virus (HIV) was widespread, but other STIs were less known. Almost half of the participants had never heard of chlamydia, 10.8% knew the HPV vaccination, and only 2.2% were aware that no cure exists for HPV infection. While boys were more likely to describe their knowledge as good, there was no general gender superiority in factual knowledge. Overall, children of immigrants and students in the least academic schools had less knowledge. It seems that adolescents suffer from suboptimal levels of knowledge on STIs beyond HIV. Urgent efforts are needed to improve adolescent STI knowledge in order to improve the uptake of primary and secondary prevention.

Ninsiima et al. [4] went deep into the gender aspect in developing countries with their report from Uganda and wrote a paper titled "Girls Have More Challenges; They Need to Be Locked

Up": A Qualitative Study of Gender Norms and the Sexuality of Young Adolescents in Uganda. Unequal power and gender norms expose adolescent girls to high risks of HIV, early marriages, pregnancies and coerced sex. In Uganda, almost half of the girls below the age of 18 are already married or pregnant, which poses a danger to the lives of young girls. This study explores, in a very good way, the social construction of gender norms from early childhood, and how it influences adolescents' agency. Adolescents' agency appears constrained by context-specific obstacles. Programs targeting behavioral change need to begin early in the lives of young children. They should target teachers and parents about the values of gender equality and strengthen the legal system to create an enabling environment to address the health and wellbeing of adolescents.

Pradhan et al. [5] published a paper titled Factors Associated with Pregnancy among Married Adolescents in Nepal: Secondary Analysis of the National Demographic and Health Surveys from 2001 to 2011. They still find higher risk associated with living in the least resourced region, early sexual debut, and older husband. Despite national efforts to reduce pregnancies among married adolescent women in Nepal, prevalence remains high. Integrated and cross-sectoral prevention efforts are urgently required. A reduction in poverty and an improvement in infrastructure may also lead to lower rates of adolescent pregnancy.

Contributions to international health science from Russian authors are rapidly increasing. Usynina et al. [6] discuss adverse pregnancy outcomes among adolescents in Northwest Russia. The study is based on the upcoming and rapidly developing Arkhangelsk Birth Registry, aiming to assess whether adolescents have an increased risk of adverse pregnancy outcomes (APO), compared to adult women. Adolescents were more likely to be underweight, smoke, have infections of the kidney and the genital tract, compared to adult women. Compared to adults, adolescents were at lower risk of low birth weight, a 5 min Apgar score <7, and need for neonatal transfer. Adolescents had no increased risk of other APO studied in the adjusted analysis, suggesting that a constellation of other factors, but not young age per se, is associated with APO in the study setting.

Lafontan el al. state that it is very simple and easy to use electronic baby monitoring in Tanzania [7]. They carried out semi-structured individual interviews post-labor at two hospitals in Tanzania. The results indicated that the use of the monitor positively affected the women's birth experience. It provided much-needed reassurance about the wellbeing of the child. The women considered that wearing the Moyo improved care due to an increase in communication and attention from birth attendants. However, the women did not fully understand the purpose and function of the device and overestimated its capabilities.

Scientific literature from Kazakhstan is increasing and improving. The paper from Dauletyarova et al. [8] discusses if Kazakhstani women are satisfied with antenatal care, implementing the WHO tool to assess the quality of antenatal services. Ninety percent of the women were satisfied with the antenatal care. Women who were dissatisfied had lower education. These women would have preferred more checkups, shorter intervals between checkups, more time with care providers and shorter waiting times. The overall dissatisfaction was associated with long waiting time and insufficient information on general health in pregnancy, results of laboratory tests, treatment during pregnancy and breastfeeding.

Abortion policies are very important in teenager health in all parts of the world. Frederico et al. [9] discuss factors influencing abortion decision-making of young women in Mozambique. The study found determinants at different levels, including the low degree of autonomy for women, the limited availability of health facilities providing abortion services and a lack of patient-centeredness of health services. Strategies are suggested to increase knowledge of abortion rights and services, and to improve the quality and accessibility of abortion services in Mozambique.

Tsikouras et al. [10] describe ten years of experience in contraception options for teenagers in a family planning center in Greece, comparing its situation with developing countries. They conclude that during adolescence, the existence of a family planning center and participation in family planning programs play a crucial role in helping the teenagers to improve their knowledge and choose an effective contraception method. This is a very important and general finding.

Back in Africa, Odland et al. [11] discuss a serious reduction of the use of manual vacuum aspiration (MVA) in hospitals in Malawi. It is a cheap and safe method, included in national strategies, but with variable use in daily routines. However, there was a major increase in MVA application at one district hospital, probably because of good education and dedicated leadership. Even with national guidelines, the implementation and follow up is highly depending on local engagement and leadership.

Kemigisha et al. [12] deliver a very interesting report on adolescents' sexual wellbeing in Southwestern Uganda. The objective of the study was to assess sexual wellbeing in a broad sense (i.e., body image, self-esteem, and gender equitable norms) and associated factors in young adolescents in Uganda. The study with 58% females was carried out in 2016. Self-esteem and body image scores were high in both genders, but girls had higher scores, compared to boys for all outcomes. A higher age and being sexually active were associated with lower scores on gender equitable norms. Gender equitable norms scores decreased with increased age of adolescents. Comprehensive and timely sexuality education programs focusing on gender differences and norms were recommended.

Clarke et al. [13] have the only US study in the Special Issue. They discuss the histories of maltreated adolescents in treatment programs in Oregon, through a qualitative study. The results highlight the need for providing adolescent girls with reliable and practical information about risky sexual behavior and drug use from reliable and trustworthy helping professionals. Strategies for developing and maintaining trust and delivering specific content are important in all programs and their implementation.

Finally, Sharma and Nam [14] describe the condom use at last sexual intercourse and its correlates among males and females aged 15–49 Years in Nepal. Being unmarried was the most important predictor of condom use among males. Higher education was associated with increased likelihood of condom use in females. However, mobility, having multiple sexual partners and HIV knowledge were not significant correlates of condom use in both sexes. A big difference was observed in the variance accounted for males and females; indicating use of condoms was poorly predicted by the variables included in the study among females. Condom use was more associated with sociodemographic factors than with sexual behaviors and HIV knowledge.

There is a very important public health aspect in all the published papers in this Special Issue. Another good development is that young scientists are using the *International Journal of Environmental Research and Public Health* as a starting point in their career. All papers have been through a thorough review process, and many of them are now basis for the study towards academic degrees and introduction to further studies. Due to the age connection, young scientists are writing about health issues for young people. Let us hope for a new Special Issue soon, with contributions from other parts of the world. Teenagers have special health concerns in a very important transition period from child to adult. This is independent of geography, culture and religion. In total, this Special Issue provides very useful information for all parts of the world, even for those who are not presented in this nice collection of papers.

References

1. Oppong-Darko, P.; Amponsa-Achiano, K.; Darj, E. "I Am Ready and Willing to Provide the Service. Though My Religion Frowns on Abortion"—Ghanaian Midwives' Mixed Attitudes to Abortion Services: A Qualitative Study. *Int. J. Environ. Res. Public Health* **2017**, *14*, 1501. [CrossRef] [PubMed]
2. Grossman, J.M.; Jenkins, L.J.; Richer, A.M. Parents' Perspectives on Family Sexuality. Communication from Middle School to High School. *Int. J. Environ. Res. Public Health* **2018**, *15*, 107. [CrossRef] [PubMed]
3. Von Rosen, F.T.; von Rosen, A.J.; Müller-Riemenschneider, F.; Damberg, I.; Tinnemann, P. STI Knowledge in Berlin Adolescents. *Int. J. Environ. Res. Public Health* **2018**, *15*, 110. [CrossRef] [PubMed]
4. Ninsiima, A.B.; Leye, E.; Michielsen, K.; Kemigisha, E.; Nyakato, V.N.; Coene, G. "Girls Have More Challenges; They Need to Be Locked Up": A Qualitative Study of Gender Norms and the Sexuality of Young Adolescents in Uganda. *Int. J. Environ. Res. Public Health* **2018**, *15*, 193. [CrossRef] [PubMed]

5. Pradhan, R.; Wynter, K.; Fisher, J. Factors Associated with Pregnancy among Married Adolescents in Nepal: Secondary Analysis of the National Demographic and Health Surveys from 2001 to 2011. *Int. J. Environ. Res. Public Health* **2018**, *15*, 229. [CrossRef] [PubMed]

6. Usynina, A.A.; Postoev, V.; Odland, J.Ø.; Grjibovski, A.M. Adverse Pregnancy Outcomes among Adolescents in Northwest Russia: A Population Registry-Based Study. *Int. J. Environ. Res. Public Health* **2018**, *15*, 261. [CrossRef] [PubMed]

7. Lafontan, S.R.; Sundby, J.; Ersdal, H.L.; Abeid, M.; Kidanto, H.L.; Mbekenga, C.K. "I Was Relieved to Know That My Baby Was Safe": Women's Attitudes and Perceptions on Using a New Electronic Fetal Heart Rate Monitor during Labor in Tanzania. *Int. J. Environ. Res. Public Health* **2018**, *15*, 302. [CrossRef] [PubMed]

8. Dauletyarova, M.A.; Semenova, Y.M.; Kaylubaeva, G.; Manabaeva, G.K.; Toktabayeva, B.; Zhelpakova, M.S.; Yurkovskaya, O.A.; Tlemissov, A.S.; Antonova, G.; Grjibovski, A.M. Are KazakhstaniWomen Satisfied with Antenatal Care? Implementing the WHO Tool to Assess the Quality of Antenatal Services. *Int. J. Environ. Res. Public Health* **2018**, *15*, 325. [CrossRef] [PubMed]

9. Frederico, M.; Michielsen, K.; Arnaldo, C.; Decat, P. Factors Influencing Abortion Decision-Making Processes among Young Women. *Int. J. Environ. Res. Public Health* **2018**, *15*, 329. [CrossRef] [PubMed]

10. Tsikouras, P.; Deuteraiou, D.; Bothou, A.; Anthoulaki, X.; Chalkidou, A.; Chatzimichael, E.; Gaitatzi, F.; Manav, B.; Koukouli, Z.; Zervoudis, S.; et al. Ten Years of Experience in Contraception Options for Teenagers in a Family Planning Center in Thrace and Review of the Literature. *Int. J. Environ. Res. Public Health* **2018**, *15*, 348. [CrossRef] [PubMed]

11. Odland, M.L.; Membe-Gadama, G.; Kafulafula, U.; Jacobsen, G.W.; Kumwenda, J.; Darj, E. The Use of Manual Vacuum Aspiration in the Treatment of Incomplete Abortions: A Descriptive Study from Three Public Hospitals in Malawi. *Int. J. Environ. Res. Public Health* **2018**, *15*, 370. [CrossRef] [PubMed]

12. Kemigisha, E.; Nyakato, V.N.; Bruce, K.; Ruzaaza, G.N.; Mlahagwa, W.; Ninsiima, A.B.; Coene, G.; Leye, E.; Michielsen, K. Adolescents' Sexual Wellbeing in Southwestern Uganda: A Cross-Sectional Assessment of Body Image, Self-Esteem and Gender Equitable Norms. *Int. J. Environ. Res. Public Health* **2018**, *15*, 372. [CrossRef] [PubMed]

13. Clark, M.; Buchanan, R.; Leve, L.D. Young Women's Perspectives of Their Adolescent Treatment Programs: A Qualitative Study. *Int. J. Environ. Res. Public Health* **2018**, *15*, 373. [CrossRef] [PubMed]

14. Sharma, B.; Nam, E.W. Condom Use at Last Sexual Intercourse and Its Correlates among Males and Females Aged 15–49 Years in Nepal. *Int. J. Environ. Res. Public Health* **2018**, *15*, 535. [CrossRef] [PubMed]

© 2018 by the author. Licensee MDPI, Basel, Switzerland. This article is an open access article distributed under the terms and conditions of the Creative Commons Attribution (CC BY) license (http://creativecommons.org/licenses/by/4.0/).

International Journal of
*Environmental Research
and Public Health*

MDPI

Article

Condom Use at Last Sexual Intercourse and Its Correlates among Males and Females Aged 15–49 Years in Nepal

Bimala Sharma [1,2] and Eun Woo Nam [1,2,*]

1   Yonsei Global Health Center, Yonsei University, Wonju 03722, Korea; bimalasharma@gmail.com
2   Department of Health Administration, Graduate School, Yonsei University, Wonju 03722, Korea
*   Correspondence: ewnam@yonsei.ac.kr; Tel.: +82-33-760-2413; Fax: +82-33-762-9562

Received: 14 December 2017; Accepted: 13 March 2018; Published: 16 March 2018

Abstract: This study aimed to assess the prevalence and correlates of condom use at last sexual intercourse among people aged 15–49 years in Nepal. Secondary data analysis was performed using the Nepal Demographic and Health Survey 2011. The study was restricted to the respondents who reported ever having had sexual intercourse; 9843 females and 3017 males were included. Condom use was assessed by asking if respondents used condoms in their most recent sexual intercourse. Chi-square test and multivariate logistic regression analysis were performed using Complex Sample Analysis Procedure to adjust for sample weight and multistage sampling design. Overall, 7.6% of total, and 16.3% of males and 6.2% of females reported using condoms in their last sexual intercourse. Living in Far-Western region, age and wealth quintile were positively associated with condom use in both males and females. Being unmarried was the most important predictor of condom use among males. Higher education was associated with increased likelihood of condom use in females. However, mobility, having multiple sexual partners, and HIV knowledge were not significant correlates of condom use in both sexes. A big difference was observed in the variance accounted for males and females; indicating use of condoms is poorly predicted by the variables included in the study among females. Condom use was more associated with sociodemographic factors than with sexual behavior and HIV knowledge.

Keywords: condom use; correlates; sociodemographic factors; gender; multiple sexual partners; HIV knowledge; Nepal

1. Introduction

The shift towards later marriage in most countries has led to an increase in premarital sex. The prevalence of condom use has increased almost everywhere, but rates remain low in many developing countries [1]. Condoms, one method of family planning (FP), provide substantial protection against human immunodeficiency virus (HIV) infection [2]. Although the South Asian Region still has a low prevalence of HIV, the highest number of people with HIV outside Africa resides in India, a bordering country of Nepal. The importance of maintaining the low prevalence status in the region cannot be overemphasized [3].

Previous studies found that condom use was associated with a large number of community factors such as type of residence [4,5], socio-demographic factors such as age and sex [5–7], marital status [8–10], education [4,9], occupation [6,9,11], and economic status [1,5,7]. Previous studies show mixed evidences regarding the relationship between multiple sexual partners and condom use [11,12]. Greater knowledge of sexually transmitted infections (STIs) was also found to be associated with increased likelihood of condom use during the last sexual encounter [11].

The potential for HIV infection is increasing with the changing social and economic environment in Nepal. Increasing internal and international migration of the population, modernization, and development of transportation and communication networks are creating more favorable environments for social interactions between people. This is providing the opportunity for pre-marital, extramarital, and unsafe sexual activity among them, thereby increasing their risk of acquiring HIV and unwanted pregnancies [13–16]. Different studies conducted among young people have reported that unsafe sexual behavior is prevalent and increasing [15–18]. In addition, extramarital sexual intercourse is also not uncommon among adult population in Nepal [19,20]. The vulnerability of HIV infection among low risk population such as wives is expected to increase, which might bridge the infection to the general population [21]. Condoms are effective in preventing both pregnancy and STI/HIV [22]. Condom use varies by marital status, with unmarried individuals more likely to use them while married couples tend to choose hormonal or permanent FP methods to prevent unwanted pregnancies [23]. However, as both populations, unmarried and married individuals may be at risk of STIs and HIV, promoting condom use among both groups is one of the recommended strategies for dual protection; and this was the basis for conceiving the study.

The FP program is one of the priority programs of the Nepalese government. The Ministry of Health distributes condoms free of charge through all health facilities, including outreach clinics and Female Community Health Volunteers. However, their utilization seems low as compared to other birth spacing methods in Nepal [24]. Global trend analyses of sexual behavior recommend that public health interventions should address the broader determinants of sexual behavior, such as gender, poverty, and mobility, in addition to individual behavioral change [1]. Thus, a conceptual framework for action on the social determinants of health of the World Health Organization was considered to examine the factors associated with condom use in the study. This model highlights the importance of socioeconomic factors as determinants of behaviors [25]. Existing efforts to address HIV/STI vulnerability and risk in the population focus primarily on risk-taking behavior, and largely fail to address contextual issues that create and facilitate risky behavior and situations in Nepal [26]. Although existing literature shows that unsafe sexual practices conducive to transmitting HIV infection are prevalent, there is limited evidence regarding condom use among the general population. This study aimed to assess the prevalence and correlates of condom use at last sexual intercourse among males and females aged 15–49 years in Nepal.

2. Methods

2.1. Study Area, Study Design, and Sampling

Nepal is a developing country in Southeast Asia with a human development index of 0.548, and a life expectancy of 69.6 years [27]. Geographically, the country is divided into three ecological belts: the Northern Range Mountain, the Mid-range Hill, and the Southern Range Terai (flat land). An analytical, cross-sectional study was conducted from the secondary data of the Nepal Demographic and Health Survey (NDHS) 2011. A publicly available dataset was obtained from the MEASURE DHS website [28]. The dataset was created by merging relevant information from the women's questionnaire and the men's questionnaire. The details of the questionnaire and procedures can be found in the website and survey report [28,29].

The NDHS used a multistage cluster sampling procedure for data collection. In the first stage, a total of 95 urban and 194 rural enumeration areas (wards in the village development committees and sub wards in the municipalities) were selected using a proportionate probability sampling method. In the second stage, households within each enumeration area (EA) were selected using systematic sampling technique. In this stage, 35 households in each urban EA and 40 households in each rural EA were randomly selected. The NDHS 2011 completed a survey of 12,674 females and 4121 males. The study was restricted to the respondents who reported ever having had a sexual encounter in the past; 9843 females and 3017 males were selected for the analysis. Therefore, total sample size for the study was 12,860 individuals.

2.2. Measurement of Variables

2.2.1. Condom Use

Condom use was measured by the question, "Was a condom used the last time you had sexual intercourse?" The responses were categorized as (i) "yes = 1" and (ii) "no= 0" for the analysis, as measured in previous studies [6,8,11].

2.2.2. Explanatory Variables

The explanatory variables are shown in Table 1. Ethnicity was categorized into three groups: upper caste (Hill Brahmin, Hill Chhetri, Terai Brahmin, and Terai Chhetri), lower caste (Hill Dalit and Terai Dalit), and others (all other recorded ethnicities) [30]. Economic status was evaluated by NDHS 2011 using principal component analysis of more than 40 assets as variables [31]. The calculated score was divided into 5 quintiles and provided in the NDHS dataset ranging from poorest to richest. Most of the other variables were categorized as they were measured by the NDHS 2011 [29]. HIV knowledge was measured using ten relevant questions selected from the NDHS survey questionnaire (Table A1). Correct responses were coded as "1" and incorrect or uncertain responses were coded as "0". The items were summed to create an HIV knowledge score, with higher scores indicating more knowledge about HIV transmission and prevention [32].

2.3. Data Analysis Methods

The data were analyzed using SPSS version 24.0 (IBM Corp., Armonk, NY, USA). Descriptive statistics were used to describe the characteristics of the study population and the prevalence of condom use. The chi-square (χ^2) test was used to analyze the association between the explanatory variables and condom use. Multivariable logistic regression analysis was conducted in a hierarchical order adapting the concept from a previous study using the NDHS 2011 [33]. Model 1 comprised community factors, model 2 included the factors of model 1 and sociodemographic factors, model 3 included the factors of model 2 and behavioral factors, and model 4 comprised the factors of model 3 and HIV knowledge. The analyses were conducted separately for males and females. Adjusted odds ratios (AORs), 95% confidence intervals (CIs), and p values were presented. The level of significance was set at 5%. Based on the sample weights, strata, and cluster given in the survey dataset, a Complex Sampling Plan File was prepared. All the analyses were performed using the Complex Sample Analysis procedure, which is recommended to adjust for sample weight and multistage sampling using the DHS data [34].

2.4. Ethical Approval

The NDHS 2011 was approved by the Nepal Health Research Council and Ethical Review Board of ICF Macro International. The dataset is completely anonymous and distributed in the public domain. Therefore, an independent ethical approval was not required.

3. Results

Of a total of 12,860 respondents, 76.6% were females, 19.1% were in the age group of 25–29 years, and 93.9% respondents were married. Of the total number of participants, 41.1% had no formal schooling, 52.6% were involved in agriculture, and 17.0% respondents were from the poorest groups. In the study, 34.5% of the respondents were from the upper caste, and 84.6% were Hindus. The majority of the respondents were from the Terai region; 33.9% respondents were from Central development region; and 86.0% were from rural areas. In the last 12 months, 14.0% of the total respondents reported being away from home for more than one month. Of the total respondents, 12.3% had multiple sexual partners in their lifetime. Lifetime multiple sexual partnership was 28.7% among currently unmarried and 11.2% among married. The mean HIV knowledge score was 7.5 out of a maximum of 10. The mean age at first sex was 17.8 years. During their last sexual intercourse, 7.6% of the respondents, 16.3% of males, and 6.2% of females used condoms with their partners (Table 1).

Table 1. Sociodemographic Characteristics of the Study Population (*N* = 12,860).

Variables		Number	Percentage/Mean#
Sex	Male	3017	23.4
	Female	9843	76.6
Age group (in years)	15–24	3151	24.9
	25–29	2494	19.1
	30–34	2142	16.8
	35–39	2068	15.9
	40–49	3005	23.3
Ethnicity	Lower caste	1812	14.6
	Others caste	5846	50.9
	Uppers caste	5202	34.5
Religion	Others	802	7.0
	Buddha	1064	8.4
	Hindu	10,994	84.6
Current marital Status	Others	790	6.1
	Married	12070	93.9
Education	No education	5167	41.1
	Primary	2559	20.0
	Secondary	4030	30.9
	Higher	1104	8.0
Occupation	Did not work	2167	18.4
	Skilled/unskilled manual	1368	10.7
	Agriculture	6803	52.6
	Service *	2522	18.3
Wealth quintile	Poorest	2565	17.0
	Poorer	2334	18.7
	Middle	2399	21.0
	Richer	2540	21.3
	Richest	3022	21.9
Ecological region	Mountain	2094	6.5
	Hill	5000	39.8
	Terai	5766	53.7
Development region	Eastern	2971	23.6
	Central	3065	33.9
	Western	2292	20.6
	Mid-western	2445	12.2
	Far-western	2087	9.6
Type of residence	Urban	3639	14.0
	Rural	9221	86.0
Mobility	No	7826	60.2
	Yes	1821	14.0
	Missing	3360	25.8
Multiple sexual partners **	Yes	1627	12.3
HIV knowledge Score	Mean	11,009	7.5
Age at first sex	Mean	12,756	17.8
	Missing	1851	16.8
Condom use ***	No	10,193	79.5
	Yes	1106	7.6
	Missing	1561	12.9

* Professional/technical/managerial; ** 28.7% among currently unmarried and 11.2% among married; *** 16.3% of males and 6.2% of females; #Percentage was adjusted for sample weight, multistage sampling and cluster weight. Thus, the percentage is not equal to unweighted count.

Table 2 shows the proportions of condom use by explanatory variables. Condom use at last sexual intercourse was more than double among males than among females (16.3% vs. 6.2%). The percentage of people using condoms was found decreased along with the increase in age, ranging from 14.0% in the age group of 15–24 years to 4% in the age group of 40–49 years. The highest proportion of condom use (11.3%) was found in the upper caste and the lowest (4.2%) in the lower caste. Condom use percentage was almost similar across different religious groups ranging from 7.6% among other religious group to 8.9% among Hindus. The percentage of people who used condoms at last sexual episode was 62.3% among respondents currently unmarried, and 7.3% among those married. The frequency of condom use was 3.2% in the no schooling group and 24.3% among the respondents with higher education. Similarly, the proportion of condom use was lowest (5.5%) among agricultural workers and the highest (15.8%) among service holders. Use of condoms was 4% in the poorest and 16.1% in the richest wealth quintile. The highest proportion of condom use (10%) was found in the Hill region, while the lowest (5.9%) in the Mountain region. Regarding the development region, condom use percentage was highest (14.0%) in the Far-Western region and the lowest (7.3%) in the Central region. Condom use was 15.0% among the individuals from urban area and 7.7% from rural area. The frequency of condom use was double among participants with multiple sexual partners than among those who did not have (14.6% vs. 7.9%).

Among the currently unmarried sample also, more males used condoms than females (68.3% vs. 20.9%). Use of condoms at last sexual intercourse was 69.1% among respondents of 15 to 24 years where as it was 0% among those who were in the age group of 40 to 49 years. Similarly, condom use frequency was 70.7% among respondents with higher education where as it was 19.8% among those who did not have formal education. The proportion of condom use was lowest (46.0%) among agricultural workers and highest (74.4%) among service holders. Condom use percentage was highest (80.3%) among the respondents belonging to richer group and the lowest (39.5%) among those who were from the poorest group. Ethnicity, religion, place of residence (by region and type), mobility, having multiple sexual partners did not have significant association with condom use among currently unmarried respondents.

Table 2. Condom Use by Sociodemographic and Behavioral Characteristics.

Variables	Categories	Total Sample (N = 11,299)				Unmarried Sample (N = 284)			
		n	%#	χ^2 Value	*p* Value	*n*	%#	χ^2 Value	*p* Value
Gender	Male	2837	16.3	268.67	<0.001	245	68.3	30.23	0.000
	Female	8462	6.2			39	20.9		
Age group (in years)	15–24	2780	14.0	182.55	<0.001	215	69.1	NA	NA
	25–29	2187	9.8			39	61.6		
	30–34	1907	7.9			15	30.3		
	35–39	1817	7.0			6	41.7		
	40–49	2608	4.0			9	0.0		
Ethnicity	Lower caste	1593	4.2	75.77	<0.001	32	53.2	1.59	0.581
	Others caste	5084	8.3			146	64.4		
	Uppers caste	4622	11.3			106	62.6		
Religion	Others	680	7.6	1.54	0.764	24	62.3	0.207	0.930
	Buddha	876	8.7			31	66.7		
	Hindu	9743	8.9			229	61.9		
Marital status	Others	284	62.3	1084.91	<0.001	NA	NA	NA	NA
	Married	11,015	7.3			NA	NA		
Education	No schooling	4428	3.2	614.72	<0.001	25	19.8	41.68	<.001
	Primary	2259	5.3			34	35.9		
	Secondary	3590	13.9			145	73.2		
	Higher	1022	24.3			80	70.7		
Occupation	Did not work	1911	10.0	216.76	<0.001	64	63.4	14.08	<0.008
	Manual	1225	9.8			50	58.5		
	Agriculture	5870	5.5			70	46.0		
	Service *	2293	15.8			100	74.4		

Table 2. *Cont.*

Variables	Categories	Total Sample (N = 11,299)				Unmarried Sample (N = 284)			
		n	%#	χ^2 Value	*p* Value	*n*	%#	χ^2 Value	*p* Value
Wealth quintile	Poorest	2243	4.3	258.43	<0.001	28	39.5	18.84	0.006
	Poorer	2047	5.7			45	47.5		
	Middle	2093	6.6			47	57.9		
	Richer	2189	9.4			62	80.3		
	Richest	2727	16.1			102	64.8		
Ecological region	Mountain	1872	5.9	18.491	0.018	36	52.9	0.715	0.597
	Hill	4347	10.0			112	61.3		
	Terai	5080	8.2			136	64.0		
Development region	Eastern	2515	8.2	50.406	0.001	63	72.8	10.04	0.058
	Central	2751	7.3			72	58.1		
	Western	1936	8.8			60	63.4		
	Mid-western	2215	9.5			53	43.8		
	Far-western	1882	14.0			36	73.5		
Type of residence	Rural	8043	7.7	93.80	<0.001	182	62.0	0.070	0.068
	Urban	3256	15.0			102	63.9		
Mobility	No	6604	8.8	22.99	<0.001	149	61.3	0.902	0.389
	Yes	1568	12.7			91	67.4		
Multiple sexual partners	No	9779	7.9	72.85	<0.001	137	60.6	0.342	0.621
	Yes	1520	14.6			147	63.9		

n = number, % = percentage, χ^2 chi-square; * Professional/technical/managerial; #Percentage was adjusted for sample weight, multistage sampling and cluster weight. Thus, the percentage is not equal to unweighted count.

Table 3 shows the logistic regression analysis of factors associated with condom use among males. In model 1, all three variables: ecological region, development region, and residence were significantly associated with condom use. In model 2, development region, age group, marital status, education, and wealth quintile were significantly associated with it. In model 3, all significant variables in model 2 except education and age at first sexual intercourse were significant. In model 4, all significant variables in model 3 remained significant, and HIV knowledge did not have any significant effect on condom use. Table 4 shows the logistic regression analysis of factors associated with condom use among females. In model 1, all three variables were significantly associated with condom use. In model 2, ecological region, development region, age group, ethnicity, marital status, education, and wealth quintile were significantly associated with it. In model 3, all significant variables in model 2 except ethnicity and marital status were significant. In model 4, all significant variables in model 3 remained significant, and HIV knowledge did not have any significant effect on condom use.

In the adjusted analysis (model 4), as compared to the Eastern region, males living in the Far-Western region and females living in the Mid-Western and the Far-Western region had increased probability of using condoms. Older age group was statistically associated with lower use of condoms in both sexes, but the association was significant only for those belonging to 40–49 years as compared to the respondents of 15–24 years among females. Occupation and religion were not associated with condom use in both males and females. However, belonging to higher wealth quintile was associated with higher condom use in both sexes. Males belonging to richer and richest group were 110% and 225%, respectively, more likely to use condoms as compared to the poorest males. Females belonging to poorer, middle, richer, and richest group were 99%, 119%, 183%, and 383%, respectively, more likely to use them as compared to the poorest females. Mobility, multiple sexual partners, and HIV knowledge did not have association with use of condom in both sexes (Tables 3 and 4).

Unmarried males were more likely (AOR, 12.8; CI, 8.2–20.0) to use condoms in their last sexual intercourse as compared to married males. Similarly, higher age at first sexual intercourse was associated with higher use of condoms among them (Table 3).

Table 3. Logistic Regression Analysis of Factors Associated with Condom Use among Males.

Factors	Variables		Adjusted OR (95% CIs)		
		Model 1	Model 2	Model 3	Model 4
Community factors	Ecological region	$p = 0.011$	$p = 0.147$	$p = 0.099$	$p = 0.037$
	Mountain	1	1	1	1
	Hill	1.89 (1.24–2.87)	1.58 (0.96–2.59)	1.48 (0.85–2.58)	1.54 (0.88–2.69)
	Terai	1.70 (1.11–2.62)	1.30 (0.78–2.16)	1.04 (0.58–1.87)	1.01 (0.55–1.82)
	Development region	$p = 0.027$	$p < 0.001$	$p < 0.001$	$p < 0.001$
	Eastern	1	1	1	1
	Central	0.74 (0.48–1.15)	0.75 (0.47–1.19)	0.81 (0.48–1.38)	0.82 (0.48–1.40)
	Western	1.06 (0.68–1.67)	1.07 (0.66–1.72)	1.48 (0.86–2.54)	1.55 (0.88–2.73)
	Mid-Western	1.08 (0.67–1.74)	1.44 (0.84–2.49)	1.53 (0.82–2.85)	1.63 (0.87–3.06)
	Far-Western	1.61 (0.94–2.76)	2.57 (1.46–4.52)	3.77 (2.08–6.82)	4.28 (2.31–7.93)
	Type of residence	$p < 0.001$	$p = 0.109$	$p = 0.679$	$p = 0.823$
	Rural	1	1	1	1
	Urban	1.98 (1.50–2.61)	1.33 (0.93–1.91)	1.08 (0.73–1.60)	0.95 (0.64–1.41)
	Age group (in years)		$p < 0.001$	$p < 0.001$	$p < 0.001$
	15–24		0.67 (0.45–0.99)	0.52 (0.33–0.81)	0.50 (0.32–0.80)
	25–29		0.47 (0.29–0.75)	0.45 (0.26–0.76)	0.45 (0.26–0.77)
	30–34		0.53 (0.34–0.81)	0.43 (0.26–0.70)	0.44 (0.27–0.72)
	35–39		0.32 (0.20–0.51)	0.27 (0.15–0.50)	0.26 (0.14–0.48)
	40–49				
	Ethnicity		$p = 0.092$	$p = 0.197$	$p = 0.215$
	Lower caste		1	1	1
	Others		1.56 (0.94–2.59)	1.60 (0.92–2.77)	1.57 (0.90–2.72)
	Upper caste		1.75 (1.05–2.92)	1.64 (0.93–2.90)	1.63 (0.92–2.89)
	Religion		$p = 0.945$	$p = 0.774$	$p = 0.527$
	Others		1	1	1
	Buddha		1.14 (0.50–2.61)	1.13 (0.46–2.76)	1.17 (0.47–2.92)
	Hindu		1.09 (0.60–1.98)	0.92 (0.47–1.80)	0.85 (0.44–1.66)
Sociodemographic factors	Marital status		$p < 0.001$	$p < 0.001$	$p < 0.001$
	Married		1	1	1
	Others		10.71 (7.28–15.77)	11.88 (7.67–18.36)	12.88 (8.27–20.05)
	Education		$p = 0.007$	$p = 0.116$	$p = 0.178$
	No schooling		1	1	1
	Primary		0.77 (0.39–1.50)	0.81 (0.36–1.83)	0.99 (0.41–2.39)
	Secondary		1.49 (0.85–2.61)	1.50 (0.73–3.09)	1.67 (0.77–3.63)
	Higher		1.74 (0.94–3.20)	1.30 (0.60–2.83)	1.39 (0.60–3.19)

Table 3. *Cont.*

Factors	Variables		Adjusted OR (95% CIs)		
		Model 1	Model 2	Model 3	Model 4
Occupation	Did not work		$p = 0.638$	$p = 0.650$	$p = 0.826$
	Manual		1	1	1
	Agriculture		0.70 (0.31–1.56)	0.78 (0.30–2.03)	0.76 (0.29–2.00)
	Service *		0.66 (0.29–1.50)	0.60 (0.22–1.64)	0.67 (0.24–1.87)
			0.80 (0.36–1.79)	0.78 (0.30–2.04)	0.81 (0.31–2.15)
Wealth quintile	Poorest		$p = 0.003$	$p = 0.001$	$p < 0.001$
	Poorer		1	1	1
	Middle		0.74 (0.43–1.27)	0.64 (0.33–1.22)	0.74 (0.39–1.41)
	Richer		1.18 (0.67–2.08)	1.09 (0.54–2.20)	1.28 (0.65–2.52)
	Richest		1.50 (0.88–2.55)	1.68 (0.91–3.10)	2.10 (1.18–3.74)
			2.21 (1.19–4.11)	2.41 (1.15–5.06)	3.25 (1.59–6.64)
Behavioral factors	Mobility			$p = 0.907$	$p = 0.566$
	No			1	1
	Yes			1.02 (0.71–1.45)	1.11 (0.77–1.60)
	Multiple sex partners			$p = 0.743$	$p = 0.916$
	No			1	1
	Yes			1.05 (0.78–1.41)	1.01 (0.74–1.38)
	Age at first sex			$p = 0.015$	$p = 0.009$
				1.07 (1.01–1.14)	1.08 (1.02–1.15)
HIV knowledge	HIV knowledge				$p = 0.163$
					0.90 (0.79–1.04)
Cox and Snell R^2		0.018	0.191	0.211	0.220

p indicates p value and is placed before the reference value for each variable, CIs: confidence intervals, OR: odds ratio; * Professional/technical/managerial.

Table 4. Logistic Regression Analysis of Factors Associated with Condom Use among Females.

Factors	Variables		Adjusted OR (95% CIs)			
			Model 1	Model 2	Model 3	Model 4
Community factors	Ecological region		*p* = 0.034	*p* = 0.003	*p* = 0.012	*p* = 0.010
		Mountain	1	1	1	1
		Hill	1.63 (1.08–2.47)	1.22 (0.81–1.82)	1.01 (0.65–1.56)	0.99 (0.63–1.54)
		Terai	1.30 (0.86–1.98)	0.78 (0.51–1.20)	0.66 (0.41–1.07)	0.65 (0.40–1.06)
	Development regions		*p* < 0.001	*p* < 0.001	*p* < 0.001	*p* < 0.001
		Eastern	1	1	1	1
		Central	0.83 (0.56–1.23)	0.80 (0.55–1.15)	0.96 (0.62–1.49)	0.87 (0.58–1.31)
		Western	1.02 (0.69–1.53)	1.02 (0.70–1.49)	1.09 (0.71–1.67)	1.05 (0.68–1.62)
		Mid-western	1.34 (0.90–1.99)	1.92 (1.33–2.78)	1.99 (1.25–3.14)	1.91 (1.21–3.01)
		Far-western	2.21 (1.56–3.12)	3.89 (2.69–5.62)	4.21 (2.64–6.69)	3.83 (2.40–6.10)
	Type of residence		*p* < 0.001	*p* = 0.330	*p* = 0.711	*p* = 0.473
		Rural	1	1	1	1
		Urban	2.23 (1.75–2.84)	1.13 (0.88–1.45)	1.05 (0.80–1.38)	1.10 (0.83–1.47)
	Age group (in years)			*p* < 0.001	*p* = 0.001	*p* = 0.001
		15–24		1	1	1
		25–29		0.90 (0.68–1.19)	0.84 (0.61–1.14)	0.84 (0.61–1.15)
		30–34		0.82 (0.60–1.11)	0.75 (0.52–1.07)	0.71 (0.49–1.04)
		35–39		0.68 (0.46–0.99)	0.65 (0.41–1.03)	0.65 (0.41–1.03)
		40–49		0.41 (0.28–0.61)	0.34 (0.20–0.56)	0.29 (0.16–0.51)
	Ethicality			*p* = 0.013	*p* = 0.149	*p* = 0.071
		Lower caste		1	1	1
		Others		1.95 (1.25–2.06)	1.64 (0.98–2.74)	1.82 (1.08–3.06)
		Upper caste		1.73 (1.13–2.64)	1.58 (0.97–2.56)	1.61 (0.97–2.68)
	Religion			*p* = 0.255	*p*=0.124	*p* = 0.326
		Other		1	1	1
		Buddha		1.16 (0.59–2.25)	1.10 (0.54–2.25)	1.04 (0.48–2.22)
		Hindu		0.82 (0.50–1.33)	0.71 (0.42–1.22)	0.76 (0.41–1.41)
Sociodemographic factors	Marital status			*p* = 0.037	*p* = 0.132	*p* = 0.078
		Married		1	1	1
		Others		2.96 (1.06–8.26)	2.29 (0.77–6.81)	2.85 (0.88–9.25)
	Education			*p* < 0.001	*p* < 0.001	*p* = 0.001
		No schooling		1	1	1
		Primary		1.25 (0.90–1.73)	1.07 (0.73–1.58)	1.00 (0.67–1.49)
		Secondary		2.41 (1.71–3.41)	1.93 (1.30–2.87)	1.66 (1.14–2.42)
		Higher		3.96 (2.66–5.88)	2.76 (1.70–4.49)	2.57 (1.56–4.24)

Table 4. *Cont.*

Factors	Variables		Adjusted OR (95% CIs)		
		Model 1	Model 2	Model 3	Model 4
	Occupation				
	Did not work		$p = 0.833$	$p = 0.998$	$p = 0.999$
	Manual		1	1	1
	Agriculture		0.86 (0.42–1.76)	0.98 (0.41–2.29)	0.98 (0.45–2.10)
	Service *		0.90 (0.67–1.19)	0.97 (0.70–1.33)	1.01 (0.71–1.42)
			0.88 (0.66–1.17)	0.98 (0.71–1.36)	1.01 (0.73–1.41)
	Wealth quintile		$p < 000$	$p < 0.001$	$p < 0.001$
	Poorest		1	1	1
	Poorer		1.97 (1.31–2.98)	2.25 (1.43–3.52)	1.99 (1.27–3.11)
	Middle		2.09 (1.34–3.27)	2.28 (1.34–3.88)	2.19 (1.25–3.83)
	Richer		2.61 (1.63–4.18)	3.20 (1.87–5.46)	2.83 (1.63–4.90)
	Richest		4.31 (2.55–7.28)	5.51 (3.09–9.82)	4.83 (2.63–8.87)
	Mobility				
	No			$p = 0.938$	$p = 0.989$
	Yes			1	1
				0.98 (0.67–1.42)	0.99 (0.68–1.45)
Behavioral factors	Multiple sex partners				
	No			$p = 0.908$	$p = 0.967$
	Yes			1	1
				0.95 (0.45–2.03)	0.98 (0.45–2.11)
	Age at first sex			$p = 0.186$	$p = 0.229$
				1.03 (0.98–1.07)	1.02 (0.97–1.07)
Knowledge	HIV knowledge				$p = 0.554$
					1.03 (0.92–1.15)
Cox and Snell R^2		0.012	0.053	0.055	0.054

p indicates p value and is placed before the reference value for each variable, CIs: confidence intervals, ORs: odds ratios; * Professional/technical/managerial.

Females from the upper caste were more likely to use condoms than the females of the lower caste. Similarly, education was significantly associated with condom use only in females. Females belonging to primary and secondary education were 66% and 157%, respectively, more likely to use condoms in their last sexual intercourse as compared to the females from no formal schooling (Table 4).

The Cox and Snell R^2 was 1.8% in model 1, 19.1% in model 2, 21.1% in model 3, and 22.0% in model 4 among males (Table 3). Similarly, Cox and Snell R^2 values of 1.2%, 5.3%, 5.5%, and 5.4% were obtained in model 1, model 2, model 3, and model 4, respectively, among females (Table 4). These meant that 22.0% and 5.4% variation in the frequency of condom use was determined by the factors of model 4 among males and females, respectively, in Nepal. It shows that condom use is mostly affected by sociodemographic factors than behavioral factors and HIV knowledge. In addition, the variation of the Cox and Snell R^2 values among males and females shows that, unlike among males, condom use among females was less likely to be determined by the factors included in the models.

4. Discussion

The study identified the prevalence of condom use at last sexual intercourse and associated factors among 15–49 years male and female population in Nepal. A low prevalence of condom use at last sexual intercourse was found, and sociodemographic factors were significantly associated with condom use among a large sample of general population. Being male, being unmarried, and being young were most important. Unlike this study, most of the previous studies on condom use in Nepal dealt with particular type of people, especially high-risk population for HIV and among small samples.

The prevalence of condom use was further low among females as compared to males in the study. We found a shortage of evidence on condom use prevalence among the general population in Nepal. Small scale studies show low and irregular use of condoms even among casual partners [15–17,35]. In India, 4.8% of ever married women of 15–49 years reported condom use at their last sexual intercourse; and condom use was 32% with husband and 38% with boyfriend among young urban women [6,36]. As condoms are recognized as birth control, married heterosexual people may be reluctant to use them for HIV prevention. Although family planning services have emphasized condom use, this method represented only 3.5% in total contraceptive prevalence rate in Nepal. Use of other FP methods such as hormonal contraceptives and sterilization are most popular among women in Nepal [24]. In Nepal, men who reported a desire to have no more children were more likely to choose permanent methods [37]. Couples in which either husband or wife have been sterilized or women using other hormonal methods usually do not consider using condoms [23]. Therefore, low use of condoms might be because most of the participants were married and condoms are less likely to be used in such relationships, that they are not even considered as methods of family planning. Low perceived susceptibility for HIV infection and low felt need for FP could be why condoms were not used.

The chi-square test showed that males were more likely to report condom use during their most recent sexual intercourse. The gender difference of condom use exists in total as well as unmarried samples in the study. Thus, we conducted gender-disaggregated analysis to find out correlates of condom use. There is a gender difference around sex, with women having fewer opportunities and less freedom than young men in Nepal [38]. This situation affects women's possibility of asking for and using condoms with partners. A similar result was found in a previous study, where gender played a significant role in decision making in condom use; men were more likely to take decisions on condom use than women [39]. A study among female sex workers reports that violence from partners, resistance from partners, and lack of negotiation capacity were the important reasons for non-use of condoms with husbands and clients [40]. Condom use is with linked with commercial sex work; if a woman suggests or insists that her husband use condoms, he may believe that she suspects him of having a STD or being HIV positive [23]. Thus, it seems more unlikely to suggest or insist condom use with husbands and regular partners. Greater emphasis must be given to addressing the gender discrimination embedded in Nepalese culture to vulnerability to HIV/STI infection [26]. In the study, difference in the variance accounted for males and females in models notably reflects the issue related to gender power relation; perhaps the most important determinant of condom use among women might be their partners' interest or decision than the factors included in the study.

Older age was associated with a lower frequency of condom use in the study. Age is linked with awareness, marital status, and opportunity of having multiple sexual partners, which might influence condom use. Marital status was one of the most important determinants of condom use at last sexual episode among males. Condoms are more preferred with casual sexual partners than with a regular sex partner [10,23]. However, marital status did not influence condom use among females. The global trend shows that married women find negotiation of safer sex and use of condoms for FP more difficult than do single women [1]. A low proportion of unmarried females in the study might have influenced the association. In India, most married women have societal pressure to prove their fertility and they might not see any reason to use condoms as contraception. In addition, women may not consider condoms because they believe condoms interfere with their efforts to establish their relation with husbands or partners [23]. Likewise, a study in South Africa found widespread disapproval of condom use within marriage [4]. Type of sexual partner was the strongest predictor of condom use; it was higher among men who reported last sex with a casual partner [10]. It shows condom use is linked with casual sex and not considered within marital union. The misconception and reasons of non-use of condoms in marital relation need to be explored and addressed in Nepal.

Living in an urban or rural area did not influence use of condoms; rather there might be other factors which determine their use or non-use. However, development region had a significant effect on condom use in both sexes and ecological region among females. It indicates that some administrative regions and ecological regions are better for using condoms. In Nepal, a large number of health indicators are better in urban areas, and Central and Western development regions [23,25], but this was not true for condom use. As compared to the Eastern region, males living in Far-Western, and females living in Far-Western and Mid-Western regions had a significantly higher likelihood of condom use. The Far-Western region is considered as the most vulnerable region for HIV due to labor migration to India. The disease is commonly known as Mumbai disease in the region, because labor migrants who returned from Mumbai, a city of India, carry the infection with them [41,42]. Higher condom use in the region is a positive finding, but it is not sufficient to prevent new HIV infection [43].

The majority of the people in Nepal are Hindus. However, religion did affect use of condoms among males and female. Regarding ethnicity, condom use was significantly higher among the upper caste females as compared to the lower caste females. However, ethnicity did not have any effect on condom use among males. In general, use of condoms was not affected by religious as well as caste affiliation in Nepal. The condom promotion program should equally focus across people from all religion and ethnicity.

This study revealed that education did not have any significant association with condom use among males; but there was a significant association among females. This shows that formally educated women might have better negotiation power and skill for condom use with their partners. Higher education had higher odds of condom use in previous studies in different study settings [5,10]. Although there was a statistically significant association between education and condom use, total variance predicted by the analysis models was very low in females. This clearly shows that there are other factors not included in the study that determine use of condoms among females. The probability of condom use was higher among respondents belonging to poorer, middle, richer, and the richest groups as compared to the poorest group. Higher economic status might be associated with other factors such as awareness level and affordability of condoms at the time of need. Although condoms are provided free of charge through all government health facilities in Nepal [24], economic status might be associated with the capacity to afford condoms from private pharmacies due to issues regarding quality, confidentiality, or getting them at the time of need. Low condom use was also observed in the poor and middle wealth quintiles in a previous study from other countries [5]. However, use of condoms was not affected by the type of job people did in the study. Some studies in other countries show that occupation was correlated with condom use [9,11]. Thus, condom promotion should focus more on people of poor socioeconomic status.

In Nepal, both internal and international migration has been increasing in the last 2 decades; this is linked to the possibility of HIV transmission. In a study among returnee labor migrants from overseas in Nepal, 49% of respondents had sex with paid/unpaid partners, and only 61% used condom always [13]. The current study shows mobility was not significantly associated with condom use in both sexes in the adjusted analysis. This indicates increasing vulnerability of HIV transmission to the general population. In addition, both the married and unmarried population had had multiple sexual partners in their lifetimes. In the multivariable analysis, having multiple sexual partners was not statistically associated with condom use among both males and females. In Nepal, condoms are not usually considered among married couples. As most of the respondents were married, the last sexual intercourse might not have been with a casual partner. This might be one reason of insignificant association. However, the chi-square test shows having multiple sexual partners was also not significant with condom use among unmarried respondents. This shows both married and unmarried people are at risk of HIV transmission in Nepal. Older age at first sex was associated with increased likelihood of reporting condom use among male respondents. A study conducted in Botswana also reported that age at first sex was positively correlated to condom use for both males and females [9]. This might indicate responsible sexual behavior among those whose sexual debut was delayed.

It is supposed that use of condoms is increased along with an increase in HIV related knowledge among people. However, higher HIV knowledge was also not associated with condom use in both sexes in the study. In a study conducted in India, knowledge on HIV prevention was significantly associated with condom use during last sex with husband [6]. Greater knowledge of STIs was also found to be associated with increased likelihood of condom use during the last sexual encounter in Jamaica [11]. Despite a high level of knowledge, reported condom use was very low among young migrant factory workers in Nepal, as reported in a previous study [15]. This finding may indicate that providing knowledge about HIV infection alone is not sufficient to promote condom use in Nepal.

4.1. Limitation of the Study

The study is based on the large national survey conducted using standard questionnaire and survey procedure. The study still has some limitations. First, the survey type may induce behavioral desirability bias. Individuals may be reticent or embarrassed to express their real sexual behavior. It is challenging to validate the respondents' answers. Second, due to cross-sectional nature of the survey, cause and effect relationships could not be established. Third, as there was limited literature, some references are compared and discussed from non-similar settings in spite of different HIV risk and contexts.

4.2. Implication of the Study

Gender, age, marital status, education, economic status, and place of residence are important factors associated with condom use among general population of Nepal. The study also shows that condom use is mostly affected by sociodemographic factors than multiple sexual partnership and HIV knowledge. Thus, condom promotion is a multi-dimensional issue. The government of Nepal should consider these social determinants to promote condom use for dual protections: unwanted births and HIV infection. The Ministry of Health should collaborate with other social sectors such as gender development, education, finance, and local development etc. In addition, the difference in variance accounted for males and females shows that condom use among females is mostly affected by the factors other than included in the study models; perhaps it would be their partner's willingness and decision. Further studies, especially qualitative studies are required to explore reasons of non-use of condoms among females.

5. Conclusions

The prevalence of condom use at last sexual intercourse was low in Nepal. Living in the Far-Western region, younger age, upper caste, and belonging to a higher wealth quintile were significantly associated with the increased likelihood of condom use in both sexes. However, religion, occupation, and residence type were not significant correlates of condom use. Similarly, HIV knowledge, having multiple sexual partners, and mobility also did not have significant association with condom use in both males and females. Being currently unmarried was the most important predictor of using condoms at most recent sexual encounter in males. Higher education was significantly associated with an increased probability of condom use in females. The study shows that condom use was more predicted by sociodemographic factors rather than mobility, multiple sexual partnership, and HIV knowledge. However, as low variance was predicted among females, condom use might be more determined by the willingness of their partners and gender power relation. A condom promotion program should consider social determinants such as gender, age, marital status, ethnicity, education, and economic status. Condom promotion should equally focus on both urban and rural areas. Geographical accessibility of condoms and knowledge of HIV infection might not be sufficient to make people use condoms.

Acknowledgments: We are grateful to the USAID, Ministry of Health, Nepal, and New Era for conducting the survey and making the data publicly available. We thank all participants and organizations involved directly and indirectly for the conduction of this survey. No funding sources received for reporting of this study.

Author Contributions: Bimala Sharma and Eun Woo Nam conceived and designed the study. Bimala Sharma analyzed the data and prepared the manuscript. Eun Woo Nam critically reviewed and revised the manuscript. All authors approved the final version of the manuscript.

Conflicts of Interest: The authors declare no conflict of interest.

Appendix A

Table A1. Assessment of HIV Knowledge.

Number of Questions	Questions Asked	Coding
1	Have you heard of about other infections that can be transmitted through sexual contact (STI)?	Yes = 1 No = 0
2	Have you ever heard of an illness called AIDS?	Yes = 1 No = 0
3	Can people reduce their chances of acquiring the AIDS virus by having just one uninfected sex partner who has no other sex partners?	Yes = 1 No/Do not know = 0
4	Can people reduce their chances of acquiring the AIDS virus by using a condom every time they have sex?	Yes = 1 No/Do not know = 0
5	Can people acquire the AIDS virus from mosquito bites?	No = 1 Yes/Do not know = 0
6	Is it possible for a healthy looking person to have the AIDS virus?	Yes = 1 No/Do not know = 0
7	Can one get HIV by sharing food with a person who has AIDS?	No = 1 Yes/Do not know = 0
8	Can HIV be transmitted from a mother to her baby during delivery?	Yes = 1 No/Do not know = 0
9	Can HIV be transmitted from a mother to her baby by breastfeeding?	Yes = 1 No/Do not know = 0
10	Are there any special drugs that a doctor or nurse can give to a woman infected with the AIDS virus to reduce the risk of transmission to the baby?	Yes = 1 No/Do not know = 0

References

1. Wellings, K.; Collumbien, M.; Slaymaker, E.; Singh, S.; Hodges, Z.; Patel, D.; Bajos, N. Sexual behaviour in context: A global perspective. *Lancet* **2006**, *368*, 1706–1728. [CrossRef]
2. Pinkerton, S.D.; Abramson, P.R. Effectiveness of condoms in preventing HIV transmission. *Soc. Sci. Med.* **1997**, *44*, 1303–1312. [CrossRef]
3. Rodrigo, C.; Rajapakse, S. Current Status of HIV/AIDS in South Asia. *J. Glob. Infect. Dis.* **2009**, *1*, 93–101. [CrossRef] [PubMed]
4. Maharaj, P.; Cleland, J. Condom use within marital and cohabiting partnerships in KwaZulu-Natal, South Africa. *Stud. Fam. Plan.* **2004**, *35*, 116–124. [CrossRef]
5. Kingbo, M.H.K.A. Association of Socio Demographic Characteristics with Condom Used at Last Sexual Intercourse among Adults 15 to 49 Years between Côte D'Ivoire and Senegal an Examination of Measure Demographic Health Survey Data 2005. Master's Thesis, Georgia State University, Atlanta, Georgia, 2013. Available online: http://scholarworks.gsu.edu/iph_theses/275 (accessed on 2 June 2017).
6. Marak, B.; Bhatnagar, T. Sexual behaviours and condom use among young urban women in a town in northeast India: Implications for prevention and control of sexually transmitted infections. *Clin. Epidemiol. Glob. Health* **2015**, *3*, S43–S48. [CrossRef]
7. Chimbindi, N.Z.; McGrath, N.; Herbst, K.; San Tint, K.; Newell, M.L. Socio-Demographic Determinants of Condom Use Among Sexually Active Young Adults in Rural KwaZulu-Natal, South Africa. *Open AIDS J.* **2010**, *4*, 88–95. [CrossRef] [PubMed]
8. Hendriksen, E.S.; Pettifor, A.; Lee, S.J.; Coates, T.J.; Rees, H.V. Predictors of condom use among young adults in South Africa: The Reproductive Health and HIV Research Unit National Youth Survey. *Am. J. Public Health* **2007**, *97*, 1241–1248. [CrossRef] [PubMed]
9. Malema, B.W. Determinants of Condom use in Botswana: An empirical Investigation of the Role of Gender. *Botsw. J. Econ.* **2012**, *10*, 59–78.
10. Agha, S. Factors associated with HIV testing and condom use in Mozambique: Implications for programs. *Reprod. Health* **2012**, *9*, 20. [CrossRef] [PubMed]
11. Nnedu, O.N.; McCorvey, S.; Campbell-Forrester, S.; Chang, J.; Salihu, H.M.; Jolly, P.E. Factors Influencing Condom Use among Sexually Transmitted Infection Clinic Patients in Montego Bay, Jamaica. *Open Reprod. Sci. J.* **2008**, *1*, 45–50. [CrossRef] [PubMed]
12. Calazans, G.; Araujo, T.W.; Venturi, G.; Ivan França, J. Factors associated with condom use among youth aged 15–24 years in Brazil in 2003. *AIDS* **2005**, *19*, S42–S50. [CrossRef] [PubMed]
13. Dahal, S.; Pokharel, P.K.; Yadav, B.K. Sexual Behaviour and Perceived Risk of HIV/AIDS among Returnee Labour Migrants from Overseas in Nepal. *Health Sci. J.* **2013**, *7*, 218–228.
14. Regmi, P.; Simkhada, P.; Van Teijlingen, E.R. Sexual and reproductive health status among young peoples in Nepal: Opportunities and barriers for sexual health education and services utilization. *Kathmandu Univ. Med. J.* **2008**, *6*, 248–256.
15. Puri, M.; Cleland, J. Sexual behavior and perceived risk of HIV/AIDS among young migrant factory workers in Nepal. *J. Adolesc. Health* **2006**, *38*, 237–246. [CrossRef] [PubMed]
16. Acharya, D.R.; Regmi, P.; Simkhada, P.; Van Teijlingen, E. *Modernization and Changes in Attitudes towards Sex and Relationships in Young People*; Social Science Baha: Kathmandu, Nepal, 2015; pp. 63–94.
17. Upreti, D.; Regmi, P.; Pant, P.; Simkhada, P. Young people's knowledge, attitude, and behaviour on STI/HIV/AIDS in the context of Nepal: A systematic review. *Kathmandu Univ. Med. J.* **2009**, *7*, 383–391. [CrossRef]
18. Adhikari, R.; Tamang, J. Premarital sexual behavior among male college students of Kathmandu, Nepal. *BMC Public Health* **2009**, *9*, 241. [CrossRef] [PubMed]
19. Bhatta, D.N. Shadow of domestic violence and extramarital sex cohesive with spousal communication among males in Nepal. *Reprod. Health* **2014**, *11*, 44. [CrossRef] [PubMed]
20. Thapa, S.; Thapa, D.K.; Buve, A.; Hannes, K.; Nepal, C.; Mathei, C. HIV-Related Risk Behaviors Among Labor Migrants, Their Wives and the General Population in Nepal. *J. Community Health* **2017**, *42*, 260–268. [CrossRef] [PubMed]

21. Karki, S. HIV/AIDS Situation in Nepal: Transition to Women. Master's Thesis, Department of Medical and Health Sciences, Linkoping University, Linkoping, Sweden, 2008.
22. Meekers, D.; Silva, M.; Klein, M. Determinants of condom use among youth in Madagascar. *J. Biosoc. Sci.* **2006**, *38*, 365–380. [CrossRef] [PubMed]
23. Bhattacharya, G. Sociocultural and behavioral contexts of condom use in heterosexual married couples in India: Challenges to the HIV prevention program. *Health Educ. Behav.* **2004**, *31*, 101–117. [CrossRef] [PubMed]
24. Department of Health Service. *Annual Report, Department of Health Service, 2015/2016*; Government of Nepal, Ministry of Health: Kathmandu, Nepal, 2016.
25. World Health Organization. *A Conceptual Framework for Action on the Social Determinants of Health*; World Health Organization: Geneva, Switzerland, 2010. Available online: http://www.who.int/sdhconference/resources/ConceptualframeworkforactiononSDH_eng.pdf (accessed on 19 October 2017).
26. Smith-Estelle, A.; Gruskin, S. Vulnerability to HIV/STIs among rural women from migrant communities in Nepal: A health and human rights framework. *Reprod. Health Matters* **2003**, *11*, 142–151. [CrossRef]
27. UNDP (United Nations Development Program). Human Development Report 2015. 2015. Available online: http://hdr.undp.org/sites/default/files/2015_human_development_report.pdf (accessed on 20 October 2017).
28. Measure DHS: Demographic and Health Surveys. Available online: http://www.measuredhs (accessed on 2 April 2017).
29. *Nepal Demographic and Health Survey 2011*; Ministry of Health and Population (MoHP): Kathmandu, Nepal; New ERA and ICF International: Calverton, MD, USA, 2012. Available online: http://dhsprogram.com/pubs/pdf/FR257/FR257%5B13April2012%5D.pdf (accessed on 7 October 2017).
30. Karkee, R.; Lee, A.H.; Khanal, V. Need factors for utilization of institutional delivery services in Nepal: An analysis from Nepal Demographic and Health Survey, 2011. *BMJ Open* **2014**, *4*, e004372. [CrossRef] [PubMed]
31. Rutstein, S.O.; Johnson, K. *The DHS Wealth Index*; DHS Comparative Reports No. 6; ORC Macro: Calverton, MD, USA, 2004.
32. Yaya, S.; Bishwajit, G.; Danhoundo, G.; Seydou, I. Extent of Knowledge about HIV and its Determinants among Men in Bangladesh. *Front. Public Health* **2016**, *4*, 246. [CrossRef] [PubMed]
33. Khanal, V.; Adhikari, M.; Karkee, R.; Gavidia, T. Factors associated with the utilization of postnatal care services among the mothers of Nepal: Analysis of Nepal demographic and health survey 2011. *BMC Women Health* **2014**, *14*, 19. [CrossRef] [PubMed]
34. West, B.T. Statistical and methodological issues in the analysis of complex sample survey data: Practical guidance for trauma researchers. *J. Trauma. Stress* **2008**, *21*, 440–447. [CrossRef] [PubMed]
35. Adhikari, R. Are Nepali students at risk of HIV? A cross-sectional study of condom use at first sexual intercourse among college students in Kathmandu. *J. Int. AIDS Soc.* **2010**, *13*, 7. [CrossRef] [PubMed]
36. Sogarwal, R.; Bachani, D. Awareness of women about STDs, HIV/AIDS and condom use in India: Lessons for preventive programmes. *Health Popul. Perspect. Issues* **2010**, *32*, 148–158.
37. Dahal, G.P.; Padmadas, S.S.; Hinde, P.A. Fertility-limiting behavior and contraceptive choice among men in Nepal. *Int. Fam. Plan. Perspect.* **2008**, *34*, 6–14. [CrossRef] [PubMed]
38. Regmi, P.R.; Simkhada, P.; Van Teijlingen, E. "Boys Remain Prestigious, Girls Become Prostitutes": Socio-Cultural Context of Relationships and Sex among Young People in Nepal. *Glob. J. Health Sci.* **2010**, *2*, 60. [CrossRef]
39. Subba, T. Women's Vulnerability to HIV Risk: Decision Making on Condom Use among Migrant Spouses. Master's Thesis, University of Eastern Finland, Kuopio, Finland, 2017.
40. Ghimire, L.; Smith, W.C.S.; van Teijlingen, E.R.; Dahal, R.; Luitel, N.P. Reasons for non-use of condoms and self-efficacy among female sex workers: A qualitative study in Nepal. *BMC Women Health* **2011**, *11*, 42. [CrossRef] [PubMed]
41. Bam, K.; Thapa, R.; Newman, M.S.; Bhatt, L.P.; Bhatta, S.K. Sexual behavior and condom use among seasonal Dalit migrant laborers to India from Far West, Nepal: A qualitative study. *PLoS ONE* **2013**, *8*, e74903. [CrossRef] [PubMed]

42. Poudel, K.C.; Okumura, J.; Sherchand, J.B.; Jimba, M.; Murakami, I.; Wakai, S. Mumbai disease in far western Nepal: HIV infection and syphilis among male migrant-returnees and non-migrants. *Trop. Med. Int. Health* **2003**, *8*, 933–939. [CrossRef] [PubMed]
43. Vaidya, N.K.; Wu, J. HIV epidemic in Far-Western Nepal: Effect of seasonal labor migration to India. *BMC Public Health* **2011**, *11*, 310. [CrossRef] [PubMed]

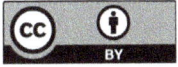

© 2018 by the authors. Licensee MDPI, Basel, Switzerland. This article is an open access article distributed under the terms and conditions of the Creative Commons Attribution (CC BY) license (http://creativecommons.org/licenses/by/4.0/).

International Journal of
*Environmental Research
and Public Health*

MDPI

Article

Young Women's Perspectives of Their Adolescent Treatment Programs: A Qualitative Study

Miriam Clark [1], Rohanna Buchanan [1,*] and Leslie D. Leve [2]

[1]   Oregon Social Learning Center, Eugene, OR 97401, USA; miriamc@oslc.org
[2]   College of Education, University of Oregon, Eugene, OR 97403, USA; leve@uoregon.edu
*   Correspondence: rohannab@oslc.org; Tel.: +1-541-485-2711

Received: 29 January 2018; Accepted: 19 February 2018; Published: 22 February 2018

Abstract: The perspectives of at-risk adolescent clients can play an important role in informing treatment services. The current study examines qualitative interview data from 15 young women with histories of maltreatment. Using a semi-structured qualitative interview approach, we asked the women to think retrospectively about their treatment experiences as adolescent girls. Results highlight the need for providing adolescent girls with reliable and practical information about risky sexual behavior and drug use from relatable and trustworthy helping professionals. We discuss strategies for developing and maintaining trust and delivering specific content.

Keywords: teenage pregnancies; unwanted pregnancies; child abuse; substance use; health risking sexual behavior; mental health; services for adolescents

1. Introduction

Childhood maltreatment is associated with an elevated risk of adolescent drug use and risky sexual behavior [1]. Both adolescents and adults with histories of maltreatment are more likely to have sex while drinking or using drugs, which often results in unprotected casual sex—leading to sexually transmitted infections and unwanted pregnancies [2–4]. Additionally, adults with histories of childhood trauma are more likely to exchange sex for drugs or money [5,6], be arrested for prostitution, have unprotected sex with casual partners [1], and have a high sensitivity to social rejection which leads to more risky sexual encounters [7].

Several evidence-based treatment programs have demonstrated effectiveness in reducing the probability of adolescents with histories of maltreatment engaging in drug use and risky sexual behavior (see Multisystemic Therapy, Treatment Foster Care Oregon, Functional Family Therapy, and Trauma-Focused Cognitive–Behavioral Therapy) [8]. However, one area that has received little attention in developing and refining treatment programs is the importance of directly soliciting clients' opinions and input [9]. Client input can provide valuable insight into the client/clinician or client/intervention relationship. In fact, Hodgetts and Wright [10] argue that researchers cannot fully understand the impact of treatment without learning about and incorporating the clients' experiences and perspectives.

Numerous studies have explored adolescents' views of their interactions with helping professionals including mental health therapists, mentors, doctors, nurses, or other treatment providers [10–16]. However, these studies often lack specific information about how client-clinician relationships are developed and built over time. For example, in a review of 54 qualitative studies examining adolescents' views on their relationships with helping professionals, Freake and colleagues [12] identified 12 important themes that regularly emerge in qualitative data. The 12 themes include confidentiality, giving advice, listening, kindness, trustworthiness, being qualified, being non-patronizing, being non-judgmental, being easy to talk to, consistency, being treated as an individual, and—for medical issues specifically—that adolescent girls prefer a female doctor. Although these themes have been examined broadly in prior research, Freake and colleagues identified a need for researchers to look deeper into these factors and examine how adolescents' perceptions about treatment develop over time. Specifically, Freake and colleagues report that prior research shows that helping professionals often lack an understanding about how clients want professionals to explain things, what being "easy to talk to" means, and how trust can be developed and sustained.

The Current Study

One strategy to gain insight into how the adolescent client/clinician relationship changes over time is to ask young adults how they viewed the treatment programs they attended and to solicit their suggestions for future programs. The retrospective nature of this type of inquiry brings added insight that is not possible when questions are asked during treatment [17]. Retrospective inquiry is a critical tool in the current study because research has shown that impulsivity and sensation seeking behaviors are at their peak during adolescence, that adolescents often feel invincible, that futuristic thinking is uncommon (adolescents live in the moment), and that the adolescent brain continues to develop well into the mid-20's [18,19]. Because of these features of human development, most adolescents are not able to accurately perspective-take and reflect on their own current behaviors and associated risks and needs. Waiting until individuals are in their 20's, and then asking them about their teen years, means that most individuals have developed a greater capacity to reflect on their choices and what was/was not helpful during adolescence and decisions they wished they had made, yet they are still close enough to the period of adolescence to have a deep understanding of what it is like to be a teen in today's world. Following this approach, we conducted 15 semi-structured, open-ended qualitative interviews with young women with a history of maltreatment and placement in out-of-home care. During the interviews, we asked the women to reflect on their experiences with treatment programs. Three research questions guided the qualitative interviews and analyses:

1. What types of treatment services did young women with histories of maltreatment experience as adolescents?
2. What feedback do young women with histories of maltreatment have that relates to both positive and negative characteristics of helping professionals and treatment programs for adolescent girls with histories of maltreatment?
3. What feedback do young women with histories of maltreatment have to inform treatment program content and delivery related to drug use, risky sexual activity, and partner choice for adolescent girls with histories of maltreatment?

2. Materials and Methods

2.1. Participants

Young women (n = 15) with maltreatment histories who had participated in treatment programs as adolescents were recruited for the current study. The women were identified from two completed, randomized, controlled trials in which they had participated during adolescence [20,21] and from a local community mental health center. Recruitment included an initial telephone call to determine interest and eligibility for participation followed by an in-person, individually administered IRB-approved informed consent procedure. The IRB protocol number is 10312013.040 from the University of Oregon. Interview content was examined after each interview and we determined that we reached sufficient data saturation [22] with the sample of 15 women. All recruitment and interview activity took place between November of 2013 and April of 2014.

2.2. Measures

Interview guide. We used an individually administered, semi-structured, and open-ended qualitative interview format and conducted one interview with each participant. We designed the questions in the interview guide to prompt respondents to think retrospectively about treatment programs they attended during their adolescent years and to solicit information about the topics most important to them. Asking participants retrospectively about the programs in which they had participated allowed them to think critically about how these programs might have influenced their lives. The treatment-related questions in the interview guide were general in order to allow respondents to formulate their own unbiased responses. Questions asked participants to think retrospectively about their treatment experiences as adolescents and explain the treatment elements that were helpful or not helpful for them. Example questions included: "What parts of the program did you find helpful?", "What was helpful about those parts?", "Were there any parts of the program you did not think were helpful?", "Why did you not think they were helpful?". Interviewers were trained in techniques to elicit information from participants, remain neutral to a range of responses, and move the discussion through the semi-structured format.

Demographic survey. Each participant completed a demographic survey prior to the interview. The demographic survey included items related to the participants' age, race/ethnicity, current relationship status, and education.

2.3. Analysis

Interviews were conducted by two graduate research assistants. Both interviewers were trained in qualitative interview techniques which allowed participants to feel comfortable to express their opinions naturally while moving through the semi-structured interview guide. All interviews were audio recorded and transcribed verbatim. The interviewers then reviewed each transcript for accuracy. We assigned participants, other individuals, and treatment programs identified in the transcripts an identification number prior to analysis to protect confidentiality and reduce subjectivity in the analyses [22]. After reviewing all of the interviews, the authors met and discussed broad themes identified across all transcripts. The first author coded all of the interview transcripts. Using NVIVO software [23], she completed an initial coding of the broad themes for each interview. Next, a codebook emerged as the first author coded sections of text (ranging in size from short phrases to long discussions) by hand into more specific emergent sub-themes, then compared the coded content across each interview. The coder grouped codes into themes and subthemes using the method of constant comparison [24]. All authors met to thoroughly review the first author's analysis, discuss findings related to the broad themes and sub-themes, and to agree on representative quotes.

2.4. Reflexivity Statement

The first author and coder for the study is a research assistant with a MS in sociology. She is trained in qualitative research methodology including developing interview questions, conducting interviews, and coding and analyzing qualitative data. She has 9 years of experience conducting qualitative and quantitative interviews and assessments in English and Spanish with children, adolescents, and parents from racially and economically diverse populations. She has assisted with the development of research protocols and procedures for multiple research studies with children and adolescents. The second author has a Ph.D. in school psychology. She is clinically trained in behavioral treatment models and has been involved in the mental health treatment of children and adolescents for 18 years. Her experience includes serving as a clinician, clinical supervisor, and principal investigator on a number of research studies with children and adolescents involved with juvenile justice, child welfare, and special education systems. She has significant experience developing and implementing treatments for adolescent girls. The third author has a Ph.D. in developmental psychology and has been studying both typical and atypical child and adolescent development for the past 20 years. For the past 15 years, she has been part of a research team evaluating developmental pathways and intervention outcomes for girls with child welfare and juvenile justice involvement. Her roles have included theoretical conceptualization, assessment development, data analysis, and manuscript development (she is not clinically trained and does not serve clients).

3. Results

3.1. Quantitative Results: Participants and Interviews

The young women in the current study were 18–24 years of age (M = 20.93, SD = 2.09) at the time of the interview. Participants identified as White or Caucasian (60%), American Indian/Alaska Native (7%), or more than one race (33%). Overall, 20% of the sample identified as Hispanic/Latino. Participants reported that they were married (n = 1), living with a partner and unmarried (n = 6), or were dating or seeing someone but not living together or married (n = 8). Participants reported a range of education attainment including having completed the 8th grade (n = 1), having completed some high school (n = 4), having received a GED (n = 3), having received a high school diploma (n = 5), and having completed some college (n = 2). The sample was generally unemployed and low income, with only four women employed for pay and a median income range of $5000–$9999.

Interviews were scheduled for two hours. The average interview length was 102 min (range = 66–136 min).

3.2. Broad Themes from the Qualitative Interviews

When talking about their prior treatment experiences, the women told highly detailed and lengthy stories that were sometimes directly related to the interview questions and sometimes more tangential to the focus of the question. The stories focused on a range of programs including sex education classes in school, day-treatment programs, treatment foster care, independent living programs, and residential treatment programs. Three broad themes emerged from the interviews: positive experiences from past programs, negative experiences from past programs, and suggestions for developing effective treatment programs. We grouped subthemes within these broad themes.

3.3. Positive Experiences from Past Programs

All 15 women identified positive past experiences in treatment programs, sex education, and/or other means of gaining information about risk and prevention related to sexual behavior and drug use. Participants' positive experiences were grouped into five sub-themes: (a) traits of the helping professional, (b) knowledge gained, (c) positive social activities, (d) social support from the helping professional and (e) specific resources found helpful.

Traits of the helping professional. Fourteen participants discussed positive qualities they noticed in the helping professionals they had interacted with as adolescents. The women identified a range of positive qualities regarding the helping professional's approach including being non-judgmental, being understanding, being honest, keeping information confidential, being interested in the adolescent, having similar past experiences as the adolescent, and rewarding positive behavior. The women also identified positive qualities that made the helping professional easier to connect with including being down to earth, funny, young, a friend, kind, outgoing, female, easygoing, and interested in specific activities such as art or sports. One participant summed up many of these characteristics when she discussed her favorite counselor fondly:

> "My counselor . . . was the epitome of an overachieving counselor. She was absolutely amazing. She was really young . . . She dressed like a teenager, and she went through a lot of traumatic events herself growing up. So she not only did she, like, sympathize, she empathized. She went through it. So being able to talk to someone that had already had experience in the matters that I was going through, that really helped . . . She was like a big sister, and that's what I think teen girls need if they don't have an older sister or something they can look up to."

Another participant highlighted the importance of a non-judgmental and understanding approach, "Cuz she um she knew about everything that I had done but she didn't . . . criticize me for it or, or made me feel like I was being judged. She was just always kind of um uh, understanding I guess".

Knowledge gained. Twelve participants identified specific things they remembered learning that they said have helped them. Topics they identified included sex education, coping skills, values such as patience and positivity, and the negative effects of drugs. One of the women highlighted that she had learned specific coping skills, saying, "They went into great length with coping skills. And really great ways to take my anger out in a positive manner: Crocheting, knitting, painting".

Positive social activities. Nine participants identified social and active aspects of programs as valuable. Most of the social experiences discussed by the young women happened with a mentor in a therapeutic program, though some occurred at school or with other helping professionals (e.g., counselor, therapist). Activities mentioned included art, hiking, work experience, sports, hanging out, movies, music, and school activities. The women talked about the importance of having fun and doing exciting things to replace the desire for drugs and alcohol. One of the young women stated, "That's what's good about the BSS [behavior support specialist]. Cuz they like took you out of the situation and taught you, 'you know, we can go rollerblading, instead of going to smoke crack.'" Another woman identified that she had a history of substance use as an adolescent but she was sober when she engaged in social activities, "I did, uh, youth group, campus life is what it was called. And I did basketball; I did volleyball".

Social support from the helping professional. The opportunity to talk to or spend time with a helping professional was something ten participants said they enjoyed and found helpful. While most of the women simply said that it was nice to have someone to talk to, one participant talked about the help she received saying, "Counseling really helped me. Like just being able to talk to someone and them, like, not judge me and to be able to talk back to me, is like, I dunno, I feel like an equal when I talk to a counselor, a lot of the time." Another participant described the support she received from her mentor in more detail,

"It was just nice to have somebody to kind of hang out with and talk to that wasn't my grandma because I was living with her at the time. And um, yeah, it was just it was nice having somebody to go to. Definitely just hang out with ... it was weird how it helped out ... it kind of boost my self-esteem a little bit ... I think how to kind of to cope a little more with not being able to see my family that much. And being able to see her [mentor] kind of took my mind off of, kind of, the sad parts of my life back then."

Specific resources found helpful. Nine participants listed specific resources they found helpful from various treatment and education programs. These resources included medication; food; shelter; birth control; help with resumes; help obtaining a driver's license; financial help; help with college tuition; classes in budgeting, cooking, and shopping; STI testing; support groups for LGBT adolescents; clothing; bus passes; washing machines; and a place to hang out for adolescents. One participant expressed her appreciation for these resources, "I was in [an] independent living program ... And we would ... do resumes and, um, talk about, like, getting food stamps and drivers licenses ... They gave me $600 a month. They helped out with college. That was an awesome program".

3.4. Negative Experiences from Past Programs

All 15 women talked about past negative experiences in treatment programs or sex education; these were grouped into seven sub-themes: (a) lack of information about sex and drugs, (b) negative qualities of the helping professional, (c) adolescent did not participate in or appreciate program, (d) adolescent did not like characteristics of the facility or program, (e) high turnover rate of helping professionals, and (f) worries about confidentiality.

Lack of information about sex and drugs. One sub-theme that emerged in 13 of the interviews was that adolescents lack information about safe sex practices and the risks of drug use. The women emphasized that prior treatment and education programs had not provided sufficient practical information for them to make healthy and safe choices. The women talked about how adolescents' lack of such information is a result of misinformation, not receiving information in the first place, or not believing the information they did receive. For example, one respondent said, "definitely some people aren't aware of how some sexual transmitted diseases [STIs] aren't protected from things like condoms, and they don't think about things like blowjobs and things like that and how you could receive it [an STI] orally." Another participant described that some adolescents do not know where to obtain information about safe sex, saying:

> "I just feel that and with their [adolescents] age being so young now I think that they're embarrassed to talk to their parents [about sex]. I think that they, um, just they don't know what their parents will say. They don't know what their friends will say. Um, sometimes, they don't ... have that much information ... , but they don't know where to start ... "

Negative qualities of the helping professional. Ten participants discussed negative qualities they remembered in their relationship with their helping professional. Negative qualities in the relationships varied in nature, but all contributed to an environment where the adolescents had difficulty building rapport. Participants mentioned things such as feeling judged unfairly, feeling a lack of trust, feeling that meetings with the helping professional were not frequent enough, and feeling that the helping professional was hard to relate to due to an age difference. One participant described her difficulty building rapport with counselors this way, "They just didn't, they seemed so unattached to the situation. ... they had no idea they didn't even really wanna be there it seemed like with some of 'em. And they were just doing it kinda for a job ... " Another participant discussed how she felt that her helping professional did not trust her,

> " ... the things I told them about my parents and stuff, they didn't believe any of it, pretty much. That, that was a pretty big deal, cuz my dad was very, my dad was abusive and stuff and I had a lotta issues at home and nobody heard that, so and they acted like I'm the problem."

Another participant explained, when asked if she felt comfortable talking to her mentor about sex, how she felt that she would have been judged had she gone into too much detail, "I felt comfortable talking to her about the idea of sex, but not like actual. Cuz she's an adult and sometimes it's just awkward because you feel like they're going to judge you".

Adolescent did not participate in or appreciate program. Ten participants reported feeling that treatment was not a good fit for them as an adolescent because of their own feelings toward the program. They talked about how they refused to participate (by either not attending or remaining silent in treatment), not liking the program, feeling that they were forced into treatment, or feeling that they were not ready for treatment. For example, one participant said, "Um, it, um [sighs] well, I wasn't ready for services. Um, that is the main reason why it didn't work, was because I wasn't ready to quit [using drugs]." Another participant described her negative experience in a residential program,

> "I did not like being around a bunch of people that I didn't want to be around, that I was forced to be around. Like the girls in the programs that had issues and stuff. It made it harder and what else? I didn't like not having my own stuff and being told what to do every day."

Half of these women who expressed negative feelings toward the program also expressed regret that they had had these negative feelings. For example, one woman expressed her regret for not attending, saying, "I wish I would have gone more [to therapy] ... I had to actually go down there and I just never [did,] I would rather hang out with my friends." Another participant said, "I wished I had been more open with him [her therapist]. I probably would've gotten better treatment".

Adolescent did not like characteristics of the facility or program. Eight of the women mentioned specific things they did not like about the facility or the program. Six women said they did not like being in a group treatment program and gave examples related to the structure, the classes, the lack of funding, feeling forced to be there, or the location of services. One of the women highlighted the lack of funding by saying, "I feel that [the program] isn't being given enough money and I know that just this whole economy sucks, but they are doing a lot for us [clients], and um, they just don't have the adequate supplies they need. I mean, they don't even have a stove in their kitchen." Three of the women said they did not like being in therapy in general because they felt that they did not have enough say in the therapy received, their family did not come to family therapy, or they did not like being forced to open up to a stranger (e.g., new therapist). Two women mentioned that they felt like they were over medicated. One of these women described her frustration with the treatment program by saying, "I just didn't appreciate the fact that they tried to get me to take things [medication] that I didn't need".

High turnover rate of helping professionals. Five respondents discussed the high turnover rate of the helping professional (e.g., mentor, worker, therapist) they had been assigned as an adolescent. Some of the women talked about their experience with therapist turnover being due to the high turnover at the agency, while others talked about how they moved often and had to change helping professionals as a result of the move. One woman described her experience with turnover this way:

> "I wished that they had made a contract with ILP [independent living program] workers that they had to work, they couldn't just quit. They had to work for a set period of time. . . . I went through about four or five ILP workers because they found different jobs, or they just randomly decided to switch their caseload, and then they wouldn't really tell me about it or anything, and it just kind of happened."

Regardless of the reason for the turnover, the women reported that the high turnover rate made it difficult to build rapport and open up to a new helping professional. The women talked about how they felt they needed to be more guarded over time as they experienced more therapist turnover and had difficulty putting trust in someone that might leave. Another participant talked about moving and her experience with turnover, saying:

> " . . . once I turned . . . fourteen I was like, "I'm not doing counseling anymore." And they'd make me go and I'd just sit there. And I wouldn't say nothing, cuz I was just like, I'm, I'm tired of connecting with somebody, and like, everything switches every time I move, you know what I mean? It's pointless."

Worries about confidentiality. Three participants said that they had not wanted to open up to a helping professional out of fear the helping professional would break confidentiality. The way the women talked about their concerns related to confidentiality suggested that, as adolescents, they were unclear about mandatory reporting rules. One participant shared her story like this:

> "I didn't really feel comfortable really talking about drugs to a counselor cuz they say in the beginning you know, this is confidential unless we feel like you're harming yourself or others. And you kinda are when you do those. So, like you like feel like you're—you can't really say anything at all."

Two other participants said that their counselor did break confidentiality and one explained her story this way:

> "I did not like the fact that every time we talked, she would, you know, she would write down everything I said. And then she'd go off and show it to my parents. I don't like the breaking of, you know, trust, and confidentiality. I hate that crap."

3.5. Ideas for Developing Effective Treatment Programs for Adolescent Girls with Maltreatment Histories

In addition to questions about their prior intervention experiences, we asked the women about their ideas for effective treatment programs. We asked participants what an ideal program would look like for adolescent girls related to helping professionals and program content.

Characteristics of the ideal helping professional. When asked who should deliver specific types of programs or services, participants identified qualities related to age, gender, experience, and personality. These characteristics seemed indicative of the desire to have a helping professional to whom they could relate. For example, one participant said,

"Definitely having someone close to age or the same age ... someone who's just close to the same personality sometimes is very helpful or like interested in the same activities and uh, yeah, I think that would be really helpful. Because I know the girl I was seeing she was into art and music and that was my big thing and it was nice being able to talk about it or do some art projects."

Age. Nine of the women mentioned the importance of having a young program facilitator, mentor, or therapist. Their definitions of young varied slightly, but all mentioned ages that ranged in the 20s and 30s. When discussing age of helping professionals, one participant said, "I didn't want someone to act motherly towards me." Another participant expanded on the same idea when she said,

"Having older people can sometimes make some girls feel judged because, um, that person grew up a little bit different than how girls are growing up now and it might make it, it might make them feel like they are talking to their parents more than talking to a friend. So someone just younger."

The other six participants did not identify age as an important characteristic of the treatment personnel.

Gender. Seven participants said that the gender of the treatment personnel was important. Six out of these seven said that they preferred female mentors or program facilitators. One of those six said that although she preferred a female mentor, there should be a mix of genders for facilitators of treatment groups. Another one of those six said that she would prefer either a woman or a gay male. One participant said that she felt sex education would best be taught by someone of the opposite gender. Another participant said that both sexes should teach adolescents about sex. The remaining seven participants did not list gender as an important characteristic of mentors, sex education teachers, or other helping professionals.

Experience. Eight of the respondents discussed the importance of having someone who has "been through it." They wanted helping professionals who had experience with drugs, risky sexual behavior, or had experienced traumatic events. One participant described it this way:

" ... it's hard to tell someone that you know where they're coming from when you've never dealt with anything like that before. I know that had I had someone who had actually been through stuff that I had been through, maybe not everything, maybe just one or two things, or maybe just one, I think that would have helped me realize, cuz they know and they've, you know, at that point what I would say is they've survived. You know, they've gotten out. And they, they can do it, obviously I can too."

Another participant put it this way: "Yeah, personal experience. Um somebody who can relate easily and um, just kind of give, give some sort of hope you know to them whoever they are. Wherever they're at in their stage, you know, of life." A different participant explained why having someone who lacked such experience was not helpful:

"Cuz if you've never done drugs, you can't sit there and be like, 'Do not use drugs, they're really bad for you,' because that's all you hear. ... some girl comes up and says, 'Well why are they really bad? How do they taste? You know, what do they smell like when you're around them?' ... Then you're gonna be like, 'I don't know.'

Personality traits. The women mentioned a variety of personality traits that they found important for treatment personnel. These included things such as being happy, a good friend, committed, nice, logical, relatable, persistent, mature, comfortable, knowledgeable, fun, understandable, helpful, able to listen, fun, honest, and positive. By far the most common theme that came up (in 13 of the interviews) was how much adolescents need to feel understood and accepted. They wanted someone who is understanding, non-judgmental, or open-minded. One participant put it this way, " ... what you could do is just uh, make 'em feel like you're on their side, I guess with everything and that you're doing it to help them." Another participant furthered this idea when she said, "non-judgmental person. Ideal .... Somebody who's not a cop. [laughs], I mean nothing against cops, officers, policemen. Um, you know but not someone who's going to make them feel like threatened or make them feel like they're going to be [threatened]".

Ideal program content. When asked about ideal treatment program content, participants shared ideas that included both information and skills. Themes included consequences of risky sexual behavior and drug use, skills to talk with partners about sex and/or drugs, resources, use of protection during sex, and that it is okay to abstain from sex and/or drugs.

Potential consequences of risky sexual behavior and drug use. Thirteen of the 15 women mentioned the importance of teaching about risks involved with sex and drugs and how engaging in risky behavior can impact their current and future lives. Specifically, the women highlighted potential consequences related to risky sexual behavior and drug use individually, as well as those associated with drug use combined with risky sexual behavior.

Eleven of the women talked about the importance of teaching about potential consequences associated with risky sexual behavior. The specific risks the women identified were physical, social, and emotional. Physical risks included STI transmission (e.g., transmission via oral sex, potential of STI transmission with unprotected sex), pregnancy (e.g., sore breasts, morning sickness, cravings, labor, mood swings), and sexual assault. When the women talked about social risks, they emphasized how potential male partners might not want female partners who had been sexually promiscuous. The emotional risks they highlighted included experiences where male and female partners did not have the same feelings about the sexual relationship. Their stories included situations where the male partners lied to get sex, or where the female was in love but the male was just interested in sex. One participant talked about gender differences she had noticed in adolescent views of sex, "Cuz for girls it's emotional bonding ... for boys it's just getting in your pants. That's what I've experienced anyway. It's really sad but it's the truth." Another participant warned, "Just because he says he cares about you before doesn't mean that he still will afterwards." The participants also warned that pressure from a partner to have sex means you are not being respected by the partner.

Many of the women expressed how important it was for treatment programs to provide in-depth information about these potential consequences. One participant explained how to talk about the realities of pregnancy,

> "Like telling them the pros and cons of getting pregnant and having a baby. And tell them that it's worth waiting. It is hard to do school and raise a kid, but I think if they really just talk about some of the unpleasant stuff about being pregnant that a lot of the girls would really be okay to wait. Yeah, once I got pregnant there was a lot of stuff I did not know about. I took health and family's class and I didn't know that you could get hemorrhoids. And you're just very uncomfortable especially once you get bigger and your mood swings really do go up and down."

Six women talked about teaching adolescent girls about the potential consequences associated with drug use. The specific risks identified focused on incarceration (detention or jail), social effects (e.g., intoxicated friends might steal your things), physical effects, and safety. When talking about the physical effects of drug use, the women highlighted both long- and short-term health effects (e.g., damage to the heart, looking older than their age).

Most respondents suggested that explaining the risks associated with drug use would deter adolescent girls from using. For example, one woman said, "Show them the really bad adverse side effects of using any amount of, you know, alcohol, drugs, hallucinogenics." Another participant said,

> "I mean, let them know the risks, really. I mean, if half of the girls knew what some of the drugs could do to your body, I think a lot of people wouldn't use 'em. What it can do to you. I mean it can completely change you and you can become someone who you never thought you would. .... if I could tell people, you know, a life story and have them not use ... I just, it's not worth it."

Some participants gave suggestions for how to be safe when using drugs such as obtaining drugs from a trusted source to avoid impurities/contamination and using in a private space because it is easier for people to take advantage of you when you are in a public place. One woman said,

*"Like just don't just do it from some stranger or, you know, somebody you don't know that well. . . .
you have to be in a really safe environment. Um, my advice . . . have like someone who at least is
like somewhat sober or all the way sober. To, like, you know like if something did happen that they
could actually take care of the situation instead of being oblivious to everything."*

When asked what advice they would give to adolescent girls, four women talked about teaching
the risks associated with drug use combined with sexual activity and relationships. The women's
stories illustrated three specific types of risks: (1) risks associated with men who use drugs, (2) risk
of judgement being impaired when under the influence of drugs/alcohol during sex, and (3) drugs
having consequences that affect your relationships—both current relationships and future relationships.
For example, one participant said she would, "Recommend the girl get away from that situation and
that area because it's usually the area you know, her sense of home that's keeping her there in the first
place. It's not just the boyfriend and girlfriend."

Skills to talk with partner about sex and/or drugs. Ten women discussed the importance of teaching
adolescents how to talk to their partner about sex and/or drugs. One woman talked about how
programs should teach adolescent girls skills to talk to partners so the men listen and understand them,
saying, " . . . like figure out how guys wanna hear what they're [girls] trying to say and teach 'em how
to say it." Another participant explained what programs can teach adolescent girls to say to partners
this way,

*"Tell the girl, "Hey, when you, if you're gonna decide to do something with somebody, you guys
should sit down and talk about it first. You know, like, 'Do you want to use protection?...' Talk
about what it is you're gonna do before you do it. You know, try to get the guy to, you know, be more
sensitive to your needs, you know and don't just hop into it. Be like, 'Hey wait, can we talk about
this first?' You know. 'Maybe can we wait?'"*

Resources. Eleven women suggested teaching adolescents how to find resources (e.g., condoms,
medical services, social support, housing). Four participants talked about the need to connect
adolescents to resources for STI and pregnancy prevention, and three talked specifically about getting
information and medical care from a community health clinic ("go to Planned Parenthood . . . They're
a really good resource with condoms or Plan B or whatever you need"). Three participants said it was
important to teach adolescents to utilize their parents or other trusted adults as resources about healthy
and safe sex practices ("Maybe to encourage 'em maybe to talk to their parents about it [sex]"). Related
to housing, one participant talked about the need for adolescents to learn how to find safe housing.
Her experience illustrated that adolescent girls often stay in unhealthy relationships because they are
living with their partner. She emphasized the need for adolescents to find alternative housing in order
to escape unhealthy or unsafe relationships ("people should always have . . . a little piece of paper . . .
that they always have access to that has certain phone numbers on there so they can always . . . call for
help"). Another participant talked about the connection between sex and access to resources such as
housing, food, and security. This participant wanted programs to teach adolescents how to ask for
help because there are alternatives to using sex to access resources. She suggested " . . . going to your
nearest DHS office and asking for help. Explaining to them your situation or going to [facility A] or
[facility B] and explaining to them. Cuz . . . there's a lot of resources to help them."

Use of protection during sex. Eleven participants said that adolescents need to be taught to
think about and use protection during sex. Specific examples included teaching adolescent girls
to think about the importance of safe sex practices; and to obtain, use, and store different types of
birth control/STI prevention (e.g., "condoms," "Plan B"). For example, one woman explained why
adolescents need to know how to correctly use a condom,

*" . . . like a condom, with people is like, when are you gonna stop? And then you have to put it on,
you know? And if a girl doesn't know how to put it on, then she's not gonna try right in front
of the person. So definitely learning how to put a condom on. Learning you know how to keep
yourself clean."*

It is okay to abstain from sex and/or drugs. Eleven participants said that adolescents need to learn to choose for themselves when to use drugs or have sex. Related to drugs, one participant said, "Just teach them as best you can about peer pressure." She went on to say, "And that your friends are either gonna be your friends or their not really gonna, or their not your friends at all." Related to sex, the main sentiment expressed by the women was that adolescent girls should not feel pressure to have sex if they are in a relationship or their friends are sexually active. The women wanted adolescent girls to learn that they should not feel shame for not being ready to have sex, to not worry about being mocked for abstaining from sex, and "that it shouldn't be a race" to lose their virginity. One participant talked about " … not doing it until they're ready and not feeling ashamed if they realize they weren't ready." Another participant expressed her regret that she had had sex so young and advocated teaching adolescent girls to make their own decisions about sex, saying,

> "Try and go to abstinence. Yeah … sex at an early age, I, I regret it. Um, I, that's just how it is. You do it and then you go, 'wow that wasn't great, I regret it.' And you will regret it for the rest of your life, or most of it … oh I think it might help out a lot of girls. Cuz they'll be like, 'okay, I don't have to do it if I don't want to.' Um, it'll teach girls more about … having an opinion and having their own free will."

Throughout the interviews, the women emphasized that adolescent girls should learn that it is worth waiting to have sex until they are ready.

4. Discussion

The women in the sample were highly engaged in the interviews as evidenced by the detail of their responses and length of the interviews. Participants provided lengthy, in-depth insights into their prior treatment experiences and suggestions for improving treatment programs and relationships with helping professionals. Though some of the feedback is less feasible to implement (e.g., hiring young, skilled therapists who have recovered from prior drug abuse), much of the women's feedback can be readily implemented and is consistent with recommendations from the treatment literature.

This study adds to the current body of literature in two important ways. First, asking young adults retrospectively about their treatment programs provides insight into how their perceptions related to program effectiveness have developed over time. Second, asking women with histories of maltreatment about their treatment experiences provides insight into an at-risk population. While our participants identified desired characteristics of helping professionals that are consistent with findings in prior studies [12], this study further develops those themes and helps to fill the gaps in the extant literature by examining how helping professionals can develop and maintain relationships over time.

4.1. Implications for Practice

The comments reflected by the women in the sample illustrated the juxtaposition between adolescents as thrill seekers while simultaneously seeking stability and consistency. Their stories repeatedly demonstrated a desire for stability (represented by being taken care of by male partners and frustration with therapist turnover) contrasted with serious thrill-seeking behavior (represented by things that are potentially harmful e.g., risky sex and/or drug use; or things that are prosocial e.g., sports, art, clubs). This juxtaposition is consistent with literature showing that adolescents are both thrill seekers [18,19] and positively respond to structure and stability [25].

Participants emphasized the importance of giving adolescent girls information. They repeatedly made suggestions about what treatment programs should tell adolescent girls about the risks of sex and drugs and how to access community resources. To a lesser extent, their stories highlight the importance of teaching safety and refusal skills or skills for accessing family or community support. The current literature shows that information, skills, and social support are necessary to reduce risk and promote healthy behavior in adolescents. For example, the Centers for Disease Control and Prevention (CDC) identified that effective HIV/STD [26,27] prevention programs for adolescents include skill-building components and support from family in addition to knowledge gained. Additionally, because there has been an increased use of technology by adolescents, smart phone applications or other digital methods might be an effective strategy for improving access to information. Current research suggests that there is a lack of an effective strategy to provide such information using technology [28] and that even advanced high school students struggle to judge the quality and accuracy of information they find online [29].

The women's stories indirectly highlight the importance of having agency over one's body. Their experiences show that they felt like they did not exert control over their own sexual behavior and/or substance use as adolescents, which was directly linked to not having agency over their lives in a broader sense. The women's suggestions for treatment programs largely stemmed from not wanting other maltreated adolescents to be taken advantage of (the way they were) and therefore wanting to provide adolescents with knowledge and skills to make healthy choices.

Characteristics of the helping professional. Consistent with findings from prior research [12], the women's reports of positive experiences with helping professionals were linked to trusting relationships with providers they could relate to and who had empathy for them and their experiences. The women highlighted qualities such as being non-judgmental, understanding, honest, and maintaining confidentiality as positive qualities of helping professionals. They found the support from helping professionals from their prior treatment programs to be helpful and enjoyed spending time talking and doing activities with them.

Many of the participants described their ideal helping professional as a young female who could relate to teen clients because she had overcome adversity in her own life (e.g., childhood maltreatment, drug use). Their stories showed that the women wanted a helping professional who would have empathy for them and that it was more difficult to relate to someone with a different background than themselves. Providing female clients with female mentors or therapists to enhance client-helping professional relatability is a common strategy for several existing treatment programs [30–32].

In addition to positive characteristics, the participants in this study also provided examples of negative characteristics of providers or programs. For example, high counselor turnover, misunderstandings about limits to confidentiality, feeling judged, feeling that the helping professional was not educated about sex and/or drugs, a lack of personal connection to the helping professional, feeling like they were forced into treatment, and not having a say in the treatment received were the main sources of the women's negative prior experiences. The majority of the women talked about their own lack of participation in treatment as adolescents stemming from negative experiences with providers and programs.

These findings point to clear opportunities to increase client participation in treatment, specifically, the relatability and consistency of helping professionals. The women recommended that helping professionals be selected who are fun, kind, and show that they are listening and positive regardless of what the client shares. In addition, while there are myriad reasons for turnover in helping professionals, strategies such as improving the organizational climate by reducing stress [33,34] and increasing salaries [34] have been shown to reduce turnover.

Specific content. One of the more revealing aspects of the interviews was the lack of practical information the women had as adolescents, and their impressions of the lasting negative impact of this on their lives. Most of the women talked about specific and practical helpful things they remembered learning in prior programs such as healthy coping skills, emotion regulation, sex education, and the risks of drug use. They said that learning about accessing practical resources such as medication, food, shelter, education, money, and social support were invaluable to reducing their dependence on partners. In addition, the women reflected on the value of learning to participate in healthy, safe, and exciting activities (such as sports, art, and clubs). In fact, they stated that these activities directly replaced their time and desire to use drugs or alcohol. The women also talked about how they wished they had been taught more about the consequences of risky sexual behavior and drug use, how to talk to their partner about safe sex and drug use, and that it is okay to abstain from sex and/or drugs. They also wished they had been taught how to find practical resources (e.g., condoms, housing). For example, when they talked about wishing they had understood the risks of sex and drugs, they went into detail about specific risks on these issues (prevalence and consequences of STIs, side effects of pregnancy, financial burdens of having a child, and physical and emotional consequences of drugs use). They felt they needed to learn in hands-on ways, such as role-playing talks with partners and specifics on how a condom actually works and how to put it on. These findings point to the importance of pairing practical information with skills. This is consistent with a review of federal policies and programs showing that adolescents benefit from sex education that includes abstinence and harm-reduction strategies [35], and that information alone is not effective [36,37].

4.2. Limitations and Future Directions

This study was conducted in one Pacific Northwest city with limited racial diversity and had a sample of 15 women. Although findings provide insights into a topic that has not been extensively explored and has very tangible implications, findings may not be generalizable on a large scale. Due to the retrospective nature of this study, the women might not have remembered information that is important to understanding their experiences as adolescents. Future research could add to our findings in two specific ways. First, future studies should ask similar questions to more ethnically and gender diverse populations to see whether the current pattern of findings is generalizable. Learning the perspectives of men in similar circumstances would provide insight into how sex education and intervention programs can be implemented on a broad scale. Learning the perspectives of a more ethnically diverse population would also provide insight into how to implement these programs in more ethnically diverse cities. Second, future research could follow a similar population from childhood through adulthood to note changes over time. If adolescents were asked questions about their experiences while in treatment programs and then followed up with as young adults, researchers could gain valuable insight into how an adolescent's opinion during adolescence is likely to change and develop as they age out of the program and enter adulthood.

5. Conclusions

Results from the interviews consistently illustrated that the women in this study want adolescent girls with maltreatment histories to be given practical, reliable, and understandable information and skills. In addition, the women suggest that such information should be provided by a helping professional who the adolescent relates to and trusts. The women had many suggestions for ways in which helping professionals can build trust and be relatable to adolescent clients, such as maintaining confidentiality, being non-judgmental, allowing sufficient time to build rapport, and engaging them in positive, fun activities. The women's stories suggest that adolescent girls armed with information and skills will feel more confident to not only respond effectively to social pressure, but also to think critically about the impact of risky behavior on their own lives.

Acknowledgments: Support for this research was provided by the following grants: R01 DA024672, R01 DA032634, R21 DA027091, and P50 DA035763 from the Division of Epidemiology, Services, and Prevention Research, National Institute on Drug Abuse, U.S. PHS. The opinions expressed are those of the authors and do not represent views of the National Institute on Drug Abuse. The authors thank the women who participated in the interviews; Lawrence Palinkas for support on the development of the interview guide and training protocol; Danielle Guerrero for project coordination; Rachel Kovensky and Aliya Khan for conducting the interviews; Michelle Baumann, Sadie Baratta, Amala Shetty, Emily Kavanagh-Martin, Sophie Kreitzberg, Mariam Admasu, and Tim Matthews for transcribing the interviews; and Katie Lewis for editorial support.

Author Contributions: Leslie Leve conceived of and designed the research study and reviewed and edited the manuscript. Miriam Clark led the data coding and analysis. Miriam Clark and Rohanna Buchanan authored the paper.

Conflicts of Interest: The authors declare no conflict of interest.

References

1. Banducci, A.N.; Hoffman, E.M.; Lejuez, C.W.; Koenen, K. The impact of childhood abuse on inpatient substance users: Specific links with risky sex, aggression, and emotion dysregulation. *Child Abuse Negl.* **2014**, *38*, 928–938. [CrossRef] [PubMed]
2. Oshri, A.; Tubman, J.G.; Burnette, M.L. Childhood maltreatment histories, alcohol and other drug use symptoms, and sexual risk behavior in a treatment sample of adolescents. *Amer. J. Public Health* **2012**, *102*, S250–S257. [CrossRef] [PubMed]
3. Parkhill, M.R.; Norris, J.; Cue Davi, K. The role of alcohol use during sexual situations in the relationship between sexual revictimization and women's intentions to engage in unprotected sex. *Violence Victims* **2014**, *29*, 492–505. [CrossRef] [PubMed]
4. Walsh, K.; Latzman, N.E.; Latzman, R.D. Pathway from child sexual and physical abuse to risky sex among emerging adults: The role of trauma-related intrusions and alcohol problems. *J. Adolesc. Health* **2014**, *54*, 442–448. [CrossRef] [PubMed]
5. Kaestle, C.E. Selling and buying sex: A longitudinal study of risk and protective factors in adolescence. *Prev. Sci.* **2012**, *13*, 314–322. [CrossRef] [PubMed]
6. Kramer, L.A.; Berg, E.C. A survival analysis of timing of entry into prostitution: The differential impact of race, education level, and childhood/adolescent risk factors. *Sociol. Inq.* **2003**, *73*, 511–528. [CrossRef]
7. Woerner, J.; Kopetz, C.; Lechner, W.V.; Lejuez, C. History of abuse and risky sex among substance users: The role of rejection sensitivity and the need to belong. *Addict. Behav.* **2016**, *62*, 73–78. [CrossRef] [PubMed]
8. Weisz, J.R.; Kazdin, A.E. (Eds.) *Evidence-Based Psychotherapies for Children and Adolescents*, 3rd ed.; Guilford Press: New York, NY, USA, 2017; ISBN 9781462522699.
9. Macran, H.R.; Hardy, G.E.; Shapiro, D.A. The importance of considering clients' perspectives in psychotherapy research. *Int. J. Ment. Health* **1999**, *8*, 325–337.
10. Hodgetts, A.; Wright, J. Researching clients' experiences: A review of qualitative studies. *Clin. Psychol. Psychother.* **2007**, *14*, 157–163. [CrossRef]
11. French, R.; Reardon, M.; Smith, P. Engaging with a mental health service: Perspectives of at-risk youth. *Child Adolesc. Soc. Work J.* **2003**, *20*, 529–548. [CrossRef]
12. Freake, H.; Barley, V.; Kent, G. Adolescents' views of helping professionals: A review of the literature. *J. Adolesc.* **2007**, *30*, 639–653. [CrossRef] [PubMed]
13. Reznik, Y.; Tebb, K. Where do teens go to get the 411 on sexual health? A teen intern in clinical research with teens. *Perm. J.* **2008**, *12*, PMCID:PMC3037124. [CrossRef]
14. Gibson, K.; Cartwright, C. Agency in young clients' narratives of counseling: "It's whatever you want to make of it". *J. Couns. Psychol.* **2013**, *60*. [CrossRef] [PubMed]
15. Jobe, A.; Gorin, S. "If kids don't feel safe they don't do anything": Young people's views on seeking and receiving help from Children's Social Care Services in England. *Child Fam. Soc. Work* **2013**, *18*, 429–438. [CrossRef]
16. Van Staa, A.; Jedeloo, S.; van der Stege, H.; On Your Own Feet Research Group. "What we want": Chronically ill adolescents' preferences and priorities for improving health care. *Patient Prefer Adherence* **2011**, *5*, 291–305. [CrossRef] [PubMed]
17. Offord, A.; Turner, H.; Cooper, M. Adolescent inpatient treatment for anorexia nervosa: A qualitative study exploring young adults' retrospective views of treatment and discharge. *Eur. Eat. Disord. Rev.* **2006**, *14*, 377–387. [CrossRef]
18. Galvan, A.; Hare, T.; Voss, H.; Glover, G.; Casey, B.J. Risk-taking and the adolescent brain: Who is at risk? *Dev. Sci.* **2007**, *10*, F8–F14. [CrossRef] [PubMed]
19. Giedd, J.N. The teen brain: insights from neuroimaging. *J. Adolesc. Health* **2008**, *42*, 335–343. [CrossRef] [PubMed]
20. Kim, H.K.; Pears, K.C.; Leve, L.D.; Chamberlain, P.; Smith, D.K. Intervention effects on health-risking sexual behavior among girls in foster care: The role of placement disruption and tobacco and marijuana use. *J. Child Adolesc. Subst. Abuse* **2013**, *22*, 370–387. [CrossRef] [PubMed]
21. Leve, L.D.; Khurana, A.; Reich, E.B. Intergenerational transmission of maltreatment: A multilevel examination. *Dev. Psychopathol.* **2015**, *27*. [CrossRef] [PubMed]
22. Padgett, D.K. *Qualitative Methods in Social work Research*; Sage Publications, Inc.: Los Angeles, CA, USA, 2008.

23. *NVivo Qualitative Data Analysis Software*, Version 10 ed; QSR International Pty Ltd.: Cambridge, MA, USA, 2012.
24. Glaser, B.G.; Strauss, A.L. *The Discovery of Grounded Theory: Strategies for Qualitative Research*; Aldine de Gruyter: New York, NY, USA, 1967.
25. Violence Prevention. Youth Violence: Risks and Protective Factors (Centers for Disease Control and Prevention). Available online: https://www.cdc.gov/violenceprevention/youthviolence/riskprotectivefactors.html (accessed on 26 January 2018).
26. Effective HIV and STD Prevention Programs for Youth: A Summary of Scientific Evidence (Centers for Disease Control and Prevention). Available online: https://www.cdc.gov/healthyyouth/sexualbehaviors/effective_programs.htm (accessed on 26 January 2018).
27. Centers for Disease Control and Prevention. Guidelines for School Health Programs to Prevent Tobacco Use and Addiction. *MMWR Recomm. Rep.* **1994**, *43*, 1–18. Available online: https://www.cdc.gov/mmwr/preview/mmwrhtml/00026213.htm (accessed on 26 January 2018).
28. Levine, D. Sex in the digital age. In *Sex in the digital age*; Nixon, P.G., Dusterhoft, I.K., Eds.; Routledge: Abingdon, UK, 2017; ISBN 9781138214316.
29. Purcell, K.; Rainie, L.; Heaps, A.; Buchanan, J.; Fredrich, L.; Jacklin, A.; Chen, C.; Zickhur, K. How teens do research in the digital world. 2012. Available online: https://files.eric.ed.gov/fulltext/ED537513.pdf (accessed on 15 February 2018).
30. Buchanan, R.; Chamberlain, P.; Smith, D.K. Treatment Foster Care Oregon for Adolescents: Research and implementation. In *Evidence-Based Psychotherapies for Children and Adolescents*, 3rd ed.; Weisz, J.R., Kazdin, A.E., Eds.; Guilford Press: New York, NY, USA, 2017; pp. 177–198. ISBN 9781462522699.
31. Bhati, K.S. Effect of client-therapist gender match on the therapeutic relationship: An exploratory analysis. *Psychol. Rep.* **2014**, *115*, 565–583. [CrossRef] [PubMed]
32. Zane, N.; Ku, H. Effects of ethnic match, gender match, acculturation, cultural identity, and face concern on self-disclosure in counseling for Asian Americans. *Asian Am. J. Psychol.* **2014**, *5*. [CrossRef]
33. Glisson, C.; Schoenwald, S.K.; Kelleher, K.; Landsverk, J.; Hoagwood, K.E.; Mayberg, S. Research Network on Youth Mental Health. Therapist turnover and new program sustainability in mental health clinics as a function of organizational culture, climate, and service structure. *Adm. Policy Ment. Health* **2008**, *35*, 124–133. [CrossRef] [PubMed]
34. Sheidow, A.J.; Schoenwald, S.K.; Wagner, H.R.; Allred, C.A.; Burns, B.J. Predictors of workforce turnover in a transported treatment program. *Adm. Policy Ment. Health* **2007**, *34*, 45–56. [CrossRef] [PubMed]
35. Santelli, J.; Ott, M.A.; Lyon, M.; Rogers, J.; Summers, D.; Schleifer, R. Abstinence and abstinence-only education: A review of U.S. policies and programs. *J. Adolesc. Health* **2006**, *38*, 72–81. [CrossRef] [PubMed]
36. Clayton, R.R.; Cattarello, A.M.; Johnstone, B.M. The effectiveness of Drug Abuse Resistance Education (Project DARE): 5-year follow-up results. *Prev. Med.* **1996**, *25*, 307–318. [CrossRef] [PubMed]
37. Petrosino, A.; Turpin-Petrosino, C.; Finckenauer, J.O. Well-meaning programs can have harmful effects! Lessons from experiments of programs such as Scared Straight. *NCCD News* **2000**, *46*, 354–379. [CrossRef]

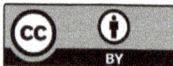

© 2018 by the authors. Licensee MDPI, Basel, Switzerland. This article is an open access article distributed under the terms and conditions of the Creative Commons Attribution (CC BY) license (http://creativecommons.org/licenses/by/4.0/).

Article

International Journal of
*Environmental Research
and Public Health*

MDPI

Adolescents' Sexual Wellbeing in Southwestern Uganda: A Cross-Sectional Assessment of Body Image, Self-Esteem and Gender Equitable Norms

Elizabeth Kemigisha [1,2,*], Viola N. Nyakato [1], Katharine Bruce [1], Gad Ndaruhutse Ruzaaza [1], Wendo Mlahagwa [1], Anna B. Ninsiima [3], Gily Coene [3], Els Leye [2,3] and Kristien Michielsen [2,*]

[1] Faculty of Interdisciplinary Studies, Mbarara University of Science and Technology, Mbarara 1410, Uganda; vnyakato@must.ac.ug (V.N.N.); kbruce2@tulane.edu (K.B.); gruzaaza@must.ac.ug (G.N.R.); wolema@must.ac.ug (W.M.)
[2] International Centre for Reproductive Health, Faculty of Medicine and Health Sciences, Ghent University, 9000 Ghent, Belgium; els.leye@ugent.be
[3] RHEA, Centre of Expertise on Gender, Diversity and Intersectionality, Vrije Universiteit Brussel, 1050 Brussels, Belgium; annekiiza2001@yahoo.com (A.B.N.); gily.coene@vub.ac.be (G.C.)
* Correspondence: ekemigisha@must.ac.ug (E.K.); Kristien.michielsen@ugent.be (K.M.); Tel.: +256-772-858818 (E.K.)

Received: 13 December 2017; Accepted: 31 January 2018; Published: 22 February 2018

Abstract: Measures of sexual wellbeing and positive aspects of sexuality in the World Health Organization definition for sexual health are rarely studied and remain poorly understood, especially among adolescents in Sub-Saharan Africa. The objective of this study was to assess sexual wellbeing in its broad sense—i.e., body image, self-esteem, and gender equitable norms—and associated factors in young adolescents in Uganda. A cross-sectional survey of adolescents ages 10–14 years in schools was carried out between June and July 2016. Among 1096 adolescents analyzed, the median age was 12 (Inter-Quartile Range (IQR): 11, 13) and 58% were female. Self-esteem and body image scores were high with median 24 (IQR: 22, 26, possible range: 7–28) and median 22 (IQR: 19, 24, possible range: 5–25) respectively. Gender equitable norms mean score was 28.1 (SD 5.2: possible range 11–44). We noted high scores for self-esteem and body image but moderate scores on gender equitable norms. Girls had higher scores compared to boys for all outcomes. A higher age and being sexually active were associated with lower scores on gender equitable norms. Gender equitable norms scores decreased with increasing age of adolescents. Comprehensive and timely sexuality education programs focusing on gender differences and norms are recommended.

Keywords: self-esteem; gender norms; body image; young adolescents; Uganda; sexuality; sexual health

1. Introduction

The World Health Organization (WHO) defines sexual health as "a state of physical, mental and social wellbeing in relation to sexuality. It requires a positive and respectful approach to sexuality and sexual relationships, as well as the possibility of having pleasurable and safe sexual experiences, free of coercion, discrimination and violence" [1]. Sexual wellbeing aspects in the current WHO definition for sexual health are rarely explored. Most scholars, country demographic surveys and international reports focus on the negative aspects of sexual health and risky sexual behavior. Understanding positive sexual health attributes is important as these empower young people to make informed choices for better sexual and reproductive health (SRH) outcomes [2]. This is particularly important among young adolescents (10–14 years) who are commonly neglected in research. Young adolescents are at a formative stage of development, but often ill-equipped with relevant knowledge and decision-making skills. This period is important to laying a foundation for positive SRH behaviors and outcomes [3,4].

As a developing country in which adolescents comprise 1/3 of the total population, Uganda is facing serious challenges related to SRH of young people [5]. These challenges include: low comprehensive Human Immunodeficiency Virus and Acquired Immune Deficiency Syndrome (HIV/AIDS) prevention knowledge at 40% with heightened risks for Sexually Transmitted Infection (STI) acquisition, high teenage pregnancy at 25% which contributes 24% of maternal mortality, and low contraceptive uptake [6]. However, there is a paucity of studies in Sub-Saharan Africa that describe positive attributes of adolescents' sexual health, which are pertinent to address prevailing SRH challenges.

Recently, there has been growing attention among scholars on the assessment of adolescent sexual wellbeing [2,7]. Recent work by Russel (2005) and Blum et al. (2014) emphasizes the need for a socio-ecological framework to assess adolescent sexuality at the individual, institutional and societal or cultural levels [3,8]. Furthermore, Harden (2014) explores the possibility of evaluating adolescent sexual wellbeing based on factors such as adolescent self-efficacy, sexual self-esteem, sexual pleasure and satisfaction, and freedom from pain and negative effects related to sexuality [9]. These aspects have been further emphasized by the European expert group on sexuality who also prioritize evaluation of aspects related to positive attitudes towards gender equality and adolescent empowerment in making informed choices [2]. Few studies have evaluated gender equitable norms, self-esteem and body image or satisfaction as they relate to positive outcomes of sexual and reproductive health [10–13]. There is no consensus on how aspects of sexual wellbeing should be assessed and reported, especially among the adolescent population, and the research on this topic is limited [2,7].

This study assessed sexual wellbeing of young adolescents in primary schools in Southwestern (SW) Uganda. We looked at several aspects related to wellbeing, namely self-esteem, gender equitable norms and body image scores, as well as their associations with socio-demographic characteristics, school and family environment, and sexual activity. We focused on individual factors such as gender, age, educational level and socio economic status as well as interpersonal and environmental factors such as school absenteeism, bullying, number of parents alive, exposure to media and sexual onset, as these have been shown to influence adolescent SRH [14]. We hypothesized that there would be a difference in scores for sexual wellbeing among younger adolescents (10–12 years compared to 13–14 years) and higher scores among boys compared to girls [15].

2. Materials and Methods

2.1. Study Design and Sample Population

This study utilized a cross-sectional design. The data was collected as part of a cluster randomized trial analyzing the effectiveness of a comprehensive sexuality education intervention among young adolescents ages 10–14 years in primary schools in SW Uganda. The sample size was 1104 adolescents in primary 5 and 6 drawn from 33 schools in urban and rural settings in Mbarara district.

2.2. Main Outcomes

The main outcomes for the study were self-esteem, body image and gender equitable norm scores, which were used independently as proxy indicators for positive aspects of sexual health. Self-esteem scores were estimated using 7 of 10 items of the Rosenberg (1965) self-esteem scale [16]. These included positively scored items such as; *"I feel that I am a person of importance"*; and negatively scored items such as *"I feel useless at times."* Item 4 *"I can do things as well as most people,"* Item 8 *"I wish I could have more respect for myself"* and Item 10, *"I take a positive attitude toward myself"* were excluded. Items 8 and 10 were excluded because they were complex and not suitable for the age group, whereas Item 4 was excluded at analysis due to poor correlation with other items in the scale. The Cronbach alpha reliability test for the items was low but acceptable at 0.60 [17]. Body image scores were estimated using 5 of the 6 items of the Body Image States Scale (BISS-6) [18]. These included items such as *"Right now, I feel extremely satisfied with my looks."* Item 5 *"Right now, I feel much worse about my looks than I usually feel"* was excluded at analysis due to poor correlation with the rest of the items on the scale, and the scale was modified from a 9 points to a 5 points Likert scale for ease of use for this age group. The Cronbach alpha reliability test for the items was 0.67. Gender equitable norms scores were estimated using 11 items. Six of these items were adapted from the Attitudes towards Women Scale for Adolescents (AWSA) [19] and 5 items were developed to suit the respondents' age and the Ugandan context. Items from the AWSA scale included, *"On average boys are cleverer than girls"* and *"Girls should be free to go out unaccompanied to meet with friends"*. The other items developed to relate to the Uganda context included, *"If there is a sick person at home, only a girl should stay home to care for the sick one as the boy goes on with school"* or *"My mother more than my father should be blamed for my mistakes."* The items were scored on a 4 point Likert scale. The Cronbach alpha reliability test for the items was 0.68. Individuals with missing data on any of the items on a scale were eliminated from that analysis.

2.3. Correlates

Information on social and demographic variables such as age and gender were collected. Pubertal or Tanner stage was estimated by self-assessment, in which respondents were shown a pictorial representation of the Tanner stages and told to select the image that best represented their own stage of development. This provided estimates of pubertal stages without requiring more invasive inspections that often make young adolescents feel uncomfortable. Studies such as Rasmussen et al. 2015 have shown that although self-assessment is not a reliable measure of exact pubertal timing, it is a sufficient estimate of relative pubertal stage for large epidemiologic studies [20]. A socio-economic score was developed based on household water source, distance from water source, household possessions and pupil possessions including shoes and pairs of school uniforms. We developed this score using a subset of items from the standard Demographic and Health Survey score so that the data could be more readily collected from young adolescents, as opposed to using other standard measurements which are administered to adults. Students self-reported on truancy and sexual activity. Truancy was defined as absence from school for any reason other than that the student was sick. Sexual activity was defined as a student reporting having had penetrative vaginal sex. Exposure to visual or audiovisual media of sexual content (pornographic content) was also assessed.

2.4. Statistical Analysis

Data analysis was done using Stata® (College Station, TX, USA). Continuous variables were summarized using means (SD) and medians (IQR) whereas categorical variables were summarized using proportions (percentages). Mean (SD) was used to summarize gender norms scores because they were normally distributed, while medians (IQR) were used to summarize body image and self-esteem because they were non-normally distributed. Among categorical variables, a bivariate analysis was conducted using odds ratios. Among continuous variables, a *t*-test was conducted for variables that were normally distributed, and a Mann–Whitney test was conducted for variables that were non-normally distributed. Multivariate logistic regression analysis with stepwise variable selection was performed on variables with a *p*-value less than 0.2 at bivariate analysis to assess the association between self-esteem scores ≤ median vs. > median, body image score ≤ median vs. > median, and gender equitable norms mean scores with socio-demographic, school and family factors and sexual behavior, respectively. A test for collinearity was done prior to multivariate analysis and for all the models the Variance Inflation Factors were less than 1.5. Odds ratios and 95% confidence intervals were calculated. A *p*-value of less than 0.05 was considered to reflect a significant association.

2.5. Ethics

The study was approved by the Mbarara University Research Ethics Committee (reference MUIRC 1/7) and the Uganda National Council for Science and Technology (reference SS 4045). We also obtained ethical approval from Ghent University as a partner institution. Written parental consent, school head teacher consent and pupils' assent were obtained prior to data collection.

3. Results

3.1. Description of the Study Population

Between June and July 2016, a total of 1104 primary school pupils ages 10–14 were interviewed. Of these, 8 were excluded because their age could not be verified, and 1096 were included in this analysis. Among the 1096 adolescents, 460 (42%) were male, the median age was 12 years (IQR: 11, 13), 635 (57.9%) were between ages of 10–12 years, and 896 (81.8%) were from schools in rural areas. A total of 79 (17.3%) pupils reported bullying and 249 (22.7%) reported truancy, as defined by absence from school for any reason other than illness. Only 83 (7.6%) reported being sexually active, 67 (80.7%) of which were boys (Table 1).

Table 1. Socio-demographic characteristics, family and school factors and sexual behavior of study participants.

	Overall, n (%) n = 1096	Male n (%) n = 460 (42.0)	Female n (%) n = 636 (58.0)	*p*-Value
Age in years				
10–12	635 (57.9)	259 (56.3)	376 (59.1)	
13–14	461 (42.1)	201 (43.7)	260 (40.9)	0.351
Pubertal age (Tanner 1–5)				
Tanner 1 or 2	509 (46.4)	217 (47.2)	292 (45.9)	1
Tanner stage >2	584 (53.6)	243 (52.8)	344 (54.1)	
Education level				
Primary 5	563 (51.4)	240 (52.2)	323 (50.8)	
Primary 6	533 (48.6)	220 (47.8)	313 (49.2)	0.650
Socio-economic status				
Low	315 (29.0)	128 (28.2)	187 (29.6)	
Medium	511 (47.1)	215 (47.4)	296 (46.8)	
High	260 (23.9)	111 (24.4)	149 (23.6)	0.871
Religion				
Moslem	101 (9.2)	48 (10.5)	53 (8.3)	
Anglican/Pentecostal	587 (53.7)	245 (53.5)	342 (53.9)	
Catholic	405 (37.1)	165 (36.0)	240 (37.8)	0.462
Family and school factors				
Location of school				
Rural	896 (81.8)	368 (80)	529 (83.2)	
Urban	199 (18.2)	92 (20)	107 (16.8)	0.178
School absenteeism (truancy)	249 (22.7)	100 (21.7)	149 (23.4)	0.510
Ever experienced bullying at school	79 (17.3)	119 (18.7)	198 (18.1)	0.528
Number of parents alive				
Both alive	905 (82.5)	378 (82.2)	527 (82.8)	
None/Single parent	124 (11.3)	48 (10.4)	76 (12.0)	0.350
Access to media (TV, Social media or Tabloids)				
Television	458 (41.8)	217(47.3)	241 (37.9)	0.002
Tabloid newspapers	222 (20.3)	125 (27.2)	97 (15.3)	<0.0001
Social media	70 (6.4)	27 (5.9)	43 (6.8)	0.558
Ever watched pornographic content	389 (35.5)	191 (41.5)	198 (31.2)	<0.0001
Sexual behavior				
Ever had sex	83 (7.6)	67 (14.6)	16 (2.5)	<0.0001

3.2. Outcomes

3.2.1. Self-Esteem

The median self-reported self-esteem score was 24 (IQR: 22, 26, range: 11–28) with a possible score range of 7–28. Girls had higher scores compared to boys, with 282 (46.4%) girls and only 153 (34.6%) boys scoring above the median. A Mann–Whitney test found that the difference in median self-esteem scores between each gender was statistically significant ($p < 0.0001$).

3.2.2. Body Image

The median self-reported body image score among respondents was 22 (IQR: 19, 24, range: 8–25) with a possible score range of 5–25. Girls reported higher scores than boys, with 302 (47.8%) girls and only 174 (38.2%) boys scoring above median. A Mann–Whitney test found that the difference between median scores for boys and girls was statistically significant ($p = 0.002$).

3.2.3. Gender Equitable Norms

The mean score for gender equitable norms was 28.1 (SD 5.2; range: 13–44), with a possible score range of 11–44. Girls had higher scores on gender equitable norms with a mean of 29.1 (SD 4.9) compared to 26.7 (SD 5.3) in boys. A *t*-test found that the difference in mean scores for boys and girls was significant ($p < 0.00001$).

3.3. Bivariate Analysis of Factors Associated with Main Outcomes

Results of bivariate analysis are presented in Table 2. Female gender was associated with higher scores for gender equitable norms, self-esteem and body image. Other characteristics associated with higher self-esteem scores included being of higher education level and religious denomination, that is, being of Catholic faith compared to Moslem or Anglican. Alternatively, pupils from urban schools and those who were truant (absent from school without clear reason) overall had lower self-esteem scores. Higher scores on gender equitable norms were reported among those with a higher socio-economic status, a higher tanner stage and a younger age. Pupils with lower gender equitable norms scores were more likely to have ever had sex. Furthermore, pupils in a higher education level and those from urban schools were more likely to have higher scores on body image.

Table 2. Bivariate analysis of self-esteem, body image and gender equitable norms with social and demographic, school and family factors and sexual behaviors.

	Self-Esteem		Body Image		Gender Equitable Norms	
	OR [†]	95% CI	OR	95% CI	Beta Coefficient	95% CI
Gender						
Male	1					
Female	1.64	(1.28–2.12) ***	1.48	(1.16–1.89) **	2.42	(1.78–3.05) ***
Age						
10–12	1					
13–14	1.06	(0.83–1.37)	1.26	(0.99–1.60)	−0.95	(−1.6--0.31) **
Pubertal age (Tanner 1–5)						
Tanner 1 and 2	1					
Tanner 3 to 5	1.06	(0.73–1.55)	1.11	(0.77–1.61)	1.52	(0.54–2.51) **
Education level						
Primary 5	1					
Primary 6	1.51	(1.19–1.94) **	1.39	(1.09–1.77) **	0.1	(−0.54–0.74)
Socio-economic status						
Low	1					
Medium	0.99	(0.74–1.32)	1.13	(0.85–1.50)	−0.05	(−0.81–0.70)
High	1.02	(0.73–1.43)	1.23	(0.88–1.71)	1.43	(0.55–2.31) **

Table 2. *Cont.*

	Self-Esteem		Body Image		Gender Equitable Norms	
	OR [†]	95% CI	OR	95% CI	Beta Coefficient	95% CI
Religion						
Moslem	1					
Anglican/Pentecostal	1.49	(0.94–2.35)	1.11	(0.73–1.71)	−0.45	(−1.58–0.68)
Catholic	1.84	(1.15–2.95) *	0.78	(0.50–1.22)	−0.017	(−1.34–0.99)
Location of school						
Rural	1					
Urban	0.62	(0.45–0.87) **	1.46	(1.07–1.99) *	0.6	(−0.21–1.44)
School absenteeism (truancy)	0.66	(0.49–0.89) **	0.87	(0.65–1.15)	−0.2	(−0.97–0.56)
Number of parents alive						
None/Single parent	1					
Both alive	1.11	(0.80–1.54)	1.23	(0.89–1.69)	−0.71	(−1.59–0.17)
Ever watched pornography	0.89	(0.69–1.15)	1.11	(0.86–1.42)	−0.56	(−1.23–0.11)
Ever had sex	0.64	(0.39–1.05)	0.63	(0.39–1.01)	−2.30	(−3.50−1.10) ***

[†] Odds Ratio * $p < 0.05$; ** $p < 0.01$; *** $p < 0.001$.

3.4. Multivariate Analysis of Factors Associated with Main Outcomes

Results of multivariate analysis are presented in Table 3. On multivariate analysis with key outcomes, female gender was associated with increased scores for self-esteem, body image and gender equitable norms. Furthermore, being in primary 6 as opposed to primary 5 was associated with higher scores for body image and self-esteem, but had no association with gender equitable norms. Older age, higher Tanner stage, lower socio-economic status, and having both parents alive compared to only one and none were associated with lower scores on gender equitable norms. Additionally, early sexual activity was associated with lower gender equitable norms scores. However, no associations were established between scores for body image or self-esteem and sexual activity. Pupils who reported school absence without a reason were more likely to have lower self-esteem scores. Students from urban schools were more likely to have lower self-esteem scores but higher body image scores.

Table 3. Multivariate analysis of self-esteem scores, body image, gender equitable norm score with socio-demographic, family and school factors and sexual behavior.

	Self-Esteem		Body Image		Gender Equality Score	
	AOR [‡]	95% CI	AOR	95% CI	Beta Coefficient	95% CI
Gender						
Female	1.65	(1.28–2.14) ***	1.52	(1.19–1.96) **	2.26	(1.62–2.92) ***
Age						
10 to 12 vs. 13 to 14	1.07	(0.82–1.40)	1.39	(1.08–1.79) *	−0.68	(−1.33−−0.03) *
Tanner age						
Tanner 1–2						
Tanner 3–5	0.89	(0.69–1.15)			−0.66	(−1.29−−0.17) *
School location						
Rural vs. Urban	0.61	(0.44–0.86) **	1.61	(1.18–2.22) **	0.58	(−0.22–1.40)
Parent alive						
One/both parents dead						
Both parents alive			1.28	(0.92–1.77)	−0.89	(−1.74−−0.03) *

Table 3. *Cont.*

	Self-Esteem		Body Image		Gender Equality Score	
	AOR [‡]	95% CI	AOR	95% CI	Beta Coefficient	95% CI
Socio-economic status						
Low						
Medium						0.05	(−0.68–0.78)
High						1.49	(0.63–2.34) **
Truancy	0.62	(0.46–0.84) **				
Ever had sex						−1.25	(−2.44−−0.05) *

[‡] Adjusted Odds Ratio * $p < 0.05$; ** $p < 0.01$; *** $p < 0.001$.

4. Discussion

Few validated measures exist for assessing positive aspects of sexual health among young adolescents, especially in the cultural context of Sub-Saharan Africa. This is one of the first studies in Uganda to measure sexual wellbeing in this subpopulation, using the proxy indicators of gender equitable norms, self-esteem, body image and relevant covariates. Overall, this research found high scores for body image and self-esteem but moderate scores for gender equitable norms among young adolescents in SW Uganda. The study also provides insight into individual and interpersonal factors at the family and school levels that are associated with body image, self-esteem and gender equitable norms. Findings illustrate diminishing gender equitable norms with increasing age and an association between low gender equitable norm scores and early sexual onset. However, we did not establish in this study any associations between scores for body image or self-esteem and sexual activity.

We found moderate scores on gender equitable norms for young adolescents. This indicates that adolescents in Uganda are already socialized at a young age to have inequitable norms, a finding which has been described in another recent study [21]. In addition, our finding that early sexual onset was associated with having lower gender equitable norms scores is of concern, as there is existing evidence that equitable gender norms promote good sexual outcomes [10,22,23]. These findings, together with the association between lower gender equitable norms scores and increasing age, are of paramount importance as they relate to the timing of educational interventions to promote gender equality. Furthermore, the finding that girls had higher gender equitable norms scores than boys has important implications for educational interventions. These gender disparities could be explained by the fact that most mainstream media and health promotion programs in schools that address adolescent SRH vulnerabilities in Uganda focus on protecting and supporting the girl child only while neglecting the needs of boys [24]. The findings of this study, along with other related research in this field, highlight the importance of addressing issues of gender and equality among both boys and girls at a young age.

Additionally, our study found that the presence of both parents compared to one or none was associated with having lower gender equity. Because equitable gender norms are clearly shaped in early childhood, parents play an important role [25,26]. This finding also highlights the fact that gender norms are influenced by multiple levels of the socio-ecological model, and interventions will therefore be most effective if they address multiple levels of the socio-ecological model. Educational interventions should involve parents as well as adolescents in order to produce meaningful and sustainable change.

We found high scores in body image and self-esteem in this age group. The findings that females were more likely than males to have higher body image and self-esteem scores contradicts much of the existing literature on gender, body image and self-esteem, which has often found that male adolescents have higher self-esteem than females [15,27]. This contradiction could be explained by the fact that our study focuses on young adolescents, while other studies on adolescents often include an older age range. It could also be related to the Ugandan context, as most research related to body image and self-esteem is conducted in Western countries [15,27,28]. It is possible that a focus on the girl child, common in many health education programs in Uganda, might contribute to higher scores in body image and self-esteem among girls compared to boys. One study conducted in seven Ugandan schools found that girls received more guidance than boys about their SRH, both in the classroom and in the home [29]. Another study of Ugandan adolescents found that boys were less likely than girls to have discussed SRH issues with their parents [30]. Whether in the classroom or at home, young boys in Uganda are less likely to discuss their SRH with adults, which may contribute to anxiety about their changing bodies and lower self-esteem.

Certain environmental and school factors were found to be associated with high self-esteem and body image scores. Living in an urban vs. a rural area was associated with lower scores on self-esteem but higher scores on body image. Economic disparities within the urban environment could explain the relatively low self-esteem scores in this group. Improving education and narrowing disparities in incomes and social amenities among people living in urban areas could reduce the gap in self-esteem. Regarding body image, it was found that being in the older age group was associated with higher body image scores, and that children from rural schools were significantly older than their counterparts in urban schools. It is therefore possible that the discrepancy in body image scores between urban and rural students may actually be explained by age and not by location. No associations between self-esteem scores or body image scores with sexual onset were established in this study. There is contradicting evidence regarding the association between self-esteem and sexual efficacy or behavior, with a few studies describing no relationship [13,27,31], whereas Ethier et al. 2006 [12] describe a positive association between the two. Studies on body image have been more or less consistent in showing associations with positive sexual outcomes [32]. The lack of an association between self-esteem or body image scores and sexual behavior in our study population could reflect a genuine lack of association. However, it may also be attributable to low variation in scores for body image and self-esteem in this group.

The study had a few key limitations. Due to the cross-sectional nature of this study, it was not possible to determine whether some of the individual or contextual factors preceded the outcome variables. Another limitation was the potential risk of social desirability bias due to self-reporting of behaviors. Whenever possible, interviewers and participants were matched on gender to try to limit this bias. Lastly, we used scales for measurement of gender norms, self-esteem and body image that have mainly been used for older adolescents. We therefore adapted these scales and piloted them. Cronbach alpha scores were slightly lower than what is generally considered acceptable, which might suggest that the results of these scores had lower reliability than would be ideal. However, because Cronbach alpha is a function of the scale length as well as the reliability, it tends to underestimate the reliability of surveys like ours which have relatively few items [33]. It is also possible that the specific items chosen from the Rosenberg self-esteem scale could have influenced the gender discrepancy in self-esteem scores. The Rosenberg scale used in this study may have limitations in its applicability because it is unidimensional. Studies that consider self-esteem from a multidimensional perspective have found that girls score higher on certain components of self-esteem, while boys score higher on others [34,35], meaning that in selecting a subset of items we may have selected items on which girls generally have higher scores. Future research should consider the multidimensionality of self-esteem.

5. Conclusions

Young adolescents in primary schools in Uganda have high scores for body image and self-esteem and moderate scores on gender equitable norms. Gender equitable norms scores reduce with increasing age, suggesting that sexuality education interventions need to start while adolescents are still young, before they have developed these harmful norms. Further research is recommended on (1) establishing causal relationships between socio-ecological variables and gender equitable norms, self-esteem or body image, and (2) validation of measurements for attributes of positive sexual health in different contexts among very young adolescents. More studies are needed in the Ugandan setting to explain possible relationships between measures of sexual wellbeing and positive sexual health outcomes in young adolescents.

Acknowledgments: We wish to thank Apolo Filomena Ojok, Clara Atuhaire, Mark Kiiza, Simeon Eloba, Derrick Nuwamanya and Amerias Arimpa for coordination activities during data collection. We thank all the research assistants who participated in the survey. We also thank Rinah Arinaitwe and her team for the data management. We acknowledge the contribution of Damazo Kadengye and Daniel Atwine for their statistical input during design of sampling procedures. We thank all the pupils who participated in the study and their parents and teachers for their cooperation. This study was funded by Flemish Interuniversity Council (VLIR UOS) under a team project, grant number ZEIN2015PR411. The funders had no role in the study design, data collection procedures or writing of the manuscript.

Author Contributions: Elizabeth Kemigisha, Viola N. Nyakato and Kristien Michielsen participated in the study design, analysis and writing of the manuscript. Katharine Bruce, Gad Ndaruhutse Ruzaaza, Wendo Mlahagwa, Els Leye, Anna B. Ninsiimaand Gily Coene participated in the writing and editing of the manuscript. All authors read and approved the final version of this manuscript.

Conflicts of Interest: The authors declare no conflict of interest.

References

1. World Health Organization (WHO). *Report on Sexual Health: Report of a Technical Consultation on Sexual Health 28–31 January 2002, Geneva*; World Health Organization: Geneva, Switzerland, 2006.
2. Ketting, E.; Friele, M.; Michielsen, K. Evaluation of holistic sexuality education: A European expert group consensus agreement. *Eur. J. Contracept. Reprod. Health Care* **2016**, *21*, 68–80. [CrossRef] [PubMed]
3. Blum, R.W.; Astone, N.M.; Decker, M.R.; Mouli, V.C. A conceptual framework for early adolescence: A platform for research. *Int. J. Adolesc. Med. Health* **2014**, *26*, 321–331. [CrossRef] [PubMed]
4. Woog, V.; Kågesten, A. *The Sexual and Reproductive Health Needs of Very Young Adolescents Aged 10–14 in Developing Countries: What Does the Evidence Show?* Guttmacher Institute: New York, NY, USA, 2017.
5. Uganda Bureau Of Statistics (UBOS). *Uganda National Population and Housing Census 2014*; Provisional Results; UBOS: Kampala, Uganda, 2014.
6. Uganda Bureau Of Statistics (UBOS); ICF. *The Uganda Demographics and Health Survey 2016: Key Indicators Report*; UBOS: Kampala, Uganda, 2017.
7. World Health Organization (WHO). *Measuring Sexual Health: Conceptual and Practical Considerations and Related Indicators*; World Health Organization: Geneva, Switzerland, 2010.
8. Russell, S.T. Conceptualizing positive adolescent sexuality development. *Sex. Res. Soc. Policy* **2005**, *2*, 4–12. [CrossRef]
9. Harden, K.P. A sex-positive framework for research on adolescent sexuality. *Perspect. Psychol. Sci.* **2014**, *9*, 455–469. [CrossRef] [PubMed]
10. De Meyer, S.; Jaruseviciene, L.; Zaborskis, A.; Decat, P.; Vega, B.; Cordova, K.; Temmerman, M.; Degomme, O.; Michielsen, K. A cross-sectional study on attitudes toward gender equality, sexual behavior, positive sexual experiences, and communication about sex among sexually active and non-sexually active adolescents in Bolivia and Ecuador. *Glob. Health Action* **2014**, *7*, 24089. [CrossRef] [PubMed]
11. Winter, V.R.; Satinsky, S. Body appreciation, sexual relationship status, and protective sexual behaviors in women. *Body Image* **2014**, *11*, 36–42. [CrossRef] [PubMed]
12. Ethier, K.A.; Kershaw, T.S.; Lewis, J.B.; Milan, S.; Niccolai, L.M.; Ickovics, J.R. Self-esteem, emotional distress and sexual behavior among adolescent females: Inter-relationships and temporal effects. *J. Adolesc. Health* **2006**, *38*, 268–274. [CrossRef] [PubMed]
13. Goodson, P.; Buhi, E.R.; Dunsmore, S.C. Self-esteem and adolescent sexual behaviors, attitudes, and intentions: A systematic review. *J. Adolesc. Health* **2006**, *38*, 310–319. [CrossRef] [PubMed]
14. Blum, R.W.; Mmari, K.N.; World Health Organization. *Risk and Protective Factors Affecting Adolescent Reproductive Health in Developing Countries*; WHO: Geneva, Switzerland, 2004.
15. Bleidorn, W.; Arslan, R.C.; Denissen, J.J.; Rentfrow, P.J.; Gebauer, J.E.; Potter, J.; Gosling, S.D. Age and gender differences in self-esteem—A cross-cultural window. *J. Pers. Soc. Psychol.* **2016**, *111*, 396–410. [CrossRef] [PubMed]

16. Rosenberg, M. *Rosenberg Self-Esteem Scale (RSE): Acceptance and Commitment Therapy*; Measures Package; University of Wollongong: Wollongong, Australia, 1965; Volume 61, p. 52.
17. Perry, R.; Charlotte, B.; Isabella, M.; Bob, C. *SPSS Explained*; Routledge: London, UK, 2004.
18. Cash, T.F.; Fleming, E.C.; Alindogan, J.; Steadman, L.; Whitehead, A. Beyond body image as a trait: The development and validation of the Body Image States Scale. *Eat. Disord.* **2002**, *10*, 103–113. [CrossRef] [PubMed]
19. Galambos, N.L.; Petersen, A.C.; Richards, M.; Gitelson, I.B. The Attitudes toward Women Scale for Adolescents (AWSA): A study of reliability and validity. *Sex Roles* **1985**, *13*, 343–356. [CrossRef]
20. Rasmussen, A.R.; Wohlfahrt-Veje, C.; de Renzy-Martin, K.T.; Hagen, C.P.; Tinggaard, J.; Mouritsen, A.; Mieritz, M.G.; Main, K.M. Validity of self-assessment of pubertal maturation. *Pediatrics* **2015**, *135*, 86–93. [CrossRef] [PubMed]
21. Vu, L.; Pulerwitz, J.; Burnett-Zieman, B.; Banura, C.; Okal, J.; Yam, E. Inequitable gender norms from early adolescence to young adulthood in Uganda: Tool validation and differences across age groups. *J. Adolesc. Health* **2017**, *60*, S15–S21. [CrossRef] [PubMed]
22. Jewkes, R.; Morrell, R. Gender and sexuality: Emerging perspectives from the heterosexual epidemic in South Africa and implications for HIV risk and prevention. *J. Int. AIDS Soc.* **2010**, *13*, 6. [CrossRef] [PubMed]
23. Rolleri, L. *Gender Norms and Sexual Health Behaviors*; Research FACTs and Findings; ACT for Youth Center of Excellence: Ithaca, NY, USA, 2013.
24. Bukenya, D.L.; Pfiffer, B. *Young Men's Health in Uganda*; Makerere University Columbia University (MUCU) Newsletter; MUCU: Kampala, Uganda, 2015.
25. Martin, C.L.; Ruble, D.N. Patterns of gender development. *Annu. Rev. Psychol.* **2010**, *61*, 353–381. [CrossRef] [PubMed]
26. McHale, S.M.; Crouter, A.C.; Whiteman, S.D. The family contexts of gender development in childhood and adolescence. *Soc. Dev.* **2003**, *12*, 125–148. [CrossRef]
27. Silva, R.N.A.; van de Bongardt, D.; Baams, L.; Raat, H. Bidirectional associations between adolescents' sexual behaviors and psychological well-being. *J. Adolesc. Health* **2018**, *62*, 63–71. [CrossRef] [PubMed]
28. Bachman, J.G.; O'Malley, P.M.; Freedman-Doan, P.; Trzesniewski, K.H.; Donnellan, M.B. Adolescent self-esteem: Differences by race/ethnicity, gender, and age. *Self Identity* **2011**, *10*, 445–473. [CrossRef] [PubMed]
29. Muhanguzi, F.K.; Ninsiima, A. Embracing teen sexuality: Teenagers' assessment of sexuality education in Uganda. *Agenda* **2011**, *25*, 54–63.
30. Muhwezi, W.W.; Katahoire, A.R.; Banura, C.; Mugooda, H.; Kwesiga, D.; Bastien, S.; Klepp, K.I. Perceptions and experiences of adolescents, parents and school administrators regarding adolescent-parent communication on sexual and reproductive health issues in urban and rural Uganda. *Reprod. Health* **2015**, *12*, 110. [CrossRef] [PubMed]
31. Wheeler, S.B. Effects of self-esteem and academic performance on adolescent decision-making: An examination of early sexual intercourse and illegal substance use. *J. Adolesc. Health* **2010**, *47*, 582–590. [CrossRef] [PubMed]
32. Winter, V.R. Toward a Relational Understanding of Objectification, Body Image, and Preventive Sexual Health. *J. Sex Res.* **2017**, *54*, 341–350. [CrossRef] [PubMed]
33. Taber, K.S. The Use of Cronbach's Alpha When Developing and Reporting Research Instruments in Science Education. *Res. Sci. Educ.* **2017**, 1–24. [CrossRef]
34. Membrilla, J.A.A.; Martínez, M.C.P. Teenagers' gender differences in self-concept. *Anal. Psicol./Ann. Psychol.* **2000**, *16*, 207–214.
35. Torres, L.H.; Mohand, M.A.-L.; Mohand, L.M. Rendimiento escolar y autoconcepto en educación primaria. Relación y análisis por género. *Int. J. Dev. Educ. Psychol. Rev. INFAD Psicol.* **2017**, *3*, 315–326.

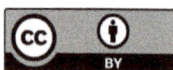

© 2018 by the authors. Licensee MDPI, Basel, Switzerland. This article is an open access article distributed under the terms and conditions of the Creative Commons Attribution (CC BY) license (http://creativecommons.org/licenses/by/4.0/).

International Journal of
Environmental Research and Public Health

MDPI

Article

The Use of Manual Vacuum Aspiration in the Treatment of Incomplete Abortions: A Descriptive Study from Three Public Hospitals in Malawi

Maria Lisa Odland [1,*], Gladys Membe-Gadama [2], Ursula Kafulafula [3], Geir W. Jacobsen [1], James Kumwenda [4] and Elisabeth Darj [1,5,6]

1   Department of Public Health and Nursing, Norwegian University of Science and Technology,
     NO-7491 Trondheim, Norway; geirjacobsen@ntnu.no (G.W.J.); elisabeth.darj@ntnu.no (E.D)
2   Queen Elizabeth Central Hospital, Blantyre, Malawi; glachime@yahoo.com
3   Kamuzu College of Nursing, Blantyre, Malawi; ursulakafulafula@kcn.unima.mw
4   Mangochi District Hospital, Mangochi, Malawi; kumwendajk@gmail.com
5   Department of Woman´s Health and Children´s Health, Uppsala University, SE-751 85 Uppsala, Sweden
6   Department of Gynecology, St. Olav´s Hospital, NO-7030 Trondheim, Norway
*   Correspondence: maria.l.odland@ntnu.no; Tel.: +47-971-255-69

Received: 1 February 2018; Accepted: 19 February 2018; Published: 21 February 2018

Abstract: Malawi has a high maternal mortality rate, of which unsafe abortion is a major cause. About 140,000 induced abortions are estimated every year, despite there being a restrictive abortion law in place. This leads to complications, such as incomplete abortions, which need to be treated to avoid further harm. Although manual vacuum aspiration (MVA) is a safe and cheap method of evacuating the uterus, the most commonly used method in Malawi is curettage. Medical treatment is used sparingly in the country, and the Ministry of Health has been trying to increase the use of MVA. The aim of this study was to investigate the treatment of incomplete abortions in three public hospitals in Southern Malawi during a three-year period. All medical files from the female/gynecological wards from 2013 to 2015 were reviewed. In total, information on obstetric history, demographics, and treatment were collected from 7270 women who had been treated for incomplete abortions. The overall use of MVA at the three hospitals during the study period was 11.4% (95% CI, 10.7–12.1). However, there was a major increase in MVA application at one District Hospital. Why there was only one successful hospital in this study is unclear, but may be due to more training and dedicated leadership at this particular hospital. Either way, the use of MVA in the treatment of incomplete abortions continues to be low in Malawi, despite recommendations from the World Health Organization (WHO) and the Malawi Ministry of Health.

Keywords: incomplete abortions; unsafe abortions; uterine evacuation; post-abortion care; manual vacuum aspiration; female health; maternal mortality; low-income countries; Malawi

---

1. Introduction

Malawi, in South East Africa, is one of the poorest countries in the world, with a population of 18 million inhabitants, limited resources and an impoverished health care system [1,2]. Consequently, it has one of the highest maternal mortality rates in the world, with 439 maternal deaths per 100,000 live births [3]. Unsafe abortion is a prominent cause of this [4] and accounts for 6–30% of all maternal mortalities in Malawi [5–8]. Even though there are ongoing discussions to liberalize the law, abortion is only legal when it is necessary to save a pregnant woman's life [9,10]. Unsafe abortions make up the majority of abortions in Malawi, with the most recent estimate being 140,000 induced abortions annually [11,12]. Products of conception retained inside the uterus is one of the most common complications after an abortion, and almost 13% of the women receiving post-abortion care in Malawi in 2009 presented with incomplete abortions [13]. Additionally, incomplete abortions can lead to more serious complications such as haemorrhage, sepsis, and in the worst-case scenario, death [14,15]. Incomplete abortions are generally treated with surgical or medical uterine evacuation [16]. In Malawi, medical evacuation is not frequently used [17]. Surgical evacuation can be carried out by using vacuum aspiration or dilatation and curettage (D&C) [16]. Curettage usually requires general anaesthesia, an operating theatre, and the efforts of a medical doctor or clinical officer [16,18]. Comparatively, manual vacuum aspiration (MVA) is a safe and cheap method that can be performed by authorized nurses without the use of general anaesthesia or access to electricity [16,18]. The World Health Organization (WHO) guidelines and a Cochrane Library review concluded that vacuum aspiration is the preferred surgical method for uterine evacuation after an incomplete abortion in the first trimester [16,18,19]. Manual vacuum aspiration is faster, less painful, and is associated with less blood loss and fewer complications than D&C [16]. A recent Malawian study showed that the median cost per D&C intervention was 29% higher than the cost per MVA ($63 versus $49 United States Dollars) [20]. This is important in a health care system with limited resources. Nevertheless, in 2014, a study showed that the use of MVA declined during the 2008 to 2012 time period, while the use of D&C increased in selected parts of the country [17]. In 2012, MVA use accounted for just under 5% of uterine evacuations, with D&C use accounting for about 95%, and medical treatment for <1% of uterine evacuations [17]. Even though MVA equipment is on the government standard equipment list, and its use is officially promoted, many health facilities do not use it to evacuate incomplete abortions [21]. A qualitative study in two hospitals with a declining use of MVA, suggested that several factors influenced post-abortion care and MVA use; lack of training, and shortage of equipment and human resources were mentioned as major limiting factors [22].

Encouraging the use of MVA could help reduce obstetric complications and optimize resources. Considering the quality of existing data, the decline in the use of MVA in the southern part of Malawi and the reasons for this decline, new and updated information is required before a larger educational intervention can be initiated [17]. Accordingly, the aim of this study was to investigate how women with incomplete abortions were treated in three public hospitals in Southern Malawi between 2013 and 2015.

2. Materials and Methods

2.1. Study Design and Setting

The study was designed to identify which methods were used to manage incomplete abortions for women seeking post-abortion care in public hospitals in the southern part of Malawi; this constitutes a follow-up to a previous survey [17]. We chose a retrospective descriptive design that involved reviewing hospital files for a chosen time-period.

The study was conducted at two district hospitals, Chiradzulu and Mangochi, and the Queen Elizabeth Central Hospital (QECH). While the majority of post-abortion care cases are treated in public hospitals [13], the QECH is the referral hospital for the whole southern region of Malawi. Hence, a large number of women with incomplete abortions are treated at the QECH.

2.2. Study Population

All records from patients admitted in the three study hospitals were routinely stored after discharge and could be accessed by the clerk in charge at each hospital. All files from the female/gynecological ward, between 1 January 2013 and 31 December 2015, at the three hospitals were retrieved and reviewed. Women who had been treated for incomplete abortions were included.

2.3. Inclusion and Exclusion Criteria

Fetal death up to 28 weeks of gestation is classified as a miscarriage in Malawi, and therefore all pregnant women in this category were included. Women admitted for all other reasons, as well as women who were not offered any post-abortion treatment at all, were excluded. Since complications after a spontaneous miscarriage and an induced abortion are hard to distinguish, and are mostly unreported, these cases were not separated. Manual vacuum aspiration should preferably only be used in the first trimester, and may potentially be used up to 14-weeks of gestation [18]. However, mothers of higher gestational ages were included, as many of these women may have had residual amounts of retained products that might have been treated with MVA if they had been examined properly prior to surgery.

2.4. Data Collection

Data were taken from the female/gynecological ward records by a team of three research assistants, including nurses and midwives familiar with medical terms. The process was managed by a medical doctor, who also served as the principal investigator. The same data extraction tools were employed at all three study sites. Demographic data (residence, age, marital status, level of education, religion, and occupation), reproductive history (gravity, parity, number of children still alive, and gestational age), length of hospital stay, and type of evacuation were retrieved for each patient.

2.5. Study Period

Data collection was conducted during the period from 1 April 2016 to 31 May 2016.

2.6. Statistical Analysis

Data were analyzed using IBM SPSS Statistics version 22 (Armonk, New York, USA). Values are given as proportions (percent) with their 95% confidence interval (CI), and age is reported as the mean and standard deviation (SD).

2.7. Ethics Statement

Ethical approval was granted by the local Malawian College of Medicine Research and Ethics Committee (COMREC) P.06/15/1748, and the Regional Committee for Medical and Health Research Ethics Central Norway (REC Central), 2015/455/REK. Permission to access individual patient records was granted by the District Health Officers at Mangochi and Chiradzulu District Hospitals, and the Head of the Department of the Obstetric and Gynecological ward at QECH. All patient information was anonymized and de-identified prior to analysis.

3. Results

Demographic characteristics of the three annual study cohorts, and for all years, are provided in Table 1. The overall mean maternal age was 24.8 (SD 6.5) years, and the average number of offspring was 1.4 (SD 1.6), with 5.6% having more than five offspring (range 1–12). About one-third of the mothers (29.5%, 95% CI, 28.4–30.7) had no previous births, 85.6% (95% CI, 83.6–87.4) were married, 4.3% (95% CI, 2.9–6.2) had a higher education, and about one-third (33.9%; 95% CI, 30.9–36.9) had gainful employment. Islam was the most common religion (30%), followed by Christian groups including Roman Catholics (18%), and members of the Church of Central Africa Pentecost (12%). There were no obvious differences in demographic characteristics over the years (Table 1).

Table 1. Available information on demographic characteristics of women treated for incomplete abortions in the three hospitals in Malawi during the period of 2013 to 2015 (*n* = 7270) [1].

Characteristics	2013 (*n* = 2307)	2014 (*n* = 2561)	2015 (*n* = 2402)	All Years (*n* = 7270)
Mean age (SD) years	24.9 (6.4)	24.8 (6.6)	24.9 (6.5)	24.8 (6.5)
Pregnancy history				
Primigravida	479 (26.6)	655 (31.9)	561 (29.8)	1695 (29.5)

Table 1. *Cont.*

Characteristics	2013 (*n* = 2307)	2014 (*n* = 2561)	2015 (*n* = 2402)	All Years (*n* = 7270)
Multigravida	1321 (73.4)	1397 (68.1)	1324 (70.2)	4042 (70.5)
Number of living children				
None	390 (36.4)	609 (40.7)	446 (39.9)	1445 (39.2)
1	238 (22.2)	303 (20.3)	232 (20.8)	773 (21.0)
2+	442 (41.4)	584 (39.0)	440 (39.3)	1466 (39.8)
Gestational length				
1st trimester	737 (34.8)	851 (36.1)	772 (35.1)	2360 (35.3)
>1st trimester	1382 (65.2)	1507 (63.9)	1429 (64.9)	4318 (64.7)
Marital status				
Unmarried [2]	38 (12.4)	68 (13.7)	88 (16.1)	194 (14.4)
Married	268 (87.6)	427 (86.3)	458 (83.9)	1153 (85.6)
Hospital Admission [3]				
Rural facility	825 (35.8)	909 (35.5)	867 (36.1)	2601 (35.8)
Urban facility	1482 (64.2)	1652 (64.5)	1535 (63.9)	4669 (64.2)
Educational level				
None	1 (1.3)	6 (2.9)	9 (2.5)	16 (2.5)
Primary	42 (53.8)	107 (51.7)	181 (50.1)	330 (51.1)
Secondary	34 (43.6)	86 (41.5)	152 (42.1)	272 (42.1)
Tertiary	1 (1.3)	8 (3.9)	19 (5.3)	28 (4.3)
Occupation				
None	74 (34.7)	158 (44.9)	159 (40.0)	391 (40.6)
Housewife	48 (22.5)	41 (11.6)	37 (9.3)	126 (13.1)
Student	634 (16.0)	37 (10.5)	49 (12.3)	120 (12.4)
Gainful employment [4]	57 (26.8)	116 (33.0)	153 (38.4)	237 (33.9)

[1] Numbers are given as *n* (%) unless otherwise indicated. [2] The unmarried group includes: being single, separated, divorced, or widowed. [3] Rural: Chiradzulu and Mangochi hospitals. Urban: Queen Elizabeth Central Hospital (QECH). [4] Gainful employment: cleaner, farmer, businesswoman, policewoman, and other.

The overall use of MVA in the three study hospitals (*n* = 7270) from 2013 to 2015 was 11.4% (Table 2). Correspondingly, surgical evacuation with D&C was used in 86.4% of the cases. Medical treatment with Misoprostol was used in 1.4 % (95% CI, 1.1–1.7) of the cases. A combination of suction and curettage was only used in cases with molar pregnancies at QECH, which included 0.5% (95% CI, 0.4–0.7) of the cases. In addition, a few cases (0.3% (95% CI, 0.2–0.4)) had laparotomy and hysterectomy. Only MVA and D&C are included in Tables 2 and 3.

Overall, there was an increase in the use of MVA at all three hospitals, from 6.9% (95% CI, 5.9–8.0) in 2013, to 17.4% (95% CI, 15.9–19.0) in 2015 (as seen in Table 2). This increase occurred mostly in the Mangochi hospital (9.1% in 2013 to 40.6%); in the other two hospitals there was a marginal increase in the use of MVA, from 8.4% to 14.4% at Chiradzulu, and 5.9% to 11.8% at QECH.

Table 2. Surgical methods used for removal of retained products of conception after incomplete abortions [1], by year and hospital in the three Malawi hospitals during 2013 to 2015 [2,3].

Year	Type of PAC	Chiradzulu (*n* = 1117)	Mangochi (*n* = 1484)	QECH [4] (*n* = 4669)	All Hospitals (*n* = 7270)
2013 (*n* = 2307)	MVA [5]	8.4 (5.5–12.0)	9.1 (6.8–12.0)	5.9 (4.7–7.2)	6.9 (5.9–8.0)
	D&C [6]	91.3 (87.6–94.2)	89.5 (86.5–92.0)	91.5 (90.0–92.9)	91.0 (89.8–92.2)
2014 (*n* = 2561)	MVA [5]	14.9 (11.5–19.0)	20.5 (17.2–24.2)	5.2 (4.2–6.4)	9.8 (8.7–11.1)
	D&C [6]	85.1 (81.0–88.5)	78.9 (75.2–82.3)	92.4 (91.0–93.6)	88.5 (87.2–89.7)
2015 (*n* = 2402)	MVA [5]	14.4 (11.2–18.0)	40.6 (35.9–45.4)	11.8 (10.2–13.5)	17.4 (15.9–19.0)
	D&C [6]	85.6 (82.0-88.8)	59.2 (54.4–63.9)	83.8 (81.9–85-7)	79.8 (78.1–81.4)
All years (*n* = 7270)	MVA [5]	12.9 (11.0-15.0)	22.4 (20.3-24.6)	7.6 (6.8–8.4)	11.4 (10.7–12.2)
	D&C [6]	87.0 (84.9-88.9)	76.9 (74.7-79.0)	89.3 (88.4–90.2)	86.4 (85.6–87.2)

[1] Gestation up to 28 weeks. [2] Numbers are given as percentages (95% CI), unless otherwise indicated. [3] Suction and curettage, laparotomy, and medical treatment were not included. [4] Queen Elizabeth Central Hospital (QECH). [5] Manual vacuum aspiration (MVA). [6] Dilatation and Curettage (D&C).

Table 3 and Figure 1 show first-trimester abortions only. Of all the incomplete abortions in the first-trimester, 21.4% (95% CI, 19.7-23.0) were treated with MVA (Table 3). However, in 2015 the Mangochi District Hospital used MVA to treat 70.9% of the patients with first-trimester abortions (Table 3 and Figure 1).

Table 3. Surgical methods used for removal of retained products of conception for first-trimester incomplete abortions [1] in three Malawi hospitals by year for the 2013 to 2015 period [2,3].

Year	Type of PAC	Chiradzulu (n = 372)	Mangochi (n = 475)	QECH [4] (n = 1513)	All Hospitals (n = 2360)
2013 (n = 737)	MVA [5]	15.3 (9.5–22.9)	19.4 (13.8–25.1)	11.2 (8.4–14.5)	13.8 (11.4–16.5)
	D&C [6]	84.7 (77.1–90.5)	80.0 (73.3–85.7)	86.3 (82.7–89.4)	84.5 (81.7–87.1)
2014 (n = 851)	MVA [5]	25.6 (18.2–34.2)	42.8 (35.1–50.7)	10.4 (8.0–13.2)	18.9 (16.3–21.7)
	D&C [6]	74.4 (65.8–81.8)	57.2 (49.3–64.9)	87.9 (84.9–90.4)	79.9 (77.1–82.5)
2015 (n = 772)	MVA [5]	21.1 (14.3–29.4)	70.9 (62.4–78.4)	23.3 (19.7–27.2)	31.2 (28.0–34.6)
	D&C [6]	78.9 (70.6–85.7)	29.1 (21.6–37.6)	70.7 (66.5–74.6)	64.8 (61.3–68.1)
All years (n = 2360)	MVA [5]	20.7 (16.7–25.2)	42.1 (37.6–46.7)	15.0 (13.2–16.9)	21.4 (19.7–23.1)
	D&C [6]	79.3 (74.8–83.3)	57.7 (53.1–62.2)	81.6 (79.5–83.5)	76.4 (74.6–78.1)

[1] Abortions in first trimester included. [2] Numbers are given as percentages (95% CI) unless otherwise indicated. [3] Suction and curettage, laparotomy and medical treatment were not included; [4] Queen Elizabeth Central Hospital (QECH). [5] Manual vacuum aspiration (MVA). [6] Dilatation and Curettage (D&C).

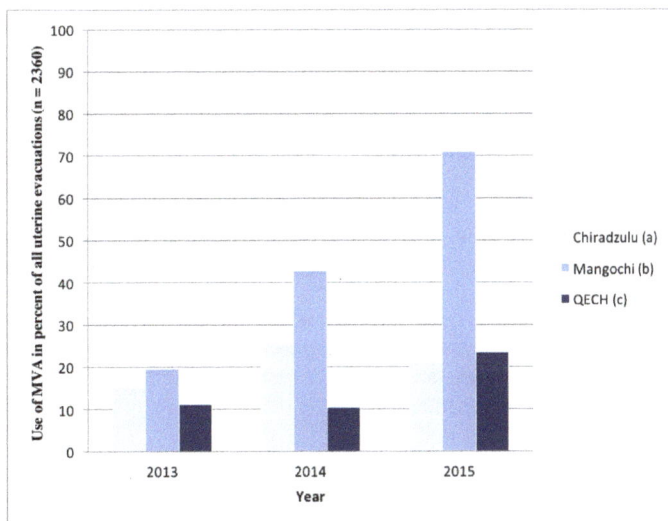

Figure 1. Use of manual vacuum aspiration (MVA) for removal of retained products of conception in first-trimester incomplete abortions, by year and specific Malawi hospital (2013 to 2015). (a) Chiradzulu District Hospital; (b) Mangochi District Hospital; (c) Queen Elizabeth Central Hospital.

During the last six months of 2015, the Mangochi District Hospital treated between 80% and 90% of all first-trimester abortions with MVA (not shown in Table 3). Furthermore, the Mangochi District Hospital experienced a 10.4% decline in hospital-based maternal mortality from 2013/2014 to 2015. In addition, the Mangochi District Hospital had no maternal deaths due to abortion in 2015. At the two other hospitals, there was no decline in hospital-based maternal mortality, and at QECH there was a slight increase in maternal deaths due to abortion.

4. Discussion

The overall use of MVA as a part of post-abortion care in the southern districts of Malawi during the 2013 to 2015 period was 11.4%, which is lower than the overall use of MVA from 2008 to 2012 [17]. Nevertheless, we found an increase in the use of MVA in all three hospitals in 2015 compared to 2013 [17]. One hospital, namely the Mangochi District Hospital, was primarily responsible for the overall study outcome, and showed more than a 50% increase in the use of MVA in the treatment of first trimester abortions.

We could not distinguish between miscarriages and induced abortions, and therefore these were not studied separately. However, there were abortion cases that showed signs of having been induced with foreign objects, and a few women admitted that they had taken drugs or local herbs to induce termination of their pregnancy. Also, several patients presented with symptoms of miscarriage in the second trimester. Considering that most miscarriages occur in the first trimester [23], and that two-thirds of the women in our study presented with symptoms of a second-trimester miscarriage, it seems reasonable to assume that most of the latter abortions were induced. Nevertheless, most women (n = 2036) were in their 13th week of gestation when they presented with symptoms.

A limitation of the present study is its retrospective nature, with the use of existing hospital files as the data source. Since all records were kept on paper, there is the possibility that some information may have been lost. In our previous study, for the 2008 to 2012 period, it was only possible to locate 5000 women that had been registered for treatment of incomplete abortions at the three hospitals [17]. In the current study, more than 7000 files were retrieved over the three-year period, which may indicate that the hospital records had been retained more effectively and accurately over the last few years. The fact that all files were sorted by month supports this. Moreover, all three hospitals had a designated clerk in charge of the records, which facilitated our task. Possibly, an increase in interest may have improved record keeping among health care personnel. Even so, we acknowledge that some files may have been lost, as there is some missing data.

A strength of retrospective data collection is the reduction of selection bias; the care providers did not know that their information would be used in research. Hence, they chose their treatment without being influenced by the researchers or any pre-study hypothesis. Furthermore, a selected team of health personnel was supervised by one principal investigator so that the same search protocol was employed throughout the data collection period. In part, our study was carried out by the same local teams as in 2012, and we believe this limited any errors due to misclassification [17].

Because our project took place in only three hospitals in Southern Malawi, our results may not be generalizable to the whole country, even though they were comparable to those in our previous study [17]. Together, these research efforts allowed for the observation of trends in the treatment of incomplete abortions over a longer period.

There was an increase in the use of MVA in all the hospitals, although the hospital of Mangochi was the only one that had a documented major improvement. In past years, there has been a general shift in policy by the Malawi Ministry of Health to encourage a reduction in maternal deaths, and MVA has been a promoted treatment, as it leads to fewer complications. The Mangochi District Hospital encouraged staff to attend MVA training sessions organized by the Ministry of Health; the staff in turn trained their colleagues. The hospital management also promoted and encouraged the use of MVA. The Mangochi District Hospital is the only hospital that adopted the guidelines fully, and treated almost 90% of first-trimester abortions with MVA by the end of 2015. The results are promising, and we speculate that this accounts for the decline in maternal mortality [16,19]. In fact, there were no maternal deaths due to abortion at this hospital in 2015. The other study hospitals did not experience a decrease in maternal mortality and had more deaths due to abortion in 2015. Even so, change in maternal mortality is not necessarily directly linked to the use of MVA, but more use of MVA could have reflected improvements in other parts of the hospital, such as improved obstetric and postnatal care.

Medical treatment with Misoprostol is increasingly being used to treat incomplete abortions and is a cheap and safe way to induce contractions of the uterus and an evacuation in a natural way [20,24,25].

However, the QECH was the only hospital that used medical treatment, in just 3.2% (95 CI, 2.6–4.5) of the cases in 2015; medical treatment was mostly used to prepare patients for surgical treatment. Low use of medical evacuation of the uterus could be due to limited resources and a fear of misuse in inducing abortions. However, medical evacuation of the uterus is more often incomplete [26–28], and patients are supposed to return for a check-up to be rescanned and ensure that the uterus is empty [27,28]. In Malawi, patients may not come back to be rescanned due to long waiting times, and lack of transportation and money, which could then lead to incomplete septic miscarriages associated with high morbidity and mortality. Hence, health personnel are more comfortable evacuating the uterus surgically to ensure that the patient will not be lost to follow-up. If surgical treatment is maintained as the best option, which seems to be the case in Malawi at the moment, then MVA is the safest and cheapest way to treat incomplete abortions in the first trimester [16,20].

Maternal mortality is still high in Sub-Saharan Africa and unsafe abortion is a major cause that in turn is closely related to the abortion laws [4,6–8]. Legalizing abortion has led to a reduction in maternal mortality in several countries, such as Romania and South Africa [29]. Fortunately, Malawi is considering moderating their restrictive abortion laws. Even so, an immediate change making abortion accessible to women is not likely to happen in the near future. In the meantime, other measures need to be taken to reduce maternal mortality. Using MVA rather than D&C can make the treatment of incomplete abortions safer and cheaper, which is important in a health care system that is already frail due to limited resources and staff.

5. Conclusions

While one of the study hospitals increased their use of MVA significantly, the other two hospitals continued to use D&C as a primary treatment for incomplete abortions. The observed trend of increased use of MVA could be due to training and better access to equipment, as seen in other developing countries [30–32], and should be investigated further in Malawi.

Acknowledgments: We would like to thank the research assistants that participated in the study. Also, we would like to thank all the staff at the College of Medicine, the QECH, the Chiradzulu District Hospital and the Mangochi District Hospital for their collaboration and contributions. The study was funded by the Programme for Global Health and Vaccination Research (Globvac), project number 244672, a part of the Norwegian Research Council. With thanks, we acknowledge Evert Nieboer, Emeritus Professor, McMaster University (Hamilton, Ontario, Canada) for his language editing.

Author Contributions: Maria Lisa Odland and Elisabeth Darj conceived and designed the study; Maria Lisa Odland performed the data collection; Maria Lisa Odland, Geir W. Jacobsen and Elisabeth Darj analyzed the data; Ursula Kafulafula, Gladys Membe-Gadama and James Kumwenda contributed with materials and tools; Maria Lisa Odland wrote the paper, and Gladys Membe-Gadama, Ursula Kafulafula., Geir W. Jacobsen, James Kumwenda and Elisabeth Darj gave substantial input.

Conflicts of Interest: Authors declare no conflict of interest.

References

1. The World Bank 2017. Country Profile: Malawi. Available online: http://databank.worldbank.org/data/Views/Reports/ReportWidgetCustom.aspx?Report_Name=CountryProfile&Id=b450fd57&tbar=y&dd=y&inf=n&zm=n&country=MWI (Accessed on 30 January 2018).
2. United Nations. Human Development Index and Its Components: United Nations Development Programme. 2015. Available online: http://hdr.undp.org/en/composite/HDI (accessed on 30 January 2018).
3. Malawi Demographic and Health Survey 2015–2016. National Statistics Office, Zomba, Malawi. Available online: https://dhsprogram.com/pubs/pdf/FR319/FR319.pdf (accessed on 13 February 2018).
4. Hord, C.; Wolf, M. Breaking the cycle of unsafe abortion in Africa. *Afr. J. Reprod. Health* **2004**, *8*, 29–36. [CrossRef] [PubMed]
5. Colbourn, T.; Lewycka, S.; Nambiar, B.; Colbourn, T.; Lewycka, S.; Nambiar, B.; Anwar, I.; Phoya, A.; Mhango, C. *BMJ Open* **2013**, *3*, e004150. [CrossRef]

6. Jackson, E.; Johnson, B.R.; Gebreselassie, H.; Kangaude, G.D.; Mhango, C. A strategic assessment of unsafe abortion in Malawi. *Reprod. Health Matters* **2011**, *19*, 133–143. [CrossRef]
7. Lema, V.M.; Changole, J.; Kanyighe, C.; Malunga, E.V. Maternal mortality at the Queen Elizabeth Central Teaching Hospital, Blantyre, Malawi. *East Afr. Med. J.* **2005**, *82*, 3–9. [CrossRef] [PubMed]
8. Geubbels, E. 2006. Epidemiology of Maternal Mortality in Malawi. *Malawi Med. J.* **2006**, *18*, 206–225. [PubMed]
9. Malawi Government. *The Law Commission Discussion Paper on Review of Abortion Law in Malawi*; Malawi Government: Lilongwe, Malawi, 2013.
10. Malawian Penal Code. *Laws of Malawi. Chapter 7:01*; Blackhall Publishing: Dublin, Ireland, 1930.
11. Polis, C.B.; Mhango, C.; Philbin, J.; Chimwaza, W.; Chipeta, E.; Msusa, A. Incidence of induced abortion in Malawi; 2015. *PLoS One* **2017**, *12*, 1–16. [CrossRef] [PubMed]
12. Levandowski, B.A.; Mhango, C.; Kuchingale, E.; Lunguzi, J.; Katengeza, H.; Gebreselassie, H.; Singh, S. The incidence of induced abortion in Malawi. *Int. Perspect. Sex. Reprod. Health* **2013**, *39*, 88–96. [CrossRef] [PubMed]
13. Kalilani-Phiri, L.; Gebreselassie, H.; Levandowski, B.A.; Kuchingale, E.; Kachale, F.; Kangaude, G. The severity of abortion complications in Malawi. *Int. J. Gynaecol. Obstet.* **2015**, *128*, 160–164. [CrossRef] [PubMed]
14. Grimes, D.A.; Benson, J.; Singh, S.; Romero, M.; Ganatra, B.; Okonofua, F.E.; Shas, I.H. Unsafe abortion: The preventable pandemic. *Lancet* **2006**, *368*, 1908–1919. [CrossRef]
15. Ahman, E.; Shah, I.H. New estimates and trends regarding unsafe abortion mortality. *Int. J. Gynecolo. Obst.* **2011**, *115*, 121–126. [CrossRef] [PubMed]
16. Tuncalp, O.; Gulmezoglu, A.M.; Souza, J.P. Surgical procedures for evacuating incomplete miscarriage. *Cochrane Database Syst. Rev.* **2010**, *9*. [CrossRef] [PubMed]
17. Odland, M.L.; Rasmussen, H.; Jacobsen, G.W.; Kafulafula, U.K.; Chamanga, P.; Odland, J.O. Decrease in use of manual vacuum aspiration in postabortion care in Malawi: A cross-sectional study from three public hospitals, 2008–2012. *PLoS One* **2014**, *9*. [CrossRef] [PubMed]
18. World Health Organization. Safe abortion: technical and policy guidance for health systems 2012. Available online: http://apps.who.int/iris/bitstream/10665/70914/1/9789241548434_eng.pdf (accessed on 30 January 2018).
19. Pereira, P.P.; Oliveira, A.L.; Cabar, F.R.; Armelin, A.R.; Maganha, C.A.; Zugaib, M. Comparative study of manual vacuum aspiration and uterine curettage for treatment of abortion. *Rev. Assoc. Med. Bras.* **2006**, *52*, 304–307. [CrossRef] [PubMed]
20. Benson, J.; Gebreselassie, H.; Manibo, M.A.; Raisanen, K.; Johnston, H.B.; Mhango, C.; Levamdowski, B.A. Costs of postabortion care in public sector health facilities in Malawi: A cross-sectional survey. *BMC Health Serv. Res.* **2015**, *15*. [CrossRef] [PubMed]
21. Malawi Ministry of Health. *Standard Equipment List for Typical District and Community Hospital and Health Centre with Generic Specifications for Some Common and General Equipment*; Malawi Ministry of Health: Lilongwe, Malawi, 2009.
22. Cook, S.; de Kok, B.; Odland, M.L. "It's a very complicated issue here": Understanding the limited and declining use of manual vacuum aspiration for postabortion care in Malawi: A qualitative study. *Health Policy Plan* **2017**, *32*, 305–313. [CrossRef] [PubMed]
23. Magowan, B.; Thompson, A.; Owen, P. *Clinical Obstetrics and Gynaecology*, 3rd ed.; Saunders Elsevier Limited: Philadelphia, PA, 2014.
24. Kiemtore, S.; Zamane, H.; Kain, D.P.; Sawadogo, Y.A.; Ouedraogo, I.; Ouedraogo, A.; Lankoandé, J. Effects of an intervention initiated by a national society to improve postabortion care in rural facilities in Burkina Faso. *Int. J. Gynaecol. Obstet.* **2017**, *136*, 215–219. [CrossRef] [PubMed]
25. Cleeve, A.; Byamugisha, J.; Gemzell-Danielsson, K.; Mbona Tumwesigye, N.; Atuhairwe, S.; Faxelid, E.; Klingberg-Allvin, M. Women's Acceptability of Misoprostol Treatment for Incomplete Abortion by Midwives and Physicians - Secondary Outcome Analysis from a Randomized Controlled Equivalence Trial at District Level in Uganda. *PLoS One* **2016**, *11*, 1–13. [CrossRef] [PubMed]
26. Sotiriadis, A.; Makrydimas, G.; Papatheodorou, S.; Ioannidis, J.P. Expectant, medical, or surgical management of first-trimester miscarriage: a meta-analysis. *Obstet. Gynecol.* **2005**, *105*, 1104–1113. [CrossRef] [PubMed]

27. Shwekerela, B.; Kalumuna, R.; Kipingili, R.; Mashaka, N.; Westheimer, E.; Clark, W.; Winikoff, B. Misoprostol for treatment of incomplete abortion at the regional hospital level: Results from Tanzania. *BJOG* **2007**, *114*, 1363–1367. [CrossRef] [PubMed]

28. Weeks, A.; Alia, G.; Blum, J.; Winikoff, B.; Ekwaru, P.; Durocher, J.; Florence, M. A randomized trial of misoprostol compared with manual vacuum aspiration for incomplete abortion. *Obstet. Gynecol.* **2005**, *106*, 540–547. [CrossRef] [PubMed]

29. Benson, J.; Andersen, K.; Samandari, G. Reductions in abortion-related mortality following policy reform: Evidence from Romania, South Africa and Bangladesh. *Reprod. Health* **2011**, *8*, 39. [CrossRef] [PubMed]

30. Begum, F.; Zaidi, S.; Fatima, P.; Shamsuddin, L.; Anowar-ul-Azim, A.K.; Begum, R.A. Improving manual vacuum aspiration service delivery, introducing misoprostol for cases of incomplete abortion, and strengthening postabortion contraception in Bangladesh. *Int. J. Gynaecol. Obstet.* **2014**, *126*, 31–35. [CrossRef] [PubMed]

31. Zaidi, S.; Yasmin, H.; Hassan, L.; Khakwani, M.; Sami, S.; Abbas, T. Replacement of dilation and curettage/evacuation by manual vacuum aspiration and medical abortion, and the introduction of postabortion contraception in Pakistan. *Int. J. Gynaecol. Obstet.* **2014**, *126*, 40–44. [CrossRef] [PubMed]

32. Tumasang, F.; Leke, R.J.; Aguh, V. Expanding the use of manual vacuum aspiration for incomplete abortion in selected health institutions in Yaounde, Cameroon. *Int. J. Gynaecol. Obstet.* **2014**, *126*, 28–30. [CrossRef] [PubMed]

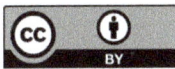

© 2018 by the authors. Licensee MDPI, Basel, Switzerland. This article is an open access article distributed under the terms and conditions of the Creative Commons Attribution (CC BY) license (http://creativecommons.org/licenses/by/4.0/).

International Journal of
*Environmental Research
and Public Health*

MDPI

Article

Ten Years of Experience in Contraception Options for Teenagers in a Family Planning Center in Thrace and Review of the Literature

Panagiotis Tsikouras [1,*], Dorelia Deuteraiou [1], Anastasia Bothou [2], Xanthi Anthoulaki [1], Anna Chalkidou [1], Eleftherios Chatzimichael [1], Fotini Gaitatzi [1], Bachar Manav [1], Zacharoula Koukouli [1], Stefanos Zervoudis [2], Grigorios Trypsianis [3] and George Galazios [1]

[1] Department of Obstetrics and Gynecology, Democritus University of Thrace, Alexandroupolis 68100, Greece; Dr.Dorelia@hotmail.com (D.D.); xanthi_vatsidou@hotmail.com (X.A.); annachalkidou@yahoo.gr (A.C.); elevchat7@med.duth.gr (E.C.); pan.bougatsou@gmail.com (F.G.); bacharmanav@windowslive.com (B.M.); harakoukouli@gmail.com (Z.K.); ggalaz@med.duth.gr (G.G.)
[2] Department of Obstetrics and Mastology, Rea Hospital, Athens 17564, Greece; natashabothou@windowslive.com (A.B.); szervoud@otenet.gr (S.Z.)
[3] Department of Medical Statistic, Democritus University of Thrace, Alexandroupolis 68100, Greece; gtryps@med.duth.gr
* Correspondence: ptsikour@med.duth.gr; Tel.: +30-6974-728-272

Received: 12 December 2017; Accepted: 12 February 2018; Published: 15 February 2018

Abstract: *Introduction*: The goal of our study was to investigate and evaluate the contraceptive behavior in teenagers from our family planning centre that services two different religious and socioeconomic populations living in the Thrace area. *Methods*: During the last 10 years 115 Christian Orthodox (group A) and 53 Muslim teenagers (group B) were enrolled in our retrospective study. Contraceptive practice attitudes were assessed by a questionnaire. Religion, demographics, socio-economic characteristics were key factors used to discuss contraception and avoid unplanned pregnancy in each group and to compare with the contraceptive method used. *Results*: The most used contraceptive method—about two times more frequently—among Christian Orthodox participants was the oral contraceptive pill ($p = 0.015$; OR = 1.81, 95% CI = 1.13–2.90), while in the other group the use of condoms and IUDs was seven and three times more frequent, respectively. Our family planning centre was the main source of information for contraception. *Conclusions*: During adolescence, the existence of a family planning centre and participation in family planning programs plays a crucial role to help the teenagers to improve their knowledge and choose an effective contraception method.

Keywords: adolescents; contraception's options; health counseling center; family planning center

1. Introduction

Reproductive health must be based on the freedom of young people to access appropriate health care services. There they can be easily informed about all the possible fertility regulation methods and make decisions for having a satisfying, safe sex life with preservation of reproductive capability [1]. The contraception choices for teenager women significantly affect their health, their school and professional education as well as their smooth transition to adulthood [2]. According to international literature, the overwhelming majority of adolescents do not want pregnancies [3]. Those who are already married also do not want childbirth and those who become pregnant do not wish the birth of another child [3]. The world population of adolescents aged 10–19 years now stands at 1.2 billion [4]. It is essential to understand and approach their sexual needs. Unfortunately, most teenagers do not have access to the counselling and services they need. More than 50% of US women have sexual contacts before the age of 18. Of these, 1/3 does not use any contraception [5].

In developing countries, most pregnancies in adolescence are unexpected and undesirable, and as a result the half of them end up with an *induced abortion* taking place, very often under unsafe conditions [6,7]. In 2011, 47% of high-school students reported having some sexual experience and 34% reported sexual contact in the last three months [8]. Annually some 750.000 teenage pregnancies are reported and 82% of these pregnancies were unplanned [9]. From these reported pregnancies observed 59% births, 14% miscarriage and 27% induced abortion. From1990 to early 2000, a significant reduction in teenage pregnancies has been observed. The majority (86%) of this decrease is due to the increased use of contraception and 14% due to abstention or delay in starting sexual contact [10]. In Greece this percentage is much smaller, but existent. Elements from the 2007 MES study in Attica are the following:

(a) Up to 16 years of age 20% of adolescents (in a 1 to 3 proportion of boys to girls) have started their sexual life,
(b) Among sexually active adolescents, 5.7%, 10.2%, 44.3%, 33% and 2.3% started sex at 12, 13, 14, 15 and 16 years of age, respectively,
(c) 40% of adolescents had some sexual experience other than vaginal sex [11].

According to the Greek data Adolescence Health Unit (AHU) Youth-health Study, among sexually active teenagers:

(a) 10% used no contraceptive method,
(b) 39% used unreliable methods, such as rhythm or withdrawal methods,
(c) 51% used condoms, and
(d) 5% the oral contraceptive pill.

Therefore, the contraception use of teenagers is a real challenge for the medical community and sometimes can be difficult, especially for those suffering from a chronic disease. This is because in several such cases, taking medication can affect the safety and effectiveness of hormonal contraception, and as a result a pregnancy with high maternal and fetal risk is unavoidable. The need for contraceptive protection of adolescents with chronic problems or special needs very often is overlooked. It is estimated that this category includes 10–20% of the population under the age of 20 [12–14]. For all the above reasons, the need for sexual education and knowledge of contraception choices and abilities of these people should not be overlooked [12–14]. Recent data showed that there are no differences in the sexual experience of these individuals. Contraception is very important factor worldwide to save and an immense amount of time, energy and money according to *prevention* of unintended pregnancies, especially in adolescents [12–14]. The use and mode of contraception is influenced from various determinants like demographic characteristics, education, occupation, religion, and social status [12–14]. The goal of this retrospective study was to investigate the contraceptive behavior of teenagers in two different ethnological and socioeconomic populations in the Thrace area.

2. Methods

From January 2006 until December 2016 we studied the different attitudes towards contraception, among females of two major community subgroups: 115 Christian Orthodox women living in Thrace, Greece (group A) and 53 Muslim women living in Thrace, Greece (group B).

All respondents were in reproductive adolescence age (from 15 to 19 years) and were randomly selected from among teenagers visiting the Family Planning Centre in the Department of Obstetrics and Gynecology of our Hospital, the University Hospital of Alexandroupolis. The study participants either in the Group A or Group B were healthy, without past diseases. They typically visited our centre with their parents for a routine gynaecologic examination and attitudes concerning contraceptive practices were assessed by means of a questionnaire. Each question was explained to the participants, who subsequently completed the questionnaire in private and finally gave it back during the next examination. For the teenagers with relatively late occurring menstruation, acne, BMI greater than 25 Kg/m² and hirsutism hormonal laboratory and vaginal ultrasound examinations were performed to investigate possible polycystic ovary (PCO) syndrome.

All teenagers who with their parents' consent were included in the study were very cooperative in answering the questions and gave anonymous detailed answers regarding their age, place of living, religion, occupation, economic and social status, menarche, and menstrual bleeding abnormalities status. As well as the main source of information offered to them about contraception, the above mentioned characteristics of each group were compared with the method of contraception used.

Statistical analysis of the data was performed using the Statistical Package for the Social Sciences (SPSS), version 19.0 (SPSS, Inc., Chicago, IL, USA). All variables were categorical and they were expressed as frequencies and percentages (%). The chi-square test was used to evaluate any potential association between the method of contraception and the participants' characteristics; odds ratios (OR) and their 95% confidence intervals (95% CI) were calculated by means of simple logistic regression analysis, as the measure of the above associations. All tests were two tailed and statistical significance was considered for $p < 0.05$.

3. Results

The demographic characteristics of the study participants are listed in Table 1. The vast majority of the participants (267 teenagers, 89.0%) used some method of contraception; the contraceptive pill (56.0%), interrupted coitus (45.7%) and the use of condoms (42.3%) were the most common methods of contraception (Table 2). The use of two different methods of contraception was observed in 41.3% of the teenagers. While35.7% of the teenagers used only one method of contraception, and three or four methods were used by 10.0% and 2.0% of the teenagers, respectively (Table 3a). The family center (47.0%) was the most usual source of information regarding contraception; a family consultant (20.3%), school (20.3%) and the sexual partner, newspaper, news or media (12.4%) were other sources of information (Table 3b).

Table 1. Epidemiologic data of the study populations.

Epidemiologic Data	No of Women	(%)
Age		
<18 years	99	33.0
≥18 years	201	67.0
Religion		
Muslims	113	37.7
Christians	187	62.3
Way of Living		
Rural	60	20.0
Urban	240	80.0
Occupation		
Student	229	76.3
Employed	39	13.0
Unemployed	32	10.7
Smoking		
No	240	80.0
Yes	60	20.0
Abnormal Bleeding		
No	200	66.7
Yes	100	33.3

Table 1. *Cont.*

Epidemiologic Data	No of Women	(%)
Disease in the Past		
No	282	94.0
Yes	18	6.0
Medication		
No	248	82.7
Yes	52	17.3
Acne		
No	221	73.7
Yes	79	26.3
Hirsutismus		
No	226	75.3
Yes	74	24.7
Diabetes Mellitus		
No	299	99.7
Yes	1	0.30
Side Effects	0	0.0
Abort/Pregnacy	0	0.0
Childern		
None	292	97.3
More than one child	8	2.7
Age of Menarche		
Median (25–75% percentile)	12 (11–13)	

Table 2. Method of contraception in the study population.

Contraception Method	No of Women	Percentage (%)
Oral contraceptives	168	56.0
Condom	137	45.7
Interrupted coitus	127	42.3
IUD	32	10.7
Spermicides	5	1.7

Table 3. (**a**) Different methods of contraception in the study population; (**b**) Source of information regarding contraception.

(a)		
Contraception Method	No of Women	Percentage (%)
None	33	11.0
One method	107	35.7
Two methods	124	41.3
Three methods	30	10.0
Four methods	6	2.0

(b)		
Source of Information	No of Women	Percentage (%)
Sexual partner	37	12.4
Family center	141	47.0
Family	61	20.3
School	61	20.3

The association of the use of different methods of contraception according to teenagers' characteristics is shown in Tables 4 and 5. The use of the contraceptive pill was almost twice more frequent among Christian Orthodox ($p = 0.015$; OR = 1.81, 95% CI = 1.13–2.90), among teenagers living in rural areas ($p = 0.012$), while a tendency towards more frequent use of the contraceptive pill was found at higher education levels ($p = 0.077$).

On the contrary, the use of condoms and IUDs were almost seven and three times more frequent among Muslims (condom: $p< 0.001$; OR = 6.73, 95% CI = 4.01–11.31; IUD: $p = 0.007$; OR = 2.71, 95% CI = 1.28–5.72), respectively. Moreover, the use of IUD and spermicide were more frequent among employed teenagers ($p = 0.087$ and $p = 0.007$, respectively). No other statistically significant associations were found.

One hundred and fourteen teenagers had clinical symptoms (late menarche, acne, hirsutism, hormone laboratory results: mean serum T levels 6915 ± 509 (0.06–0.82 ng/mL) and mean serum DHEAS of 61,957 ± 11,539 μg/dL (65.1–368)). As in the entire cohort, the use of contraceptive pill (61.8%) and the use of condom (65%) were confirmed the most common methods of contraception among the 72 Christians and the 42 Muslims with clinical symptoms, respectively (Table 6).

Table 4. Use of oral contraceptives, condom and interrupted coitus according to women's characteristics.

Epidemiologic Data	Women Using OCs (%)	p Value	OR (95% CI)
Age		0.722	
<18 years	54 (54.5)		1
≥18 years	114 (56.7)		1.09 (0.67–1.77)
Religion		0.015	
Muslims	53 (46.9)		1
Christians	115 (61.5)		1.81 (1.13–2.90)
Way of Living		0.012	
Rural	25 (41.7)		1
Urban	143 (59.6)		2.06 (1.16–3.66)
Occupation		0.077	
Student	120 (52.4)		1
Employed	26 (66.7)		1.82 (0.89–3.71)
Unemployed	22 (68.8)		2.00 (0.91–4.41)
	Women Using CONDOM (%)	**p Value**	**OR (95% CI)**
Age		0.331	
<18 years	38 (38.4)		1
≥18 years	89 (44.3)		1.28 (0.78–2.09)
Religion		<0.001	
Muslims	79 (69.9)		6.73 (4.01–11.31)
Christians	48 (25.7)		1
Way of Living		0.683	
Rural	24 (40.0)		1
Urban	103 (42.9)		1.13 (0.63–2.01)
Occupation		0.381	
Student	101 (44.1)		1
Employed	16 (41.0)		0.88 (0.44–1.76)
Unemployed	10 (31.3)		0.58 (0.26–1.27)
	Women Using C.I. (%)	**p Value**	**OR (95% CI)**
Age		0.299	
<18 years	41 (41.4)		1
≥18 years	96 (47.8)		1.29 (0.80–2.10)
Religion		0.566	
Muslims	54 (47.8)		1
Christians	83 (44.4)		0.87 (0.55–1.40)
Way of Living		0.862	
Rural	28 (46.7)		1
Urban	109 (45.4)		0.95 (0.54–1.68)
Occupation		0.927	
Student	106 (46.3)		1
Employed	17 (43.6)		0.90 (0.45–1.78)
Unemployed	14 (43.8)		0.90 (0.43–1.90)

Table 5. Use of IUD and spermicides according to women's characteristics.

Epidemiologic Data	Women Using IUD (%)	p Value	OR (95% CI)
Age		0.824	
<18 years	10 (10.1)		1
≥18 years	20 (10.9)		1.09 (0.50–2.41)
Religion		0.007	
Muslims	19 (16.8)		2.71 (1.28–5.72)
Christians	13 (7.0)		1
Way of Living		0.224	
Rural	9 (15.0)		1
Urban	23 (9.6)		0.60 (0.26–1.38)
Occupation		0.087	
Student	22 (9.6)		0.41 (0.17–1.01)
Employed	8 (20.5)		1
Unemployed	2 (6.3)		0.26 (0.05–1.32)
	Women Using SPERMICIDE (%)	p Value	OR (95% CI)
Age		0.114	
<18 years	0 (0.0)		
≥18 years	5 (2.5)		n.a.
Religion		0.299	
Muslims	3 (2.7)		1
Christians	2 (1.1)		0.40 (0.07–2.41)
Way of Living		0.260	
Rural	2 (3.3)		1
Urban	3 (1.3)		0.37 (0.06–2.25)
Occupation		0.007	
Student	2 (0.9)		0.11 (0.02–0.66)
Employed	3 (7.7)		1
Unemployed	0 (0.0)		n.a.

Table 6. Method of contraception in the participants with ance, hirsutismus and late age of menarche in relation to religion.

Contraception Method	No of Women	Percentage (%)
Muslims		
Oral contraceptives	11	47.8
Condom	15	65.2
Interrupted coitus	13	56.5
IUD	3	13.0
Spermicides	0	0.0
Christians		
Oral contraceptives	34	61.8
Condom	9	16.4
Interrupted coitus	27	49.1
IUD	2	3.6
Spermicides	0	0.0
Total		
Oral contraceptives	45	57.7
Condom	24	30.8
Interrupted coitus	40	51.3
IUD	5	6.4
Spermicides	0	0.0

IUD: Intrauterine device.

4. Discussion

Family planning services are limited by governmental programs through commercial retail sales and are trying to adopt inappropriate aspects of family planning [15]. The aim of these centers should be to provide services to all, irrespective of the country's economic situation, providing birth control methods using the medical profession and health services to adolescents to understand contraceptive options and to act quickly by choosing the most appropriate method [16,17]. There are many methods of contraception. Everyone requires education. Contraceptive methods are divided in natural, hormonal, intrauterine, spermicide, barrier methods and male contraception. Physical methods include periodic abstinence and coitus interruptus [17,18]. Effective contraceptive behaviors are not an individual achievement; on the contrary, choosing the right method depends on the increased resources that go into research and family planning services with reversible methods of contraception [17,18]. The recommend choice criteria for the individual suitable method are as follows: use of a contraceptive (CM) method in any case, no limitation on contraceptive (CM), general use CM, received benefits (of the CM) predominate over theoretical or clinically proven risks, risks override reception benefits (CM), high risk and finally use of CM only, non-existent alternative and inappropriate method for use. Information on the benefits of applying emergency contraception irrespective of the method proposed is also essential [19–21].

The oral contraceptive (OC) pill is the most prevalent form of contraception among adolescents with low compliance rates and increased interruption rates [22,23].Health care professionals should recommend the use of the male condom to reduce the transmission of sexually transmitted diseases. This specific and confidential approach of counselling increases the effectiveness with regard to the use and compliance of the contraceptive methods. It is considered essential to provide information about possible side effects that may arise from the use of various contraceptive methods, because familiarisation with the above, may significantly contribute in avoiding or interrupting the contraceptive method. It is also essential the information about the benefits of implementation of emergency contraception irrespectively of the method proposed [22,23].

The contraception method with OC effectiveness include: perfect use, avoidance of possibility of gestation when the use of the method is always fixed and correct, typical use, probability of pregnancy within one year of standard use of the method.

National studies involving multiple users with varying degrees of strictness of compliance forgotten pills, prolonged stickers and expired condoms are essential for the impact of contraception [22–25].

Regarding the use of hormonal contraception there is a clear contraindication in teenagers suffering from thrombophilia, hepatic dysfunction, systemic lupus erythematosus, cyanotic heart disease, pulmonary hypertension. Adolescents receiving antipsychotic or HIV medicines should be carefully monitored and encouraged to use injectable progestagens [25,26]. Obesity is a constantly growing health problem affecting 13% of adolescents. Obesity increases pregnancy-related morbidity because it is combined with the induction of delivery of emergency caesarean section, overweight birth, diabetes mellitus and gestational hypertension [26]. All of the above complications and especially hypertension are more common in obese teens. Concerning the use of contraception in obese patients, it should be mentioned that there is contraceptive protection regardless of the BMI size (lower rates of undesirable pregnancies) [27,28].There is limited and unclear information concerning the use of oral contraceptives in obese patients. The risk of deep vein thrombosis in obese patients is doubled. However, the additional absolute risk of venous thrombosis following the use of combined low-dose contraceptives is rather limited and certainly less than the corresponding risk due to pregnancy and periodontal disease [27–30].

There are not sufficient data about the pharmacokinetics of oral steroids in obese adolescents. As the main metabolic pathway of the EE is through the cytochrome p450 enzyme system, a reduction in EE clearance is expected in obese teenagers [30,31].

Additionally, a decrease in levonogestrel clearance is observed due to the EE-induced inhibition of the activity of the above enzyme system and consequent increase in Sex Hormone Binding Globulin (SHBG) [32]. All of the above may lead to a decrease in the contraceptive efficacy of oral contraceptives [33]. Generally, obese teenagers are more likely to become pregnant than non-obese because of a larger percentage of this population does not use contraceptive protection [32]. The effectiveness of combined hormonal contraception (pill, vaginal ring, patches) in obese patients is reduced [33]. The use of combined hormonal contraception does not affect body weight [34–36]. The use of intrauterine slow-release levodogestrel device has been associated with a slight increase in body weight [34–36]. Etonogestrel implants have little or no effect [37–42]. Regarding the use of methoxyprogesterone acetate there are conflicting data about a slight weight increase in adolescence. The use of hormonal methods of contraception is not associated with weight changes. Although in general, obesity decreases the effectiveness of oral contraceptive pills, they are superior in safety in comparison with barrier methods [41–43].

Therefore, medical information in these cases should focus on the modest reduction in efficacy and the increased but low absolute risk of vein thrombosis. The use of an intrauterine levonogestrel delivery devices may reduce the risk of obesity-related endometrial hyperplasia [44].

Despite the prevailing view, diabetes type II is more common among women of reproductive age. In puberty, the above frequency is even greater, which increases the importance of contraceptive protection. In any case, metabolic disorders may cause vascular disease.

Diabetics have a greater risk of complications in pregnancy as well as congenital disorders which makes it almost essential to seek pregnancy after restoring to normal glucose levels [45,46]. According to a recent Cochrane review comparing between hormonal and non-contraceptive diabetic women, only three studies related to this subject [47–49].

One of these was the comparison of the effect on the metabolism of women with type I diabetes of the intrauterine levonogestrel release device against the intrauterine copper device. No differences in daily insulin requirements between glycatedhaemoglobin levels and fasting glucose levels were observed over one year [50].

The other two studies referred to a comparison between progesterone contraceptive tablets and estrogen/progesterone combination contraceptive tablets. These studies showed stable glucose levels during treatment with most formulations [51]. Only high doses of contraceptives can cause a mild estrogen and progestogen disorders, having a slight adverse effect on the lipid profile whereas, tablets containing only progestogen have a correspondingly slight beneficial effect [52]. Concerning the choice of a suitable contraceptive method in diabetic adolescents, it seems that the predominance is towards the use of intrauterine devices. Oral administration of tablets is relatively safe among adolescents with type I and II diabetes without retinopathy, nephropathy and hypertension [52]. Oral contraceptive tablets are relatively safe in patients with the mild, non-antibody-presenting form of systemic lupus erythematosus. In severe cases, intrauterine devices are recommended [52–54].

In patients with HIV, the use of intrauterine devices is considered safe. The use of hormonal contraception may not adversely affect the progress of the disease or the risk of transmission [55]. However, some antiviral medications are potential modulators of hepatic enzyme activity and can therefore significantly affect the degree of hormonal contraceptive action, it is advisable in these cases to consider about prescribing of such drugs.

Women with migraines and focal neurological symptoms should prefer intrauterine devices or barrier methods because the use of hormonal methods may increase the risk of ischemic attack. It is also considered relatively safe to use hormonal contraceptives that contain only progesterone. In the case of taking antipsychotic medications, it should first be specified what type of preparation or formulations and possible interaction with combined oral hormonal contraception. Because many of them by influencing hepatic metabolism can cause a reduction in the effectiveness of contraceptive action. If there is such an interaction then either a higher 50μgE tablet (without special encouragement) should be proposed because there is more intermittent hemorrhage [56,57]. Whether applying an additional contraceptive method (e.g., a condom) or using an endometrial levonorgestel intrauterine device and finally use of injectable methoxyprogesterone acetate. The use of implants is not recommended due to low central progesterone levels [56,57].

Combined oral contraceptive pills are the most effective hormonal contraceptive method. The main principle of administration is based on the principle of using the lowest possible dose for the shortest possible time. Combined oral contraceptive pills contain estrogen and progestogen. Depending on the dose, circulating estrogens >50 μg (high dose), estrogens ≤35 μg (low dose) and estrogen = 20 μg (ultra-light dose). The beginning of combined oral contraceptive pills start on day 1 of menstrual cycle, followed by a 7-day discontinuation, and continuous contraceptives without interruption, and their mechanism of action consists of inhibiting implantation due to endometrial perforation and ovulation in cervical mucus thickening, sperm motility disorder, normal mobility disorder, and contraceptive action is exerted mainly via the progestogens of combined oral contraceptive pills. The estrogen exerts its contraceptive action but is dose-dependent through the inhibition of gonadotropin secretion (FSH, LH) causing the uterus to change the secretory capacity and cell structure of the endometrium [58–60].

Ideal progestogen pills should have strong progesterone, anti-estrogen, anti-gonadotropic action and antiglucocrticoid action. Absence of androgenic action and possible antiandrogenic action. No action similar to glucocorticoids. Lack of undesirable effects such as acne, reduction of HDL, flatulence and water retention. There are several differences regarding the hormone components contained in each formulation which can be varied depending on the type, composition, quantity and number of active tablets. The monophasic formulations contain active tablets with the same constant amount and estrogen and progestogen ratio [35,61–63]. In contrast to multiphasic, the above ratio changes. Biphasic ones contain two combinations and three-phase contain three. Recently there are also four phase contraceptive pills with a successive reduction in the estrogen ratio and a corresponding increase in the progestogen ratio.

Regarding levonorgestrel (2nd generation), desogestrel and gestodene (3rd generation) have greater affinity for progestagen receptors, they are more effective in inhibiting ovulation and ensuring the smoothness of the cycle at lower doses.

Regarding 1st generation contraceptive pills, there are side effects such as unwanted bleeding or spotting due to the fact that the dosage does not decrease at the appropriate time. The second generation ones are more effective and with a longer half-life, but with increased androgenic action that helps in sexual desire but could lead to hirsutism, acne and dyslipidaemia [64–66].

3rd generation contraceptive pills maintain efficacy of progestagen while reducing their androgenic effect and in turn, smaller androgenic effect also makes estrogen more effective. This, however, entails a greater risk for thromboembolic events.

The use of contraceptive pills results in many benefits for teenagers that are not related to contraceptive protection, such as regulating often abnormal cycles or preventing or reducing dysmenorrhoea or treating acne that is also common in teens as well as symptomatic remission of premenstrual syndrome. Continuous administration over a longer period of time (three months) is continuously gaining ground without causing particular risks. On the contrary, it improves the quality of life.

Positive effects include: restoration of a normal cycle in disorders of the cycle (hypermenorrhea, reduced blood flow, metrorrhagia, oligomenorrhea), dysmenorrhea recession through action in prostaglandin synthesis and reduction of premenstrual edema, irritability, anxiety, and depression. As far as concern ovarian and endometrial cancer can reduce the risk from 30% to 80% of endometriosis, reduce dysmenorrhoea, dysparenia and through anti-endotropic activity limit or eliminate functional, ovarian cysts. They also have a beneficial effect on the fight against acne and hirsutism by reducing androgen synthesis and specific action of estrogen and antiandrogens, causing a remission of mastodynia and many times have a positive effect on the treatment of benign breast disease.

Finally they cause an increase in bone density. The latest data shows no increase of risk of breast cancer [64,66–69].

As far as concerns the 4th generation contraceptive pills, so far there are two pharmaceutical forms. The four-phase form containing a combination of estradiol valerate as estrogen and dienogest as progestagen (E2V/DNG) and the monophasic form containing 17β-oestradiol as estrogen and norgesterol acetate as progestogen (17β-E2/NMG). There are two combinations of 4th generation contraceptives: E2V/DNG and 17βE2/NOMAC. They are characterized by their particular composition including natural estrogen and 4th generation progestagens that resemble the chemical structure with progesterone. They show greater tolerability and influence are more favorable to the metabolism of carbohydrates, lipids and homeostasis because of a more favorable interference of estrogen content in liver synthesis of proteins and the antiandrogenic action of progestogen. This is safe and effective. The combination of E2V/DNG is recommended for women who experience unwanted hemorrhages due to the better regulation of the menstrual cycle. 017βE2/NOMAC is recommended in women taking contraception for the first time (new-adolescents) because of better compliance with single-phase. The use of a combination of estrogen and progesterone as a contraceptive or hormone replacement therapy has made it possible to complete large epidemiological studies that have made it possible to assess the benefits and risks that may have arisen.

The great advantages are the reduced incidence of endometrial cancer attributed predominantly to the antimitotic activity of progesterone in the endometriomas well as reducing the incidence of ovarian cancer due to mainly in the anti-endotropic activity of the above combination [67–70].

Pill Progestogen Minipill, POPs: They contain only one progestagen (usually norethindrone or norgestrel) and are used daily. The mechanism of action based on thickening of cervical mucus. Their major disadvantage is that they do not inhibit ovulation. The are used between 4 and 22 h before contact and are considered inferior to combined oral contraceptive pills [71,72].

Copper intrauterine devices: They are the most common reversible method of contraception worldwide, with a frequency of use of 30–40% among women of childbearing age in China and only 1% in the USA (due to the risk of septic automatic abortion). Their main advantage is being an easy to use method where failure does not depend from the user. They act by preventing the passage of sperm through the endometrial cavity, and the process of fertilization within the fallopian tubes. They render the ovary less capable of being fertilized and reduce the likelihood of implantation in the endometrium, probably as a result of local inflammation. They consists of a polyethylene skeleton containing wire or copper yarn. Complications include increased blood loss during menstrual bleeding and excretion. Other complications include uterine perforation, pelvic inflammation, disease PID, expulsion of intrauterine device, and ectopic pregnancy.

Contraindications for use include pregnancy suspicion, undiagnosed genital hemorrhage, and active pelvic inflammation, history of tubal pregnancy, significant deformation of the endometrial cavity and the existence of a history of bacterial endocarditis. Uterine cavity abnormalities. It is NOT contraindication: HIV infection or immunosuppression. The existence of uterine cavity abnormalities it is NOT a contraindication: HIV infection or immunosuppression (also are not contraindicated). Data for women at high risk for STIs and IUD are unclear. Nulliparous teenagers vs mothers show higher IUD rate use, pain and discomfort. In general, IUDs are a well-tolerated method with high levels of satisfaction and continuity [73].

Barrier Methods

Male condom: It is the only reversible method of contraception for men. The average rate of failure is high (12%), while among the teenagers it is even higher (18%). It has also a significant role in limiting the transmission of sexually transmitted diseases but with some limitations. They consist of latex, polyurethane or animal membranes. New forms of male condoms made from polyurethane and their polymers seem to improve their acceptability and promise more safety. They are more protective against infections transmitted through the seminal fluid (gonococcal urethritis, chlamydia, trichomonas, HIV) than against infections transmitted through skin-to-skin contact (herpes simplex virus). Some condoms are lubricated during manufacture from the outset with the spermicide substance nanoxinol-9 which is no longer recommended due to reduced protection and higher risk for HIV. The most significant errors leading to clinical failure (ten highest among teenagers) are the rupture or displacement and the failure to use it throughout the contact [74].

Spermicides: They destroy sperm and they are available in gel, foam or cream form. They are often used simultaneously with barrier methods. The active substance is nonoxynol-9 that affects the surface of the sperm. They do not provide protection against HIV. A 2/fold to 3/fold risk of urinary tract infection during concomitant use with a barrier method is observed. They may be an appropriate option for women with sparse sexual intercourse or needing coverage for one pregnancy [75].

Polycystic ovary syndrome (PCOS): One of the most common endocrine disorders of women of reproductive age and causing hyperandrogenemia and oligo or an-ovulation. These two, lead to important psychological, social and financial consequences. Since it was found that women with PCOS manifest more often metabolic syndrome than the general population, with all its effects, there has been an increase in interest in the syndrome, both in the general population and in the medical world, in recent years. According to the currently accepted criteria include hyperandrogenism, anovulation and/or polycystic ovaries as observed by ultrasonography [76–79].

Contraceptives and PCO syndrome: Intake starts on day 1 of the menstrual cycle and it is continued for 21 days, followed by 7 days cessation. The ideal contraceptive for women with polycystic ovarian syndrome should control the development of the follicular antrum and reduce the amount of androgens, antagonise the action of androgens at the peripheral level and particularly in hair follicles and sebaceous glands and as well as restore the balance between estrogen and progestagen in the endometrium, ensuring regulation of the menstrual cycle. Administration of contraceptive tablets to women with hyperandrogenic syndrome due to PCO syndrome causes reduction in the levels of androgen circulating. The basic mechanism is the induced inhibition of maturation of follicles due to suppression of pituitary gonadotropin secretion [80–83].

In women with PCO, a contraceptive containing 30 mcg of ethinylestradiol also inhibits more effectively than lower doses of EE, steroidogenesis in adrenal glands. It also stimulates the hepatic synthesis of Sex hormone-binding globulin (SHBG). Concerning the type of progestogen, chloramandinone acetate (CMA), cyproterone acetate (CPA), dinogestor and drospirenone (DRSP) are progestagens with dynamic anandrogenicall progestagens with antiandrogenic effect. Their antiandrogenic action is mainly exerted by blocking the androgen receptors of the target organs. In addition, they reduce the action of 5α-reductase on the skin which converts testosterone to its active fraction by 5α-dihydroxytestosterone. A particular increase in SHBG is observed when using the third generation contraceptive tablets containing a combination of 30 mcg of EE with dienogest or drospirenone resulting to reduction of free testosterone by 40–50%.

The production of SHBG is to a lesser extent stimulated by second generation contraceptives containing 30 mcg of EU with levonogestrel because the androgenic action of the progestogen neutralizes the estrogenic action. Exception for the above action, some second-generation contraceptives such as the 3-phase levonogestrel, biphasic containing 30–40 mcg EU and single phase with 35 mcg EU and 2 mcg CPA. There are also studies on the efficacy of oral contraceptives containing DRSP or CPA in the treatment of hypertrichosis that show a significant reduction in circulating androgen levels after a 6–12 month treatment and a significant increase in SHBG [80–83].

Moreover, a significant decrease in the concentration of total and free testosterone was observed when the administered progestogen was CMA and DRSP. In this case the androgen concentrations are affected by those of SHBG that produce strong androgen binding. A significant decrease in dehydroandrostendione has also been observed. It is likely that this decrease is attributed to the immediate induced inhibition of adrenal androgen production. Contraceptives pills are the treatment of choice for dysfunctional bleeding in PCOS syndrome [84–86]. Many of the patients with the syndrome address from teenage age to specialists complaining for unexpected vaginal bleeding of various intensity and duration. The use of contraceptives in these cases in addition to the recession of hyperandrogenic phenomena also normalizes the woman's menstrual cycle. Also, disorders of the oligo- or amenorrhea type often appear in PCOS sufferers, although 15–30% the presence of certain oligo-ovulation is associated with normal cycles. In this case, contraceptive tablets also help to restore the normality of the cycle [87,88]. Additional benefits from the use of contraceptive pills in PCOs are: The recession of dysmenorrhoea associated with menorrhagia and polymenorrhea, iron deficiency anaemia as well as the reduction of the risk of hyperplasia and endometrial cancer. There is a remarkable positive correlation between PCOS and endometrial cancer, because risk factors for endometrial cancer such as chronic anovulation, obesity, insulin resistance and diabetes mellitus are often associated with PCOS.

Although there are not enough prospective studies, it is considered reasonable to conclude that PCOS patients also benefit from the prophylactic effect of contraceptives on endometrial cancer [86–88].

When using contraceptive pills, the potential risk of deterioration of disorders in fat metabolism or insulin resistance should not be neglected. Estrogens lead to a dose-dependent increase in insulin resistance and the progestogens modify the above effect. Since androgens are associated with disorders in fat metabolism, progestagens with androgenic effects exhibit similarly variable gravity activity. Particularly progestagens with such activity contribute to the development of excess fat. Generally, the effect of progestogens on carbohydrate metabolism depends on the degree of hyperandrogenism of the patient and the potential antiandrogenic action of the progestogen [86–88].

Genetically determined susceptibility of endogenous insulin as well as anthropometric differences potentially affecting the action of insulin from the natural history of the syndrome or environmental effects. However, it is obvious that obesity and excessively high nutrition tend to define a phenotype of PCOS more prone to metabolic disorders.

Finally, contraceptive tablets are considered as risk factors for venous thrombosis, especially in carriers of genetic mutations such as factor V Leiden. The risk of arterial thrombosis, of coronary arteries is also present particularly in 35 year old women or older. This risk is directly related to the dose of estrogen (decreases when the ethinyl estradiol dose is reduced) especially in women who smoke >25 cigarettes daily. Consequently, contraceptives should not be prescribed when there are cardiovascular disorders, history of venous thrombosis, liver disease, migraine depression obesity and presence of undiagnosed mass in the breast.

Administration of contraceptive pills to women with hyperandrogenosis due to PCO syndrome causes a great reduction in the levels of circulating androgens. In women with PCOS, a contraceptive containing 30 mcg of ethinylestradiol also inhibits adrenal steroidogenesis more effectively than lower doses of EE. Regarding the type of progestogen, chloromandinone acetate (CMA), cyproterone acetate (CPA), dienogest and drospirenone (DRSP) are progestagens with dynamic antiandrogenic action [86–88]. Contraceptive tablets are the treatment of choice for women with PCO syndrome that have menstrual disorders either in the form of amenorrhea or oligomenorrhoea or in the form of dysfunctional bleeding because they restore the balance between estrogen and progestogens in the endometrium ensuring the normal control of the genital cycle [86–88].

According to our study results, we found that the most frequently contraceptive method almost twice ($p = 0.015$; OR = 1.81, 95% CI = 1.13–2.90), with improved tendency in high education levels ($p = 0.077$) is the contraceptive pill among Christian Orthodox group A in the Thrace region. In the group B, the use of condom and IUD were almost seven and three times more frequent (condom: $p < 0.001$; OR = 6.73, 95% CI = 4.01–11.31; IUD: $p = 0.007$; OR = 2.71, 95% CI = 1.28–5.72), respectively and finally the use of IUD and spermicide were more frequent among employed teenagers ($p = 0.087$ and $p = 0.007$, respectively). The above mentioned findings were confirmed also in the total subgroup with PCO symptoms distributed with parts of the both main groups (Table 6). The unexpected high percent of the usage of oral contraceptive pills compared to relatively low percent of usage in Greece generally is based on the fact that the majority of the participants were students, who have adequate education level. Additionally the variety of activities that our family planning centre offers by

Int. J. Environ. Res. Public Health **2018**, *15*, 348

informing adolescents about the choices of contraception help them to make the best individual choice. In our family planning center the percentage of adolescents with acne and hirsutism, who already receiving OCP as a choice of contraception and receiving them both for therapeutic reasons of PCOS, is approximately 20% from the total population with PCOS. In our center the frequency of PCO according to our results is approximately 8.5% of the total adolescent population in our area.

These findings show that the teenagers in Thrace are not yet skeptical about the pill's safety, beneficial effects and correlate the pill use with serious health risks and side effects. Adolescence is a period of rapid physical development triggering the simultaneous secretion of various growth hormones and the teenagers are influential from various information sources to choose consciously for a contraception method adequate to their health condition. In the present study our family center plays a very important role and this is in accordance to literature.

5. Conclusions

Ten% of adolescents suffer from chronic diseases and need effective contraception to prevent pregnancy. There are several safe and effective methods of contraception but the choice of the most appropriate one should be personalized due to the complexity of the underlying disease.

For these reasons, proper guidance and monitoring of the implementation of the appropriate contraceptive method of the above teenagers should not be overlooked. The provision of services includes a variety of directions, bearing in mind that the needs of teenagers differ from those of adults.

It should be done in a friendly youth atmosphere in a climate of confidence, taking into account the legal specificities in different countries regarding the age of contraceptive protection. In the provision of services, it is also important to properly assess the particular needs and living conditions of each adolescent. For this reason, international models of advisory guidance have recently been published.

The correct choice of the contraceptive method involves knowing the various methods and the desire for contraception. Full understanding and proper implementation of sexual education facilitates significantly improves the use of contraception.

Typical is the example of Finland combining the application of sex education in the schools with the provision of high-quality health care. These factors have greatly contributed to reduce the rate of unwanted pregnancies and voluntary abortions. On the contrary, the cessation of implementation of the above programs has resulted in contrary trends.

Sexual behavior does not differ significantly in developed countries with respect to the age of 1st sexual intercourse, with an average of 17 years old. Also, 15% of teenage girls had their first sexual intercourse before 15 years of age, with 60% in the 18th year and 80% in the 20th year. However, the incidence of unwanted pregnancies varies, indicating with significant depending on the type of contraceptive method. A combination of a hormonal contraceptive method with male condom is preferred both for contraception and STI protection. Informing adolescent girls with a simple language about all the potential risks and benefits contributing to the proper choice of contraceptive method. The family planning centers are of great importance for organizing various social strategies not limited to formal government programmes. These strategies are based on parameters affecting the application of contraception method such as population socioeconomic status and educational background.

Acknowledgments: We would like to thank the chief and the scientific co-workers of the Pediatric and Adolescence Centre of the second Department of Obstetrics and Gynecology, Medical School of Kapodistrian University in Athens, Greece. Furthermore we would like to thank the midwife Maira Strofali of our Center in Pediatric and Adolescence Gynecology from the Department of Obstetrics and Gynecology, Democritus University in Thrace, Greece.

Author Contributions: Panagiotis Tsikouras and Georgios Galazios conceived and designed the experiments; Dorelia Deuteraiou, Anastasia Bothou, Xanthi Anthoulaki, Anna Chalkidou, Eleftherios Chatzimichael, Fotini Gaitatzi, Bachar Manav, Zacharoula Koukouli performed the experiments; Stefanos Zervoudis and Grigorios Trypsianis analyzed the data; contributed reagents/materials/analysis tools; Panagiotis Tsikouras wrote the paper.

Conflicts of Interest: The authors declare no conflict of interest. We wish to declare that all the used data in this study remain absolutely confidential and protected and were obtained with the parents' consent.

References

1. Ganatra, B.; Faundes, A. Role of birth spacing, family planning services, safe abortion services and post-abortion care in reducing maternal mortality. *Best Pract. Res. Clin. Obstet. Gynaecol.* **2016**, *36*, 145–155. [CrossRef] [PubMed]
2. Dueñas, J.L.; Lete, I.; Arbat, A.; Bermejo, R.; Coll, C.; Doval, J. L.; Serrano, I. Trends in contraception use in Spanish adolescents and young adults (15 to 24 years) between 2002 and 2008. *Eur. J. Contracept. Reprod. Health Care* **2013**, *18*, 191–198. [CrossRef] [PubMed]
3. Apter, D.; Zimmerman, Y.; Beekman, L.; Mawet, M.; Maillard, C.; Foidart, J.M.; Coelingh Bennink, H.J. Bleeding pattern and cycle control with estetrol-containing combined oral contraceptives: Results from a phase II, randomised, dose-finding study (FIESTA). *Contraception* **2016**, *94*, 366–373. [CrossRef] [PubMed]
4. Chan, S.S.; Yiu, K.W.; Yuen, P.M.; Sahota, D.S.; Chung, T.K. Menstrual problems and health-seeking behaviour in Hong Kong Chinese girls. *Hong Kong Med. J.* **2009**, *15*, 18–23. [PubMed]
5. Eaton, D.K.; Kann, L.; Kinchen, S.; Shanklin, S.; Flint, K.H.; Hawkins, J.; Harris, W.A.; Lowry, R.; McManus, T.; Chyen, D.; et al. Youth risk behavior surveillance—United States, 2011. Centers for Disease Control and Prevention (CDC). *MMWR Surveill. Summ.* **2012**, *61*, 1–162. [PubMed]
6. Martinez, G.; Copen, C.E.; Abma, J.C. Teenagers in the United States: Sexual activity, contraceptive use, and childbearing, 2006–2010 national survey of family growth. *Vital Health Stat. 23* **2011**, *31*, 1–35.
7. Finer, L.B.; Zolna, M.R. Unintended pregnancy in the United States: Incidence and disparities, 2006. *Contraception* **2011**, *84*, 478–485. [CrossRef] [PubMed]
8. Finer, L.B.; Zolna, M.R. Declines in Unintended Pregnancy in the United States, 2008–2011. *N. Engl. J. Med.* **2016**, *374*, 843–852. [CrossRef] [PubMed]
9. Blanc, A.K.; Way, A.A. Sexual behavior and contraceptive knowledge and use among adolescents in Developing countries. *Stud. Fam. Plann.* **1998**, *29*, 106–116. [CrossRef] [PubMed]
10. Henshaw, S.K.; Kost, K. Abortion patients in 1994–1995: Characteristics and contraceptive use. *Fam. Plann. Perspect.* **1996**, *28*, 140–147 & 158. [CrossRef] [PubMed]
11. VTf-v6sUk8. Available online: http://youth-health.gr/thematikes-enotites/genika-gia-tin-efibeia/seksoualikotita-kai-efibeia# (accessed on 4 June 2014).
12. Quint, E.H. Adolescents with Special Needs: Clinical Challenges in Reproductive Health Care. *J. Pediatr. Adolesc. Gynecol.* **2016**, *29*, 2–6. [CrossRef] [PubMed]
13. Quint, E.H. Menstrual and reproductive issues in adolescents with physical and developmental disabilities. *Obstet. Gynecol.* **2014**, *124 Pt 1*, 367–375. [CrossRef] [PubMed]
14. Quint, E.H. Menstrual issues in adolescents with physical and developmental disabilities. *Ann. N. Y. Acad. Sci.* **2008**, *1135*, 230–236. [CrossRef] [PubMed]
15. Cohen, R.; Sheeder, J.; Kane, M.; Teal, S.B. Factors Associated With Contraceptive Method Choice and Initiation in Adolescents and Young Women. *J Adolesc. Health* **2017**, *61*, 454–460. [CrossRef] [PubMed]
16. Papas, B.A.; Shaikh, N.; Watson, K.; Sucato, G.S. Contraceptive counseling among pediatric primary careproviders in Western Pennsylvania: A survey-based study. *SAGE Open Med.* **2017**, *5*. [CrossRef] [PubMed]
17. Beeson, T.; Mead, K.H.; Wood, S.; Goldberg, D.G.; Shin, P.; Rosenbaum, S. Privacy and Confidentiality Practices In Adolescent Family Planning Care At Federally Qualified Health Centers. *Perspect. Sex. Reprod. Health* **2016**, *48*, 17–24. [CrossRef] [PubMed]
18. Binette, A.; Howatt, K.; Waddington, A.; Reid, R.L. Ten Challenges in Contraception. *J. Womens Health (Larchmt)* **2017**, *26*, 44–49. [CrossRef] [PubMed]
19. Chen, E.; Mangone, E.R. A Systematic Review of Apps using Mobile Criteria for Adolescent Pregnancy Prevention (mCAPP). *JMIR Mhealth Uhealth* **2016**, *4*, e122. [CrossRef] [PubMed]
20. Wu, W.J.; Edelman, A. Contraceptive Method Initiation: Using the Centers for Disease Control and Prevention Selected Practice Guidelines. *Obstet. Gynecol. Clin. N. Am.* **2015**, *42*, 659–667. [CrossRef] [PubMed]
21. Apter, D. Contraception options: Aspects unique to adolescent and young adult. *Best Pract. Res. Clin. Obstet. Gynaecol.* **2017**. [CrossRef] [PubMed]

22. Lindh, I.; Skjeldestad, F.E.; Gemzell-Danielsson, K.; Heikinheimo, O.; Hognert, H.; Milsom, I.; Lidegaard, Ø. Contraceptive use in the Nordic countries. *Acta Obstet. Gynecol. Scand.* **2017**, *96*, 19–28. [CrossRef] [PubMed]

23. Black, A.; Guilbert, E.; Costescu, D.; Dunn, S.; Fisher, W.; Kives, S.; Mirosh, M.; Norman, W.V.; Pymar, H.; Reid, R.; et al. Society of Obstetricians and Gynaecologists of Canada. Canadian Contraception Consensus (Part 1 of 4). *J. Obstet. Gynaecol. Can.* **2015**, *37*, 936–942. [CrossRef]

24. Ott, M.A.; Sucato, G.S. Committee on Adolescence Contraception for adolescents. *Pediatrics* **2014**, *134*, e1257–e1281. [CrossRef] [PubMed]

25. Committee on Adolescence Contraception for adolescents. *Pediatrics* **2014**, *134*, e1244–e1256. [CrossRef]

26. Patel, R.C.; Bukusi, E.A.; Baeten, J.M. Current and future contraceptive options for women living with HIV. *Expert Opin. Pharmacother.* **2018**, *19*, 1–12. [CrossRef] [PubMed]

27. Akers, A.Y.; Cohen, E.D.; Marshal, M.P.; Roebuck, G.; Yu, L.; Hipwell, A.E. Objective and Perceived Weight: Associations with Risky Adolescent Sexual Behavior. *Perspect. Sex. Reprod. Health* **2016**, *48*, 129–137. [CrossRef] [PubMed]

28. Bhuva, K.; Kraschnewski, J.L.; Lehman, E.B.; Chuang, C.H. Does body mass index or weight perception affect contraceptive use? *Contraception* **2017**, *95*, 59–64. [CrossRef] [PubMed]

29. Sugiura, K.; Kobayashi, T.; Ojima, T. Risks of thromboembolism associated with hormonal contraceptives related to body mass index and aging in Japanese women. *Thromb. Res.* **2016**, *137*, 11–16. [CrossRef] [PubMed]

30. Nappi, R.E.; Kaunitz, A.M.; Bitzer, J. Extended regimen combined oral contraception: A review of evolving concepts and acceptance by women and clinicians. *Eur. J. Contracept. Reprod. Health Care* **2016**, *21*, 106–115. [CrossRef] [PubMed]

31. Hancock, N.L.; Stuart, G.S.; Tang, J.H.; Chibwesha, C.J.; Stringer, J.S.A.; Chi, B.H. Renewing focus on family planning service quality globally. *Contracept. Reprod. Med.* **2016**, *1*, 10. [CrossRef] [PubMed]

32. Jusko, W.J. Perspectives on variability in pharmacokinetics of an oral contraceptive product. *Contraception* **2017**, *95*, 5–9. [CrossRef] [PubMed]

33. Dragoman, M.V.; Simmons, K.B.; Paulen, M.E.; Curtis, K.M. Combined hormonal contraceptive (CHC) use among obese women and contraceptive effectiveness: A systematic review. *Contraception* **2017**, *95*, 117–129. [CrossRef] [PubMed]

34. Barlow, E. Long-Acting Reversible Contraception: An Essential Guide for Pediatric Primary Care Providers. *Pediatr. Clin. N. Am.* **2017**, *64*, 359–369. [CrossRef]

35. Francis, J.K.R.; Gold, M.A. Long-Acting Reversible Contraception for Adolescents: A Review. *JAMA Pediatr.* **2017**, *171*, 694–701. [CrossRef] [PubMed]

36. Smith, E.; Daley, A.M. A clinical guideline for intrauterine device use in adolescents. *J. Am. Acad. Nurse Pract.* **2012**, *24*, 453–462. [CrossRef] [PubMed]

37. Deshmukh, P.; Antell, K.; Brown, E.J. Contraception Update: Progestin-Only Implants and Injections. *FP Essent.* **2017**, *462*, 25–29. [PubMed]

38. Sandle, M.; Tuohy, P. 'Everyone's talking Jadelle': The experiences and attitudes of service providers regarding the use of the contraceptive implant, Jadelle in young people in New Zealand. *N. Z. Med. J.* **2017**, *130*, 40–46. [PubMed]

39. Mansour, D.; Bahamondes, L.; Critchley, H.; Darney, P.; Fraser, I.S. The management of unacceptable bleeding patterns in etonogestrel-releasing contraceptive implant users. *Contraception* **2011**, *83*, 202–210. [CrossRef] [PubMed]

40. Di Carlo, C.; Sansone, A.; De Rosa, N.; Gargano, V.; Tommaselli, G.A.; Nappi, C.; Bifulco, G. Impact of an implantable steroid contraceptive (etonogestrel-releasing implant) on quality of life and sexual function: A preliminary study. *Gynecol. Endocrinol.* **2014**, *30*, 53–56. [CrossRef] [PubMed]

41. Usinger, K.M.; Gola, S.B.; Weis, M.; Smaldone, A. Intrauterine Contraception Continuation in Adolescents and Young Women: A Systematic Review. *J. Pediatr. Adolesc. Gynecol.* **2016**, *29*, 659–667. [CrossRef] [PubMed]

42. Raymond, E.G.; Weaver, M.A.; Louie, K.S.; Tan, Y.L.; Bousiéguez, M.; Aranguré-Peraza, A.G.; Lugo-Hernández, E.M.; Sanhueza, P.; Goldberg, A.B.; Culwell, K.R.; et al. Effects of Depot Medroxyprogesterone Acetate Injection Timing on Medical Abortion Efficacy and Repeat Pregnancy: A Randomized Controlled Trial. *Obstet. Gynecol.* **2016**, *128*, 739–745. [CrossRef] [PubMed]

43. Hillard, P.J. Prevention and Management of Pregnancy in Adolescents with Endocrine Disorders. *Adolesc. Med. State Art Rev.* **2015**, *26*, 382–392. [PubMed]

44. Mansour, D. The benefits and risks of using a levonorgestrel-releasing intrauterine system for contraception. *Contraception* **2012**, *85*, 224–234. [CrossRef] [PubMed]

45. O'Brien, S.H.; Koch, T.; Vesely, S.K.; Schwarz, E.B. Hormonal Contraception and Risk of Thromboembolism in Women with Diabetes. *Diabetes Care* **2017**, *40*, 233–238. [CrossRef] [PubMed]

46. Sereika, S.M.; Becker, D.; Schmitt, P.; Powell, A.B., 3rd; Diaz, A.M.; Fischl, A.F.; Thurheimer-Cacciotti, J.; Herman, W.H.; Charron-Prochownik, D. Operationalizing and Examining Family Planning Vigilance in Adult Women With Type 1 Diabetes. *Diabetes Care* **2016**, *39*, 2197–2203. [CrossRef] [PubMed]

47. Vahratian, A.; Barber, J.S.; Lawrence, J.M.; Kim, C. Family-planning practices among women with diabetes and overweight and obese women in the 2002 National Survey For Family Growth. *Diabetes Care* **2009**, *32*, 1026–1031. [CrossRef] [PubMed]

48. Charron-Prochownik, D.; Sereika, S.M.; Falsetti, D.; Wang, S.L.; Becker, D.; Jacober, S.; Mansfield, J.; White, N.H. Knowledge, attitudes and behaviors related to sexuality and family planning in adolescent women with and without diabetes. *Pediatr. Diabetes* **2006**, *7*, 267–273. [CrossRef] [PubMed]

49. Schwarz, E.B.; Maselli, J.; Gonzales, R. Contraceptive counseling of diabetic women of reproductive age. *Obstet. Gynecol.* **2006**, *107*, 1070–1074. [CrossRef] [PubMed]

50. Manolopoulos, K.; Lang, U.; Schmitt, S.; Kirschbaum, M.; Kapellen, T.; Kiess, W. Which contraceptive methods are recommended for young women with type 1 diabetes mellitus? A survey among practitioners in Germany. *Zentralbl. Gynakol.* **1998**, *120*, 540–544. (In German) [PubMed]

51. Lauring, J.R.; Lehman, E.B.; Deimling, T.A.; Legro, R.S.; Chuang, C.H. Combined hormonal contraception use in reproductive-age women with contraindications to estrogen use. *Am. J. Obstet. Gynecol.* **2016**, *215*, 330.e1–330.e7. [CrossRef] [PubMed]

52. Powers, S.E.; Uliassi, N.W.; Sullivan, S.D.; Tuchman, L.K.; Mehra, R.; Gomez-Lobo, V. Trends in standard workup performed by pediatric subspecialists for the diagnosis of adolescent polycystic ovary syndrome. *J. Pediatr. Adolesc. Gynecol.* **2015**, *28*, 43–46. [CrossRef] [PubMed]

53. Warren-Ulanch, J.; Arslanian, S. Treatment of PCOS in adolescence. *Best Pract. Res. Clin. Endocrinol. Metab.* **2006**, *20*, 311–330. [CrossRef] [PubMed]

54. Salmi, D.J.; Zisser, H.C.; Jovanovic, L. Screening for and treatment of polycystic ovary syndrome in teenagers. *Exp. Biol. Med. (Maywood)* **2004**, *229*, 369–377. [CrossRef] [PubMed]

55. Jones, D.L.; Echenique, M.; Potter, J.; Rodriguez, V.J.; Weiss, S.M.; Fischl, M.A. Adolescent girls and young women living with HIV: Preconception counseling strategies. *Int. J. Womens Health* **2017**, *9*, 657–663. [CrossRef] [PubMed]

56. Champaloux, S.W.; Tepper, N.K.; Monsour, M.; Curtis, K.M.; Whiteman, M.K.; Marchbanks, P.A.; Jamieson, D.J. Use of combined hormonal contraceptives among women with migraines and risk of ischemic stroke. *Am. J. Obstet. Gynecol.* **2017**, *216*, 489.e1–489.e7. [CrossRef] [PubMed]

57. Weisberg, E. Contraceptive options for women in selected circumstances. *Best Pract. Res. Clin. Obstet. Gynaecol.* **2010**, *24*, 593–604. [CrossRef] [PubMed]

58. Birtch, R.L.; Olatunbosun, O.A.; Pierson, R.A. Ovarian follicular dynamics during conventional vs. continuous oral contraceptive use. *Contraception* **2006**, *73*, 235–243. [CrossRef] [PubMed]

59. Schlaff, W.D.; Lynch, A.M.; Hughes, H.D.; Cedars, M.I.; Smith, D.L. Manipulation of the pill-free interval in oral contraceptive pill users: The effect on follicular suppression. *Am. J. Obstet. Gynecol.* **2004**, *190*, 943–951. [CrossRef] [PubMed]

60. Edelman, A.; Micks, E.; Gallo, M.F.; Jensen, J.T.; Grimes, D.A. Continuous or extended cycle vs. cyclic use of combined hormonal contraceptives for contraception. *Cochrane Database Syst. Rev.* **2014**, CD004695. [CrossRef] [PubMed]

61. Shakibnia, E.B.; Timmons, S.E.; Gold, M.A.; Garbers, S. It's Pretty Hard to Tell Your Mom and Dad That You're on a Method: Exploring How an App Could Promote Adolescents' Communication with Partners and Parent(s) to Increase Self-Efficacy in Long-Acting Reversible Contraception Use. *J. Pediatr. Adolesc. Gynecol.* **2017**. [CrossRef] [PubMed]

62. Davis, S.A.; Braykov, N.P.; Lathrop, E.; Haddad, L.B. Familiarity with Long-acting Reversible Contraceptives among Obstetrics and Gynecology, Family Medicine, and Pediatrics Residents: Results of a 2015 National Survey and Implications for Contraceptive Provision for Adolescents. *J. Pediatr. Adolesc. Gynecol.* **2018**, *31*, 40–44. [CrossRef] [PubMed]

63. Smith, A.J.B.; Harney, K.F.; Singh, T.; Hurwitz, A.G. Provider and Health System Factors Associated with Usage of Long-Acting Reversible Contraception in Adolescents. *J. Pediatr. Adolesc. Gynecol.* **2017**, *30*, 609–614. [CrossRef] [PubMed]

64. Nguyen, B.T.; Elia, J.L.; Ha, C.Y.; Kaneshiro, B.E. Pregnancy Intention and Contraceptive Use among Women by Class of Obesity: Results from the 2006–2010 and 2011–2013 National Survey of Family Growth. *Womens Health Issues* **2018**, *28*, 51–58. [CrossRef] [PubMed]

65. Edelman, A.B.; Cherala, G.; Blue, S.W.; Erikson, D.W.; Jensen, J.T. Impact of obesity on the pharmacokinetics of levonorgestrel-based emergency contraception: Single and double dosing. *Contraception* **2016**, *94*, 52–57. [CrossRef] [PubMed]

66. Hopkins, B. Barriers to Health Care Providers' Provision of Long-Acting Reversible Contraception to Adolescent and Nulliparous Young Women. *Nurs. Womens Health* **2017**, *21*, 122–128. [CrossRef] [PubMed]

67. Mansour, D.; Verhoeven, C.; Sommer, W.; Weisberg, E.; Taneepanichskul, S.; Melis, G.B.; Sundström-Poromaa, I.; Korver, T. Efficacy and tolerability of a monophasic combined oral contraceptive containing nomegestrol acetate and 17β-oestradiol in a 24/4 regimen, in comparison to an oral contraceptive containing ethinylestradiol and drospirenone in a 21/7 regimen. *Eur. J. Contracept. Reprod. Health Care* **2011**, *16*, 430–443. [CrossRef] [PubMed]

68. De Leo, V.; Fruzzetti, F.; Musacchio, M.C.; Scolaro, V.; Di Sabatino, A.; Morgante, G. Effect of a new oral contraceptive with estradiol valerate/dienogest on carbohydrate metabolism. *Contraception* **2013**, *88*, 364–368. [CrossRef] [PubMed]

69. De Leo, V.; Morgante, G.; Piomboni, P.; Musacchio, M.C.; Petraglia, F.; Cianci, A. Evaluation of effects of an oral contraceptive containing ethinylestradiol combined with drospirenone on adrenal steroidogenesis in hyperandrogenic women with polycystic ovary syndrome. *Fertil. Steril.* **2007**, *88*, 113–117. [CrossRef] [PubMed]

70. Powell, A. Choosing the Right Oral Contraceptive Pill for Teens. *Pediatr. Clin. N. Am.* **2017**, *64*, 343–358. [CrossRef] [PubMed]

71. Liang, S.Y.; Grossman, D.; Phillips, K.A. User characteristics and out-of-pocket expenditures for progestin-only versus combined oral contraceptives. *Contraception* **2012**, *86*, 666–672. [CrossRef] [PubMed]

72. Hall, K.S.; Trussell, J.; Schwarz, E.B. Progestin-only contraceptive pill use among women in the United States. *Contraception* **2012**, *86*, 653–658. [CrossRef] [PubMed]

73. Jatlaoui, T.C.; Riley, H.E.; Curtis, K.M. The safety of intrauterine devices among young women: A systematic review. *Contraception* **2017**, *95*, 17–39. [CrossRef] [PubMed]

74. Upadhya, K.K.; Santelli, J.S.; Raine-Bennett, T.R.; Kottke, M.J.; Grossman, D. Over-the-Counter Access to Oral Contraceptives for Adolescents. *J. Adolesc. Health* **2017**, *60*, 634–640. [CrossRef] [PubMed]

75. Burke, A.E.; Barnhart, K.; Jensen, J.T.; Creinin, M.D.; Walsh, T.L.; Wan, L.S.; Westhoff, C.; Thomas, M.; Archer, D.; Wu, H.; et al. Contraceptive efficacy, acceptability, and safety of C31G and nonoxynol-9 spermicidal gels: A randomized controlled trial. *Obstet. Gynecol.* **2010**, *116*, 1265–1273. [CrossRef] [PubMed]

76. Ehrmann, D.A.; Liljenquist, D.R.; Kasza, K.; Azziz, R.; Legro, R.S.; Ghazzi, M.N.; PCOS/Troglitazone Study Group. Prevalence and predictors of the metabolic syndrome in women with polycystic ovary syndrome. *J. Clin. Endocrinol. Metab.* **2006**, *91*, 48–53. [CrossRef] [PubMed]

77. Azziz, R.; Marin, C.; Hoq, L.; Badamgarav, E.; Song, P. Health care-related economic burden of the polycystic ovary syndrome during the reproductive life span. *J. Clin. Endocrinol. Metab.* **2005**, *90*, 4650–4658. [CrossRef] [PubMed]

78. Carmina, E.; Rosato, F.; Jannì, A.; Rizzo, M.; Longo, R.A. Extensive clinical experience: Relative prevalence of different androgen excess disorders in 950 women referred because of clinical hyperandrogenism. *J. Clin. Endocrinol. Metab.* **2006**, *91*, 2–6. [CrossRef] [PubMed]

79. Essah, P.A.; Levy, J.R.; Sistrun, S.N.; Kelly, S.M.; Nestler, J.E. Effect of macronutrient composition on postprandial peptide YY levels. *J. Clin. Endocrinol. Metab.* **2007**, *92*, 4052–4055. [CrossRef] [PubMed]

80. Panidis, D.; Farmakiotis, D. Treatment of infertility in the polycystic ovary syndrome. *N. Engl. J. Med.* **2007**, *356*, 1999–2001. [CrossRef] [PubMed]

81. De Leo, V.; Di Sabatino, A.; Musacchio, M.C.; Morgante, G.; Scolaro, V.; Cianci, A.; Petraglia, F. Effect of oral contraceptives on markers of hyperandrogenism and SHBG in women with polycystic ovary syndrome. *Contraception* **2010**, *82*, 276–280. [CrossRef] [PubMed]

82. Diamanti-Kandarakis, E. PCOS in adolescents. *Best Pract. Res. Clin. Obstet. Gynaecol.* **2010**, *24*, 173–183. [CrossRef] [PubMed]
83. Guido, M.; Romualdi, D.; Giuliani, M.; Suriano, R.; Selvaggi, L.; Apa, R.; Lanzone, A. Drospirenone for the treatment of hirsute women with polycystic ovary syndrome: A clinical, endocrinological, metabolic pilot study. *J. Clin. Endocrinol. Metab.* **2004**, *89*, 2817–2823. [CrossRef] [PubMed]
84. Reinehr, T.; de Sousa, G.; Roth, C.L.; Andler, W. Androgens before and after weight loss in obese children. *J Clin. Endocrinol. Metab.* **2005**, *90*, 5588–5595. [CrossRef] [PubMed]
85. McCartney, C.R.; Blank, S.K.; Prendergast, K.A.; Chhabra, S.; Eagleson, C.A.; Helm, K.D.; Yoo, R.; Chang, R.J.; Foster, C.M.; Caprio, S.; et al. Obesity and sex steroid changes across puberty: Evidence for marked hyperandrogenemia in pre- and early pubertal obese girls. *J. Clin. Endocrinol. Metab.* **2007**, *92*, 430–436. [CrossRef] [PubMed]
86. Nezi, M.; Christopoulos, P.; Paltoglou, G.; Gryparis, A.; Bakoulas, V.; Deligeoroglou, E.; Creatsas, G.; Mastorakos, G. Focus on BMI and subclinical hypothyroidism in adolescent girls first examined for amenorrhea or oligomenorrhea. The emerging role of polycystic ovary syndrome. *J. Pediatr. Endocrinol. Metab.* **2016**, *29*, 693–702. [CrossRef] [PubMed]
87. Deligeoroglou, E.; Karountzos, V. Dysfunctional uterine bleeding as an early sign of polycystic ovary syndrome during adolescence: An update. *Minerva Ginecol.* **2017**, *69*, 68–74. [CrossRef] [PubMed]
88. Deligeoroglou, E.; Creatsas, G. Menstrual disorders. *Endocr. Dev.* **2012**, *22*, 160–170. [CrossRef] [PubMed]

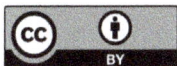

© 2018 by the authors. Licensee MDPI, Basel, Switzerland. This article is an open access article distributed under the terms and conditions of the Creative Commons Attribution (CC BY) license (http://creativecommons.org/licenses/by/4.0/).

International Journal of
*Environmental Research
and Public Health*

MDPI

Article

Factors Influencing Abortion Decision-Making Processes among Young Women

Mónica Frederico [1,2,*], Kristien Michielsen [1], Carlos Arnaldo [2] and Peter Decat [3]

[1]   International Centre for Reproductive Health (ICRH), Ghent University, 9000 Gent, Belgium;
      kristien.michielsen@ugent.be
[2]   Centro de Estudos Africanos, Universidade Eduardo Mondlane, C. P. 1993, Maputo, Mozambique;
      carlos.arnaldo@uem.ac.mz
[3]   Department of Family Medicine and primary health care, Ghent University, 9000 Gent, Belgium;
      Peter.decat@ugent.be
*   Correspondence: monica.frederico@ugent.be or mfrederico45@gmail.com; Tel.: +258-82-435-1370

Received: 29 December 2017; Accepted: 11 February 2018; Published: 13 February 2018

Abstract: *Background:* Decision-making about if and how to terminate a pregnancy is a dilemma for young women experiencing an unwanted pregnancy. Those women are subject to sociocultural and economic barriers that limit their autonomy and make them vulnerable to pressures that influence or force decisions about abortion. *Objective:* The objective of this study was to explore the individual, interpersonal and environmental factors behind the abortion decision-making process among young Mozambican women. *Methods:* A qualitative study was conducted in Maputo and Quelimane. Participants were identified during a cross-sectional survey with women in the reproductive age (15–49). In total, 14 women aged 15 to 24 who had had an abortion participated in in-depth interviews. A thematic analysis was used. *Results:* The study found determinants at different levels, including the low degree of autonomy for women, the limited availability of health facilities providing abortion services and a lack of patient-centeredness of health services. *Conclusions:* Based on the results of the study, the authors suggest strategies to increase knowledge of abortion rights and services and to improve the quality and accessibility of abortion services in Mozambique.

Keywords: abortion; decision-making; young women; Maputo; Quelimane

1. Introduction

Abortion among adolescents and youth is a major public health issue, especially in developing countries. Estimates indicate that 2.2 million unplanned pregnancies and 25% (2.5 million) unsafe abortions occur each year, in sub-Saharan Africa, among adolescents [1]. In 2008, of the 43.8 million induced abortions, 21.6 million were estimated to be unsafe, and nearly all of them (98%) took place in developing countries, with 41% (8.7 million) being performed on women aged 15 to 24 [2].

The consequences of abortion, especially unsafe abortion, are well documented and include physical complications (e.g., sepsis, hemorrhage, genital trauma), and even death [3–6]. The physical complications are more severe among adolescents than older women and increase the risk of morbidity and mortality [6,7]. However, the detrimental effects of unsafe abortion are not limited to the individual but also affect the entire healthcare system, with the treatment of complications consuming a significant share of resources (e.g., including hospital beds, blood supply, drugs) [5,8].

The decision if and how to terminate a pregnancy is influenced by a variety of factors at different levels [9]. At the individual level these factors include: their marital status, whether they were the victim of rape or incest [10,11], their economic independence and their education level [10,12]. Interpersonally factors include support from one's partner and parental support [12]. Societal determinants include social norms, religion [9,13], the stigma of premarital and extra-marital sex [14], adolescents' status, and autonomy within society [12]. At the organizational level, the existence of sex education [10,14], the health care system, and abortion laws influence the decisions if and where to have an abortion.

Those factors are related to power and (gender) inequalities. They limit young women's autonomy and make them vulnerable to pressure. Additionally, the situation is exacerbated when there is a lack of clarity and information on abortion status, despite the existence of a progressive law in this regard.

For example, Mozambican law has allowed abortion if the woman's health is at risk since the 1980s [15–18]. In 2014, a new abortion law was established that broadened the scope of the original law: women are now also allowed to terminate their pregnancy: (1) if they requested it and it is performed during the first 12 weeks; (2) in the first 16 weeks if it was the result of rape or incest, or (3) in the first 24 weeks if the mother's physical or mental health was in danger or in cases of fetus disease or anomaly. Women younger than 16 or psychically incapable of deciding need parental consent [19,20].

Notwithstanding the progressive abortion laws in Mozambique, hospital-based studies report that unsafe abortion remains one of the main causes of maternal death in Mozambique [3]. However, hospital cases are only a small share of unsafe abortions in the country. Many women undergo an abortion in illegal and unsafe circumstances for a variety of reasons [3], such as legal restrictions, the fear of stigma [21–23], and a lack of knowledge of the availability of abortion services [3,9,23].

According to the 2011 Mozambican Demographic Health Survey (DHS), at least 4.5% of all adolescents reported having terminated a pregnancy [24]. Unpublished data from the records of Mozambican Association for Family Development (AMODEFA) which has a clinic that offers sexual and reproductive health services, including safe abortion, indicate that from 2010 to 2016 a total of 70,895 women had an induced abortion in this clinic, of which 43% were aged 15 to 24. Of the 1500 women that had an induced abortion in the AMODEFA clinic in the first three months of 2017, 27.9% were also in this age group [25]. These data show the high demand for (safe) abortion among young women.

For all this described above, Mozambique is an interesting place to study this decision-making process; given the changing legal framework, women may have to navigate gray areas in terms of legality, safety, and access when seeking abortion, which is stigmatized but necessary for the health, well-being, and social position of many young women.

The objective of this study is to explore the individual, interpersonal and environmental factors behind the abortion decision-making process. This entails both the decision to have an abortion and the decision on how to have the abortion. By examining fourteen stories of young women with an episode of induced abortion, we contribute to the documentation of the circumstances around the abortion decision making, and also to inform the policymakers on complexity of this issue for, which in turn can contribute to improve the strategies designed to reduce the cases of maternal morbidity and mortality in Mozambique.

2. Materials and Methods

This is an exploratory study using in-depth interview to explore factors related to abortion decision-making in a changing context. As research on this topic is limited, we opted for a qualitative research framework that aims to identify factors influencing this decision-making process.

2.1. Location of the Study

The study was conducted in two Mozambican cities, Maputo and Quelimane. These cities were selected because they registered more abortions than other cities in the same region. According to the 2014 data from the Direcção Nacional de Planificação, 629 and 698 women, respectively, were admitted to the hospital due to induced abortion complications in Maputo and Quelimane [26]. Furthermore, the two differ radically in terms of culture, with Maputo in the South being patrilineal and Quelimane in the Central Region matrilineal, which could influence the abortion decision-making process. The fieldwork took place between July–August 2016 and January–February 2017.

2.2. Data Collection

The data were collected through in-depth interviews, asking participants about their experiences with induced abortion and what motivated them to get an abortion. To approach and recruit participants (Figure 1), we used the information collected during a cross-sectional survey with women in the reproductive age (15–49), These women were selected randomly applying multistage cluster based on household registers. The survey was designed to understand women's sexual and reproductive health and included filter questions that allowed us to identify participants who had undergone an abortion. The information sheet and informed consent form for this household survey included information about a possible follow-up study.

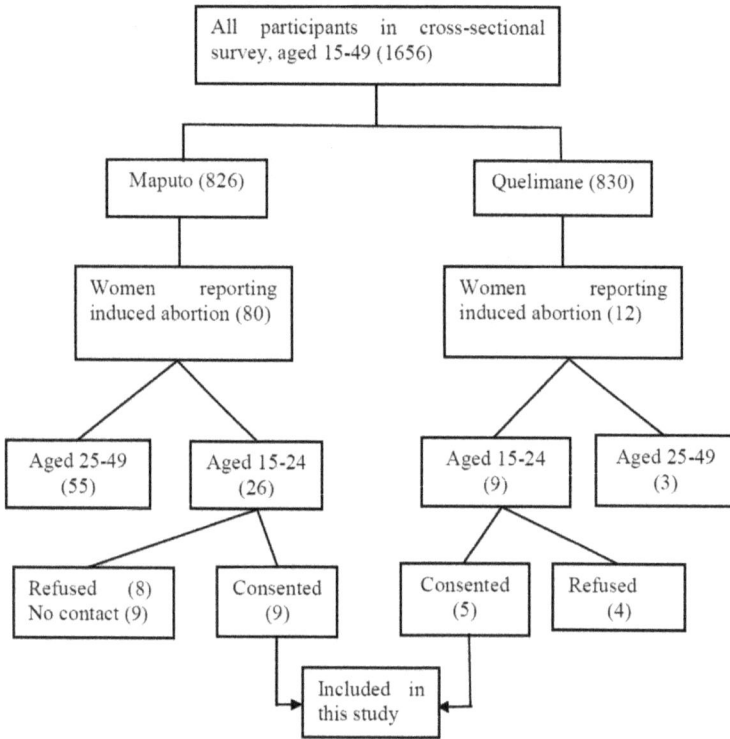

Figure 1. The process of recruitment of the participants.

Participants who were within the age-range 15–24 years and who reported having had an abortion were contacted by phone. In this contact, the researcher (MF) introduced herself, reminded the participant of the study she took part in, explained the follow-up study and asked whether she was willing to participate in this. If she did, an appointment was made at a convenient location. Before each interview, we explained to each participant why she was invited to the second interview. Participants were also informed of interview procedures, confidentiality and anonymity in the management of the data, and the possibility to withdraw from the interview at any time. In total 14, young women (15–24) agreed to participate: nine in Maputo and five in Quelimane. Six of them were interviewed twice to explore further aspects that remained unclear after the first interview. The interviews were conducted in Portuguese.

To start the interview, the participant was invited to tell her life history from puberty until the moment when the abortion occurred. During the conversation, we used probing questions to elicit more details. Gradually, we added questions related to the abortion and factors that influenced the decision process. The main questions were related to the pregnancy history, abortion decision-making, and help-seeking behaviour. The guideline was adapted from WHO tools [27,28]. Before the implementation of the guideline, it was discussed first with another Mozambican researcher to see how they fell regarding the question. After those questions were revised or removed from the guideline.

2.3. Data Analysis

The analysis consisted of three steps: transcription, reading, and codification with NVivo version 11(QSR International Pty Ltd., Doncaster, Australia). After an initial reading, one of the authors (MF) developed a coding tree on factors determining the decision-making. A structured thematic analysis was used to make inferences and elicit key emerging themes from the text-based data [29,30]. The coding tree was based on the ecological model, which is a comprehensive framework that emphasizes the interaction between, and interdependence of factors within and across all levels of a health problem since it considers that the behaviour affects and is affected by multiple levels of influence [31,32].

Next, the codes and the classification were discussed among the researchers (Mónica Frederico, Kristien Michielsen, Carlos Arnaldo and Peter Decat). Finally, the data was interpreted, and conclusions were drawn [33].

2.4. Ethical Consideration

Before the implementation of this research, we obtained ethical approval from the Institutional Committee of the Faculty of Medicine and Nacional Bioethical Committee for Health (IRB00002657). We also asked for the institutional approval of the Minister of Health and authorities at the provincial and community levels. The participants gave their informed consent after the objectives and interview procedures had been explained to them. The participants were informed that they might be contacted and invited, within six months, to participate in another interview.

2.5. Concepts

The providers are the people who carried out the abortion procedure. These may be categorized into skilled and unskilled providers: the former refers to a professional (i.e., nurse or doctor) offering abortion services to a client, while the latter is someone without any medical training. Another concept that requires further explanation is the legal procedure. This corresponds to a set of steps to be followed to comply with the law [19,20]. Specifically, this means that a committee should authorize the induced abortion and an identification document should be available, as well as an informed consent form from the pregnant woman. If the woman is a minor, consent is given by her legal guardian. An ultrasound exam is required to determine the gestational age.

3. Results

3.1. Characteristics of the Participants

The characteristics of the interviewees are summarized in Table 1. The 14 participants were aged 17 to 24 years. Eight had completed secondary school, four had achieved the second level of primary school, and two were university students. Almost all (13) were Christian. Five participants were studying, eight were unemployed, and one was working. The median age of their first sexual intercourse was 15.5 years. Participants reported living with one or both parents (12), with their uncle (1) or alone (1). They lived in suburban areas of Maputo and Quelimane, which are slums with poor living conditions. In these areas, most households earn their income through small businesses that also involve child labour (e.g., selling food or drinks).

Among the participants, five reported more than one pregnancy. One interviewee first had a stillbirth and then two abortions. Another woman gave birth to a girl and afterward terminated two pregnancies. Two interviewees reported two pregnancies, the first of which was brought to full term and the second one terminated. One woman first had an abortion and afterward gave birth to a child. In short, 14 interviewees in total reported on the experiences and decision-making of 16 abortions. One participant stated that the pregnancy was the consequence of rape. Of the 16 reported abortions, seven were performed after the new law came into force at the end of 2014, and nine were carried out before this time.

Table 1. Socio-demographic characteristics and abortion procedure.

Characteristics of Respondents	Categories	Median/Number
Age (median, range)	-	21 (min: 17; max: 24)
Age at sexual activity onset (median, range)	-	15.5 (min: 14; max: 18)
Education attainment (number)	Primary school	4
	Secondary School	8
	University	2
Religion (number)	Catholic + Evangelic	13
	Muslim	1
Occupation (number)	Studying	5
	Without occupation	8
	Vendor	1
Abortion procedure		**Number of clients**
Provider characteristics	Skilled	12
	Unskilled	2
Location of abortion	Health facility	7
	Outside of health facility	7
Treatment for abortion	Pills	5
	Aspiration/curettage	8
	Traditional medicine	1
Followed legal procedure	Yes	0
	No	14

3.2. Abortions Stories

In this study, 12 abortions were done by skilled providers and two by unskilled providers. The unskilled providers were a mother and a husband, respectively. None of the cases, whose abortion was done by a skilled provider, included in this study followed the legal procedure.

In the analysis of the interviews, we studied the personal, interpersonal and environmental factors that influenced six different types of abortion stories, see Table 2: (1) an abortion was performed because the pregnancy was unwanted; (2) an abortion was carried out although the pregnancy was wanted; (3) the abortion was done by an unskilled provider at home; (4) an abortion was carried out by a skilled provider outside the hospital; (5) a particular abortion procedure (medical or chirurgical) was chosen, and (6) the legal procedure was not followed in the hospital. Factors influencing the choice for a particular technical procedure were also examined.

Table 2. Summary of induced abortion stories. (We changed the table format, please confirm.)

Abortion Stories	Personal	Interpersonal	Environmental
Unwanted pregnancy (5 + 1 *)	Unable to be a mother Had a bad past experience Has another child Wanted to study Financial problems Felt depressed	Lack of support	The result of rape
Abortion although pregnancy is wanted (7)		Partner did not recognize the child Convinced by sister Afraid of being sent away Convinced/forced by mother Partner did not want the child Partner's behaviour changed Partner was married	
Unskilled provider (2)		Carried out by partner Carried out by mother	
Abortion outside hospital (8)	Unaware of legal obligations Lack of money	Provider told us to go to his home	Abortion services are not available in the local healthcare settings Fear of signing a document
Abortion at home (2)		Mother said that they would kill me at hospital Decided by partner	
Technical procedure		Decided by provider (aspiration, curettage **, pills ***) Husband gave traditional medicine (1)	
Why the legal procedure is not followed in the hospital (6)		Provider did not inform us about it	Information about legal procedures was not available

* The result of rape; ** Seven participants; *** six participants.

3.3. Abortion Following an Unwanted Pregnancy

In the stories about unwanted pregnancies, mostly personal factors were mentioned as reasons, with some interviewees stating that they felt unable to be a mother at the time of the pregnancy: "*(It) was at the time that I was taking pills that I got pregnant, and I induced abortion because I was not prepared (for motherhood)."* (24 years)

Some had had a bad experience in the past: "*Maybe I would be abandoned and it would be the same. (Sigh)... I learned with my first pregnancy."* (23 years)

Also, the existence of another child was mentioned as a reason to have an abortion: "*I got pregnant when I was 20, and I had a baby. When I became pregnant again, my daughter was a child, and I could not have another child."* (23 years)

For other participants, studies were the main reason why the pregnancy was not wanted: "*He was informed about it, and he said that I should keep it. However, as I wanted to continue my studies, I told him no, no (I) do not."* (17 years)

At the interpersonal level, a lack of support from the partner was often mentioned as a reason for not wanting the baby: "*He said that he recognizes the paternity, but it is not to keep that pregnancy."* (22 years)

Women frequently mentioned environmental circumstances related to their poor socio-economic situation: "*I am staying at Mom's house; it is not okay to still be having babies there."* (23 years)

"*At home, we do not have any resources to take care of this child!"* (20 years)

3.4. Abortion Following a Wanted Pregnancy

In these cases, the decision to abort the pregnancy was not made by the woman herself but imposed by others or by the circumstances.

Some participants reported that their parents/family had decided what had to be done: "*They decided while I was at school. If (it) was my decision I would keep it because I wanted it."* (18 years).

Other young women indicated the refusal of paternity as a reason to terminate the pregnancy.

"*Because my son's father did not accept the (second) pregnancy. There was a time, we argued with each other, and we terminated the relationship. Later, we started dating again, and I got pregnant. He said it was not possible."* (21 years)

"*(he) impregnated me and after that, he dumped me, (smiles) . . . I went to him, and I said that I was pregnant. He said eee: I do not know, that is not my child."* (20 years).

Some women told the interviewers that they were convinced by their boyfriend to have an abortion: "*I talked to him, and he said okay we are going to have an abortion and I accepted."* (22 years)

Others mentioned their partner's indecision and changing attitude as a reason to get an abortion, even though they did want the baby:

"*I told him I was pregnant. First, he said to keep it. (Next) He was different. Sometimes he was calling me, and other times not. I understood that he did not want me."* (20 years)

The fear of being excluded from their family due to their pregnancy was another reason reported by participants: "*So I went to talk with my older sister, and she said eee, you must abort because daddy will kick you out of our home."* (20 years)

"*As I am an orphan, and I live with my uncle, they were going to kick me out. No one would assist me."* (20 years)

3.5. Location of the Abortion: Home-Based Versus Hospital-Based

Two young women reported having had the abortion at home by an unskilled provider. It seems that these unskilled providers than the women (i.e. family members, partner) made the decisions.

"*It was mammy and my sister (who provided the induced abortion services). My sister knows these things."* (18 years)

"He (the father of the child) came to my house and took me back to his house. It was that moment when I aborted." (21 years)

Of the 16 abortions, seven were performed through health services, by a skilled provider. For some of them, the choice for a health service was influenced by the fact of knowing someone at the health facility.

"I went to talk to her (friend), and she said that "I have an aunt who works at the hospital, she can help you. Just take money"." (20 years)

"I Already knew who could induce it (abortion). No, I knew that person. I went to the hospital, and I talked to her, (and) she helped me." (22 years)

Other participants went to the health facility, but due to the lack of money to pay for an abortion at the facilities they sought help out of the health facility: *"They charged us money that we did not have. The ladies did not want to negotiate anything. I think they wanted 1200 mt (17.1 euros) if I am not wrong. He had a job, but he (boyfriend) did not have that amount of money."* (22 years)

Some participants reported that they had an abortion outside regular facilities because the health provider recommended going to his house: *"She (mother) was the one who accompanied me. She is the one who knows the doctor. We went to the central hospital, but he (the doctor) was very busy, and he told us to go to his house."* (17 years)

Others reported the fear of signing a document as a reason to seek help outside of official channels: *"I heard that to induce abortion at the hospital it is necessary for an adult to sign a consent form. I was afraid because I did not know who could accompany me. Because at that time I only wanted to hide it from others."* (22 years).

3.6. Abortion Procedure

The women were not able to explain why a particular abortion procedure (i.e., pills or aspiration, curettage) was used. It appears that they were not given the opportunity to choose and that they submitted themselves to the procedure proposed by the provider.

"The abortion was done here at home. They just went to the pharmacy, bought pills and gave them to me." (18 years)

3.7. Legal Procedure

None of those treated at the hospital stated that legal procedures were followed. They also mentioned that they had to pay without receiving any official receipt.

"First we got there and talked to a servant (a helper of the hospital). The servant asked for money for a refreshment so he could talk to a doctor. After we spoke (with servant), he went to the doctor, and the doctor came, and we arranged everything with him." (22 years)

"We went to the health center, and we talked to those doctors or nurses I mean, they said that they could provide that service. It was 1200 mt (17.1 euros), and they were going to deal with everything. They did not give us the chance to sign a document and follow those procedures." (20 years)

4. Discussion

The objective of this study was to describe abortion procedures and to explore factors influencing the abortion decision-making process among young women in Maputo and Quelimane.

The study pointed out determinants at the personal, interpersonal and environmental level. Analysing the results, we were confronted with four recurring factors that negatively impacted on the decision-making process: (1) women's lack of autonomy to make their own decisions regarding the termination of the pregnancy, (2) their general lack of knowledge, (3) the poor availability of local abortion services, and (4) the overpowering influence of providers on the decisions made.

The first factor involves women's lack of autonomy. In our study, most women indicate that decisions regarding the termination of a pregnancy are mostly taken by others, sometimes against their will. Parents, family members, partners, and providers decide what should happen. As shown in the literature, this lack of autonomy in abortion decision-making is linked to power and gender inequality [34–38]. On the one hand, *power* reflects the degree to which individuals or groups can impose their will on others, with or without the consent of those others [34,37,38]. In this case, the power of the parent/family is observed when they, directly or indirectly, influence their daughters to induce an abortion, for instance by threatening to kick them out of their home. On the other hand, gender inequality is also a factor. This refers to the power imbalance between men and women and is reflected by cases in which the partner makes the decision to terminate the pregnancy [38]. Besides this, the contextual environment of male chauvinism in Mozambique also makes it more socially acceptable for men to reject responsibility for a pregnancy [34,35,37,39,40]. Finally, women's economic dependence makes them more vulnerable, dependent and subordinated. For economic reasons, women, have no other choice but to obey and follow the family or partner's decisions. Closely linked with women's lack of autonomy is their lack of knowledge. Interviewees report that they do not know where abortion services are provided. They are not acquainted with the legal procedures and do not know their sexual rights. This lack of knowledge among women contributes to the high prevalence of pregnancy termination outside of health facilities and not in accordance with legal procedures.

Our participants often report that abortion services are absent at a local level, as has also been pointed out by Ngwena [41]. This is a particular problem in Mozambique. Not all tertiary or quaternary health facilities are authorized to perform abortions. The fact that only some tertiary and quaternary facilities are allowed to do so creates a shortage of abortion centres to cover the demand. In fact, only people with a certain level of education and a sufficiently large social network have access to legal and proper abortion procedures.

Finally, our study shows that providers mostly decide on the location, the methods used and the legality of abortion procedures. Patients are highly dependent on the health providers' commitment, professionality and accuracy and the selected procedures are not mutually decided by the provider and the patient. Providers often do not refer the client to the reference health facility or do not inform them of the legal procedures, creating a gap between law and practice that stimulates illegal and unsafe procedures. The reasons for this are unclear. It might be due to a lack of knowledge among health providers too, and, perhaps, provider saw here an opportunity to supplement the low salary [42]. Participants who seek help at the health facility they do so contacting the provider in particular, as indication given by someone.

This corroborates with studies conducted by Ngwena [41,43], Doran et al. [44], Pickles [45], Mantshi [46], and Ngwena [47], which pointed out the obstacles related to the availability of services and providers' attitudes towards safe abortion, although the law grants the population this right [41, 43–47]. As Ngwena [41,43] argues, the liberalization of abortion laws is not always put into practice and abortion rights merely exist on paper. Braam' study [48] therefore highlights the necessity of clarifying and informing women and providers of the current legislation and ensuring that abortion services are available in all circumstances described in the law.

Finally, despite cultural differences between Maputo and Quelimane, the result did not suggest differences between two areas studied regarding factors influencing the decision to terminate and how the abortion is done. However, the Figure 1 suggests that there was trend to have more participants from Maputo reporting abortion episode in her life than Quelimane. This difference maybe be because Maputo is much more multicultural and the people of this city have more access to information that gives them the opportunity to learn about matter of reproductive health including abortion, than Quelimane. So, due to this there is trend decrease the taboo relation to abortion in Maputo than in Quelimane.

These abortion stories illustrate the lack of autonomy in decision-making process given the power and gender inequalities between adults and young women, and also between man and women. They also show the lack of knowledge not only on the availability of abortion services at some health facilities, as well as, on the new law on abortion. All these lacks that women have are reinforced by poor availability of abortion services and the fact that the providers we not taking their role to help those women, as it is exposed in the next sections.

This study interviewed young women who had an induced abortion at some point in their lives (15 years up to their age at interview date). As such, it does not provide any information on the factors behind the decisions of those who did not terminate their pregnancy.

The results presented in this paper only reflect the perceptions of the young women who had an induced abortion, not those of their parents or partners. The paper is based on qualitative data that provides insights into factors influencing abortion decision-making. Since the sample included in the study is not representative for the population of young women in Mozambique, the results cannot be generalized.

5. Conclusions

Based on the results of the study, we recommend the following measures to improve the abortion decision-making process among young women:

First, strategies should be implemented to increase women's autonomy in decision-making: The study highlighted that gender and power inequalities obstructed young women to make their decision with autonomy. We reiterate the Chandra-Mouli and colleges [49] message. There is a need to address gender and power inequalities. Addressing gender inequality, and promotion of more equitable power relations leads to improved health outcomes. The interventions to promote gender-equitable and power relationships, as well as human rights, need to be central to all future programming and policies [49].

Second, patients and the whole population should be better informed about national abortion laws, the recommended and legal procedures and the location of abortion services, since, despite the decision to terminate pregnancy resulted to the imposition, if they were well informed on that, maybe they could be decide on safe and legal abortion, avoiding double autonomy deprivation. At the same time, providers must be informed about the status of national abortion laws. Additionally, they should be trained in communication skills to promote shared decision-making and patient orientation in abortion counseling.

Third, the number of health facilities providing abortions services should be increased, particularly in remote areas.

Finally, health providers should be trained in communication skills to promote shared decision-making and patient orientation in abortion counseling.

The abortion decision-making by young women is an important topic because it refers the decision made during the transitional period from childhood to adulthood. The decision may have life-long consequences, compromising the individual health, career, psychological well-being, and social acceptance. This paper, on abortion decision-making, calls attention to some attitudes that lead to the illegality of abortion despite it was done at a health facility.

Acknowledgments: Authors gratefully acknowledge the support, contribution, and comments from all those who collaborated direct or indirectly, especially Olivier Degomme, Eunice Remane Jethá, Emilia Gonçalves, Cátia Taibo, Beatriz Chongo, Hélio Maúngue and Rehana Capruchand.

Author Contributions: All authors contributed significantly to the manuscript. Mónica Frederico collected data and developed the first analysis. The themes were intensively discussed with Kristien Michielsen, Carlos Arnaldo and Peter Decat. The subsequent versions of the article were written with the active participation of all authors.

Conflicts of Interest: The authors declare no conflicts of interest.

References

1.	Guttmacher Institute. In Brief: Facts on the Sexual and Reproductive Health of Adolescent Women in the Developing World Context. Available online: http://www.guttmacher.org/pubs/FB-Adolescents-SRH.pdf (accessed on 23 October 2015).

2. Shah, I.H.; Åhman, E. Unsafe abortion differentials in 2008 by age and developing country region: High burden among young women. *Reprod. Health Matters* **2012**, *20*, 169–173. [CrossRef]

3. Ustá, M.B. O Problema do Aborto Inseguro. Outras Vozes. Available online: www.wlsa.org.mz/wp.../11/O-problema-do-aborto-inseguro.pdf (accessed on 3 March 2016).

4. Hess, R.F. Women's Stories of Abortion in Southern Gabon, Africa. *J. Transcult. Nurs.* **2007**, *18*, 41–48. [CrossRef] [PubMed]

5. Ahman, E.; Shah, I. *Unsafe Abortion: Global and Regional Estimates of the Incidence of Unsafe Abortion and Associated Mortality in 2003*, 5th ed.; World Health Organisation: Geneva, Switzerland, 2007; ISBN 978-92-4-159612-1.

6. Ahman, E.; Shah, I. *Unsafe Abortion: Global and Regional Estimates of the Incidence of Unsafe Abortion and Associated Mortality in 2000*, 4th ed.; World Health Organization: Geneva, Switzerland, 2004; ISBN 92-4-159180-3.

7. UNFPA. *Girlhood, Not Motherhood: Preventing Adolescent Pregnancy*; UNFPA: New York, USA, 2015; ISBN 978-0-89714-986-0. Available online: www.unfpa.org (accessed on 22 June 2017).

8. Ahman, E.; Shah, I. *Unsafe Abortion: Global and Regional Estimates of the Incidence of Unsafe Abortion and Associated Mortality in 2008*, 6th ed.; World Health Organization: Geneva, Switzerland, 2011; ISBN 978-92-4-150111-8.

9. Alhassan, A.Y.; Abdul-Rahim, A.; Akaabre, P.B. Knowledge, Awareness and Perceptions of Females on Clandestine Abortion in Kintampo North Municipality, Ghana. *Eur. Sci. J.* **2016**, *12*, 95–112.

10. Gbagbo, F.Y.; Amo-Adjei, J.; Laar, A. Decision-Making for Induced Abortion in the Accra Metropolis, Ghana. *Afr. J. Reprod. Health* **2015**, *19*, 34–42. [PubMed]

11. Olukoya, P. Reducing Maternal Mortality from Unsafe Abortion among Adolescents in Africa. *Afr. J. Reprod. Health* **2004**, *8*, 57–62. [CrossRef] [PubMed]

12. Plummer, M.L.; Wamoyi, J.; Nyalali, K.; Mshana, G.; Zachayo, S.; Ross, D.A.; Wight, D. Aborting and Suspending Pregnancy in Rural Tanzania: An Ethnography of Young People's Beliefs and Practices. *Stud. Fam. Plan.* **2008**, *39*, 281–292. [CrossRef]

13. Lim, L.; Wong, H.; Yong, E.; Singh, K. Profiles of Women Presenting for Abortions in Singapore: Focus on Teenage Abortions and Late Abortions. *Eur. J. Obstet. Gynecol. Reprod. Biol.* **2012**, *160*, 219–222. [CrossRef] [PubMed]

14. Kabiru, C.W.; Ushie, B.A.; Mutua, M.M.; Izugbara, C.O. Previous induced abortion among young women seeking abortion-related care in Kenya: A cross-sectional analysis. *BMC Pregnancy Childbirth* **2016**. [CrossRef] [PubMed]

15. Ustá, M.B.; Mitchell, E.M.; Gebreselassie, H.; Brookman-Amissah, E.; Kwizera, A. Who is Excluded When Abortion Access is Restricted to Twelve Weeks? Evidence from Maputo, Mozambique. *Reprod. Health Matters* **2008**, *16*, 14–17. [CrossRef]

16. Agadjanian, V. "Quasi-Legal" Abortion Services in a Sub-Saharan Setting: Users' Profile and Motivations. *Int. Fam. Plan. Perspect.* **1998**, *24*, 111–116. [CrossRef]

17. Machungo, F.; Zanconato, G.; Bergstrom, S. Reproductive Characteristics and Post- Abortion Health Consequences in Women Undergoing Illegal and Legal Abortion in Maputo. *Soc. Sci. Med.* **1997**, *45*, 1607–1613. [CrossRef]

18. Hardy, E.; Bugalho, A.; Faúndes, A.; Duarte, G.A.; Bique, C. Comparison of Women Having Clandestine and Hospital abortions: Maputo, Mozambique. *Reprod. Health Matters* **1997**, *9*, 108–115. [CrossRef]

19. Assembleia da República. Boletim da República: Lei No. 35/2014 de 31 de Dezembro. 14.o Suplemento Imprensa. Maputo, Mocambique; Report No. 105; 2014. Available online: http://www.wlsa.orgmz/wp-content/uploads/2014/11/lei-35_2014Codigo_Penal.pdf (accessed on 3 June 2015).

20. Ministério da Saúde. Boletim da República: Diploma Ministerial No. 60/2017 de 20 de Setembro. Maputo, Moçambique; (I). Report No. 147; 2017. Available online: www.wlsa.org.mz/wp-content/.../Diploma_ministerial_60-2017.pdf (accessed on 20 October 2017).

21. Cockrill, K.; Upadhyay, U.D.; Turan, J.; Foster, D.G. The Stigma of Having an Abortion: Development of a Scale and Characteristics of Women Experiencing Abortion Stigma. *Perspect. Sex. Reprod. Health* **2013**, *45*, 79–88. [CrossRef] [PubMed]

22. Kumar, A.; Hessini, L.; Mitchell, E.M.H. Conceptualising abortion stigma. *Culture Health Sex.* **2009**, *11*, 625–639. [CrossRef] [PubMed]

23. Singh, S. Hospital Admissions Resulting from Unsafe Abortion: Estimates from 13 Developing Countries. *Lancet* **2006**, *368*, 1887–1892. [CrossRef]

24. Ministério da Saude (MISAU); Instituto Nacional de Estatística (INE). *Inquérito Demográfico e de Saúde 2011*; Instituto Nacional de Estatística (INE): Maputo, Moçambique, 2013.

25. Associação Mocambiçana Para Desenvolvimento da Família (AMODEFA). *Estatisticas de Serviços Prestados em Saúde Sexual e Reproductiva*; AMODEFA: Maputo, Moçambique, 2017.

26. Direcção Nacional de Planificação. *Relatório Nacional do Ministério da Saúde*; Direcção Nacional de Planificação: Maputo, Moçambique, 2014.

27. World Health Organization. *Studying Unsafe Abortion: A Practical Guide*; World Health Organization: Geneva, Switzerland, 1996.

28. Cleland, J.; Ingham, R.; Stone, N. *Asking Young People about Sexual and Reproductive Behaviours: Illustrative Core Instruments*; Special Programme of Research, Development and Research Training in Human Reproduction; UNP: Sri Jayawardenapura, Sri Lanka; UNFPA: New York, NY, USA; WHO: Geneva, Switzerland; World Bank: Washington, DC, USA, 2001.

29. Creswell, J.W. *Research Design Qualitative Quantitative and Mixed Methods Approach*, 2nd ed.; SAGE Publications, Incorporated: London, UK, 2003; ISBN 0-7619-2441-8 (c).

30. Strauss, A.; Corbin, J. *Basics of Qualitative Research: Techniques and Procedures for Developing Grounded Theory*, 2nd ed.; Basics of Qualitative Research Grounded Theory Procedures and Techniques; SAGE: London, UK, 1998; ISBN 0-8039-5939-7.

31. Bronfenbrenner, U. Ecological Model of Human Development. In *International Encyclopedia of Education*, 2nd ed.; Elsevier: Oxford, UK, 1994; Volume 3.

32. Bronfenbrenner, U. *The Ecology of Human Development: Experiments by Nature and Design*; Harvard University Press: Cambridge, MA, USA, 1979; ISBN 0-674-22456-6.

33. Gerhardt, T.E.; Silveira, D.T. *Métodos de Pesquisa*, 1st ed.; Universidade Federal do Rio Grande do Sul: Porto Alegre, Brazil, 2009; ISBN 9788538600718.

34. John, O.L. Power Dynamics, Gender Relations and Decision-Making Regarding Induced Abortion among University Students in Nigeria. *Afr. Popul. Stud.* **2017**, *31*, 3324–3332.

35. John, O.L. Sexual Behaviour, Unwanted Pregnancy and Tripartite Levels of Decision-Making Regarding Induced. *Afr. J. Psychol. Study Soc. Issues* **2016**, *19*, 61–89.

36. Ezeah, P.; Chinyere, A. Gender Inequality in Reproductive Health Services and Sustainable Development in Nigeria: A Theoretical Analysis. *Int. J. Sociol. Anthropol.* **2015**, *7*, 46–53.

37. Letamo, G. The Influence of Gender Role Attitudes on Risky Sexual Behaviour: Evidence from the 2008 Botswana AIDS Impact Survey III. *Afr. Popul. Stud.* **2011**, *25*, 402–418.

38. Shearer, C.L.; Hosterman, S.J.; Gillen, M.M.; Lefkowitz, E.S. Are Traditional Gender Role Attitudes Associated with Risky Sexual Behavior and Condom-Related Beliefs? *Sex Roles* **2005**, *52*, 311–324. [CrossRef]

39. Rollins, B.C.; Bahr, S. A Theory of Power Relationships in Marriage. *J. Marriage Fam.* **1976**, *38*, 619–627. [CrossRef]

40. Amaro, H. Love, Sex, and Power: Considering Women's Realities in HIV Prevention. *Am. Psychol.* **1995**, *50*, 437–447. [CrossRef] [PubMed]

41. Ngwena, C. Inscribing Abortion as a Human Right: Significance of the Protocol on the Rights of Women in Africa. *Hum. Rights Q.* **2010**, *32*, 783–864. [CrossRef]

42. USAID. Avaliação da Corrupção: Moçambique. Relatório Final; December 2005. Available online: wwwpdf.usaid.gov/pdf_docs/Pnadg268.pdf (accessed on 25 October 2017).

43. Ngwena, C. Using Human Rights to Combat Unsafe Abortion: What needs to be Done? Available online: www1.chr.up.ac.za/africlaw/charles_ngwenya.pdf (accessed on 25 October 2017).

44. Doran, F.; Nancarrow, S. Barriers and facilitators of access to first-trimester abortion services for women in the developed world: A systematic review. *J. Fam. Plan. Reprod. Health Care* **2015**, *41*, 170–180. [CrossRef] [PubMed]

45. Pickles, C. Lived Experiences of the Choice on Termination of Pregnancy Act 92 of 1996: Bridging the Gap for Women in Need. *South Afr. J. Hum. Rights* **2013**, *29*, 515–535. [CrossRef]

46. Mantshi, E.T.; Laetitia, C.R. "I am all alone": Factors influencing the provision of termination of pregnancy services in two South African provinces. *Glob. Health Action* **2017**, *10*, 1–10. [CrossRef]

47. Ngwena, C. The Recognition of Access to Health Care as a Human Right in South Africa: Is It Enough? *Health Hum. Rights* **2000**, *5*, 26–44. [CrossRef] [PubMed]
48. Braam, T.; Hessini, L. The Power Dynamics Perpetuating Unsafe Abortion in Africa: A Feminist Perspective. *Afr. J. Reprod. Health* **2004**, *8*, 43–51. [CrossRef] [PubMed]
49. Chandra-Mouli, V.; Svanemyr, J.; Amin, A.; Fogstad, H.; Say, L.; Girard, F.; Temmerman, M. Twenty Years After International Conference on Population and Development: Where Are We With Adolescent Sexual and Reproductive Health and Rights? *J. Adolesc. Health* **2015**, *56*, S1–S6. [CrossRef] [PubMed]

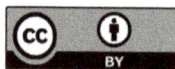

© 2018 by the authors. Licensee MDPI, Basel, Switzerland. This article is an open access article distributed under the terms and conditions of the Creative Commons Attribution (CC BY) license (http://creativecommons.org/licenses/by/4.0/).

International Journal of
Environmental Research and Public Health

MDPI

Article

Are Kazakhstani Women Satisfied with Antenatal Care? Implementing the WHO Tool to Assess the Quality of Antenatal Services

Marzhan A. Dauletyarova [1], Yuliya M. Semenova [1], Galiya Kaylubaeva [1],
Gulshat K. Manabaeva [1], Bakytkul Toktabayeva [1], Maryash S. Zhelpakova [1],
Oxana A. Yurkovskaya [1], Aidos S. Tlemissov [1], Galina Antonova [1] and Andrej M. Grjibovski [2,3,*]

[1]   Department of Public Health, Semey State Medical University, Semey 071400, Kazakhstan;
      marzick85@mail.ru (M.A.D.); yumsem@mail.ru (Y.M.S.); kail_galiya@mail.ru (G.K.);
      gulmanabaeva@mail.ru (G.K.M.); bakyt-64t@mail.ru (B.T.); 20indira04@mail.ru (M.S.Z.);
      oksanayrk@mail.ru (O.A.Y.); aidos_8668@mail.ru (A.S.T.); ssmu.univ@gmail.com (G.A.)
[2]   Central Scientific Research Laboratory, Northern State Medical University, 163000 Arkhangelsk, Russia
[3]   Department of Public Health, Health Care, Hygiene and Bioethics, North-Eastern Federal University,
      677000 Yakutsk, Russia
*   Correspondence: andrej.grjibovski@gmail.com; Tel.: +7-921-471-7053

Received: 14 January 2018; Accepted: 10 February 2018; Published: 13 February 2018

Abstract: Women's satisfaction is a part of the quality assurance process with potential to improve antenatal health services. The objective of this study was to assess the prevalence of women's satisfaction with antenatal care in an urban Kazakhstani setting and investigate associated factors. A total of 1496 women who delivered in all maternity clinics from 6 February through 11 July 2013 in Semey, East Kazakhstan, filled out a standardized pretested questionnaire on satisfaction with antenatal care. Independent associations between dissatisfaction and its correlates were studied by logistic regression. Ninety percent of the women were satisfied with the antenatal care. Women who were dissatisfied had lower education. These women would have preferred more checkups, shorter intervals between checkups, more time with care providers, and shorter waiting times. The overall dissatisfaction was associated with long waiting times and insufficient information on general health in pregnancy, results of laboratory tests, treatment during pregnancy, and breastfeeding. Although most of the women in the study setting were satisfied with the new antenatal care model, we identified the main sources of dissatisfaction that should be addressed. Given that Semey is a typical Kazakhstani city, the results can be generalized to other Kazakhstani urban settings.

Keywords: antenatal care; satisfaction; clients; determinants; Kazakhstan; Central Asia

1. Introduction

Most cases of maternal and perinatal mortality occur in women who receive no antenatal care with more than 99% of these women living in developing countries [1]. Those countries which were part of the former Soviet Union inherited the old Soviet system of antenatal care, which was accessible and affordable for nearly all pregnant women. At the same time, most pregnancies were classified as "high risk" with between 15 and 30 antenatal visits during pregnancy and frequent hospitalizations. The treatment was not considered to be evidence-based and women's satisfaction was not prioritized [2–5].

Shortly after breakup of the Soviet Union, the use of antenatal care services in the former Soviet Republics in Central Asia declined during the 1990s with a shift towards giving birth at home [6,7]. Considerable social inequalities in the use of antenatal services, limited knowledge about possible complications during pregnancy and childbirth among women, and limited capacity and knowledge of service providers have been consistently reported by international teams that promoted safe motherhood in the area [8,9].

Contrary to the other Central Asian states, 99.2% of Kazakhstani women attend a skilled antenatal care provider at least once during pregnancy. Antenatal care is provided primarily by doctors (82.6%), but also by midwives (15.3%), and in rare cases by other health professionals [10]. A pilot project on the introduction of international approaches to safe motherhood was conducted in Zhezkazgan in 2002–2003. It included a shift towards less-medicalized, more women- or family-centered care and more evidence-based approaches to antenatal care [11]. The main results of the project included a reduction in the number of prenatal visits per woman from 12 to 6, decline in the number of hospitalizations, reduction in the average length of stay in the maternity units, and a reduction in the use of non-evidence-based interventions, all leading to the fact that 98% of the women in Zheskazgan were satisfied by the care they received [11].

A nationwide reform of antenatal care had been gradually introduced between 2007 and 2010. A new Edict from the Ministry of Health regulating a reduction of the number of antenatal visits, use of evidence-based practice, and more personalized attitudes towards antenatal care was issued 7 April 2010. Maternal mortality in Kazakhstan decreased from 37.2 per 100,000 live births in 2009 to 13.6 per 100,000 live births in 2013 [12]. However, the quality of care provided by maternal institutions assessed in 2013 was considered substandard [13]. At the same time, no information on whether Kazakhstani women are satisfied and accept the new antenatal care is available in peer-reviewed literature.

Client satisfaction is an integral part of the quality assurance process and client feedback has been shown to be useful to improving health service delivery [5]. International studies on the determinants of satisfaction by antenatal care yield controversial results warranting studies in other settings [14–20]. Evaluations of women's overall satisfaction by the simplified evidence-based model of care with reduced number of antenatal visits has concluded that this model was well accepted by the women and had no long-term consequences for mothers and their children [21–26]. However, it has been emphasized that any changes in the delivery of antenatal care services should take into account women's opinions [22]. A recent qualitative study from Kazakhstan has suggested that cultural and historical aspects should be considered when adopting international models of care [27], but quantitative estimates of women's satisfaction and its determinants in Kazakhstan remain unknown.

The aim of this study was to assess women's satisfaction with antenatal care and associated factors in an urban Kazakhstani setting.

2. Materials and Methods

The study was conducted in the town of Semey (former Semipalatinsk), East Kazakhstan, which is one of the main industrial towns in the country and is known for being the Soviet nuclear weapon testing site in 1949–1991. The population of Semey was 335,400 in 2013. Obstetric services in the town are performed in two municipal maternity hospitals and a perinatal center covering the total population of Semey and adjacent rural areas. Antenatal care is provided at policlinics. Outpatient antenatal services as well as the obstetric care are free of charge.

A total of 1506 women who delivered in all municipal maternity clinics from February 6 to July 11, 2013 comprised the initial sample. Five (0.33%) of them moved to the town prior to delivery and were excluded from the study because they did not receive antenatal care in Semey. Moreover, five (0.33%) women with serious complications during delivery refused to participate in the study. Thus, the final sample consisted of 1496 women or 99.3% of the women who gave birth in Semey during the study period. Data about maternal age, parity, date of delivery, and date of the last menstrual period as well as the number of antenatal visits were obtained from the medical files.

Maternal satisfaction with the antenatal care was assessed using a 24-item questionnaire administered within three days after birth while the woman was in the maternity facility. Maternity clinics were selected as data collection sites because they do not provide antenatal care, minimizing the probability of social desirability bias. The questionnaire was developed by the WHO and used for research purposes in other countries [20,22,23]. The questionnaire was translated from English into Kazakh and Russian languages and back to ensure correctness of the translation. The Kazakh and Russian versions were then pretested on the personnel of the Department of Obstetrics and Gynecology, Semey State Medical University, and on a sample of pregnant women in one of the policlinics. Only minor changes were introduced into the formulation of the questions. Moreover, questions on education, income, ethnic background, and place of residence were added. For the purpose of this study, we used 15 questions on women's preferences on the number of antenatal visits, waiting time, and time spent with the caregiver, as well as amount and appropriateness of the information received during the visits. Given previously reported questionable validity of questions related to satisfaction with antenatal services, we used only one question ("In general, how satisfied are you with the antenatal care you have received?") to synthesize women's overall perceptions of the quality of antenatal care [28].

Women were divided into three age groups: <20 years, 20–29 years, and 30 years or older. Maternal education was classified as secondary, vocational, and higher. Income per family member was coded as below 20,000 tenge (KZT, 1 USD~330 KZT), 20,000–29,999 KZT, 30,000–49,999 KZT, and 50,000 KZT or more. The level of 20,000 KZT was considered as the poverty line in Kazakhstan in 2013. The other cut-off points correspond to the second and the third quartiles of the income distribution. Three groups were used for women's ethnic background: Kazakhs, Russians, and others. By parity, women were classified as primipara, women with 1 previous delivery, and 2 or more previous deliveries. Number of antenatal visits was dichotomized into 7 or less and 8 or more visits. Gestational age was calculated in weeks starting from the first day of the last menstruation period. Preterm birth was birth before 37 completed gestational weeks.

The overall level of satisfaction by antenatal care in the original questionnaire was coded as "very satisfied", "satisfied", and "not satisfied".

Continuous data were presented as means (M) and standard deviations (SD). Proportions of women who were satisfied with antenatal care were presented with 95% confidence intervals (CI) calculated using Wilson's method [29], which is considered to be superior to the most commonly used Wald. Bivariate relationships were assessed by Pearson's chi-squared test. Associations between independent variables and dissatisfaction with antenatal care were studied using multivariable logistic regression. Crude and adjusted odds ratios (OR) with 95% CI were calculated. The reference group for each of the variables was chosen to be what is believed to be the most favorable category. A backward elimination procedure was applied to obtain the final regression model. This method is preferable to the forward method which runs a greater risk of Type II error and has a greater statistical power than the forced entry method for the given sample size [30]. Statistical Package for the Social Sciences (SPSS, version 17.0, SPSS Inc., Chicago, IL, USA) was used for all analyses.

The study was approved by the ethical committee of the Semey State Medical University (Protocol 2 from 20 November 2012, Project Identification Code). All women were informed about the aims of the study and signed informed consent forms.

3. Results

Altogether, 30.1% of the respondents were very satisfied while 59.9% were satisfied with antenatal care. As in most other studies, we dichotomized the outcome as satisfied ("satisfied" and "very satisfied" combined) and not satisfied for further analyses to ensure international comparisons.

In our sample, most of the women were 20–29 years old, had higher education, and were ethnic Kazakhs. Primiparous women comprised nearly half of the sample. More than a quarter of the women reported their income to be below the poverty line. Altogether, 5.6% of infants in the sample were born preterm. The number of antenatal visits varied from 1 to 18 (M = 7.5, SD = 2.6). Nearly half of the women had 7 or less checkups during the index pregnancy. Socio-demographic characteristics of the sample are presented in Table 1.

Table 1. Bivariate associations between satisfaction by antenatal care and maternal socio-demographic and obstetric characteristics.

Variables	N (%)	Satisfied, N (%)	Not Satisfied, N (%)	p
Age, years				0.310
<20	96 (6.4)	85 (6.3)	11 (7.3)	
20–29	1025 (68.5)	916 (68.1)	109 (72.7)	
30+	375 (25.1)	345 (25.6)	30 (20.0)	
Education				0.231
Secondary	277 (18.5)	247 (18.4)	30 (20.0)	
Vocational	543 (36.3)	481 (35.7)	62 (41.3)	
Higher	676 (45.2)	618 (45.9)	58 (38.7)	
Income, KZT				0.209
<20,000	440 (29.4)	388 (28.8)	52 (34.6)	
20,000–29,999	359 (24.0)	332 (24.7)	27 (18.0)	
30,000–49,999	436 (29.1)	389 (28.9)	47 (31.3)	
50,000+	261 (17.4)	237 (17.6)	24 (16.0)	
Ethnic background				0.625
Kazakh	1124 (75.1)	1014 (75.3)	110 (73.3)	
Russian	305 (20.4)	274 (20.4)	31 (20.7)	
Other	67 (4.5)	58 (4.3)	9 (6.0)	
Parity				0.084
0	681 (45.5)	606 (45.0)	75 (50.0)	
1	478 (32.0)	426 (31.6)	52 (34.7)	
2+	337 (22.5)	314 (23.3)	23 (15.3)	
Gestational age, weeks				0.087
<37	84 (5.6)	71 (5.3)	13 (8.7)	
37 or more	1412 (94.4)	1275 (94.7)	137 (91.3)	
Number of visits				0.655
1–7	734 (49.1)	663 (49.3)	71 (47.3)	
8 or more	762 (50.9)	683 (50.7)	79 (52.7)	
Total	1496 (100.0)	1346 (100.0)	150 (100.0)	

Altogether, 90.0% (95% CI: 88.3–91.4) of the women were satisfied with antenatal services. No associations between any of the socio-demographic characteristics and dissatisfaction with antenatal care were observed in bivariate analyses (Table 1).

The reported waiting time at the clinic before being seen by the antenatal care provider varied between 0 and 300 min with an average of 35.7 min. For further analyses the waiting time was categorized into three groups: 0–59 min, 60–119 min, and 120 min or more. Altogether, 22.6% of the women had to wait for more than 2 h before being seen by a medical professional. The reported time usually spent with the antenatal care provider ranged from 3 to 60 min with a mean of 19.8 min (SD = 9.3). For further analyses the time spent with the care provider was classified into three categories: <15 min, 15–44 min, and 45 min or more. Both waiting time and time with the providers of antenatal care were significantly associated with dissatisfaction in crude analyses (Table 2).

Women who were dissatisfied with antenatal care were more likely to have preferred more checkups, and reported that the number of checkups was less than expected and that the time between checkups was too long ($p < 0.001$ for all questions). Moreover, they were more likely to be unhappy with the waiting time and would have preferred more time with the care provider ($p < 0.001$ for both questions). No difference between the satisfaction with the antenatal care and either the gender of the provider or his/her professional background within the given categories was observed (Table 2).

Table 2. Bivariate associations between satisfaction by antenatal care and answers to the questions on the antenatal visits.

Questions	N (%)	Satisfied, N (%)	Not Satisfied, N (%)	p
Are you happy about the number of antenatal checkups you have had, or would you have preferred:				
more checkups	23 (15.8)	190 (14.1)	47 (31.3)	<0.001
fewer checkups	60 (4.0)	52 (3.9)	8 (5.3)	
number of checkups was right	1199 (90.1)	1104 (82.0)	95 (63.3)	
Have the number of antenatal checkups been:				
More than you expected	186 (12.4)	172 (12.8)	14 (9.3)	<0.001
Less than you expected	205 (13.7)	154 (11.4)	51 (34.0)	
About the same as you expected	1105 (73.9)	1020 (75.8)	85 (56.7)	
Has the time between checkups been:				<0.001
Too short	107 (7.2)	97 (7.2)	10 (6.7)	
Too long	153 (10.2)	110 (8.2)	43 (28.7)	
About right	1236 (82.6)	1139 (84.6)	97 (64.7)	
How long do you usually have to wait at the clinic before being seen by a doctor/nurse/midwife who provides you antenatal care?				<0.001
0–59 min	1158 (77.4)	1058 (78.6)	100 (66.7)	
60–119 min	248 (16.6)	219 (16.3)	29 (19.3)	
120 or more min	90 (6.0)	69 (5.1)	21 (14.0)	
Are you happy with the time you normally have to wait?				<0.001
No	485 (32.4)	397 (29.5)	88 (58.7)	
Yes	1011 (67.6)	949 (70.5)	62 (41.3)	
How much time do you usually spend with the doctor/nurse/midwife who provides you antenatal care?				0.005
<15 min	334 (22.3)	285 (21.2)	49 (32.7)	
15–44 min	1137 (76.0)	1039 (77.2)	98 (65.3)	
45 min or more	25 (1.7)	22 (1.6)	3(2.0)	
Do you have enough time with the doctor/nurse/midwife during your checkups, or would you prefer:				<0.001
A lot more time	175 (11.7)	146 (10.8)	29 (19.3)	
A little more time	198 (13.2)	158 (11.7)	40 (26.7)	
Time is about right	1123 (75.1)	1042 (77.4)	81 (54.0)	
If you had a choice, would you prefer to be seen by:				0.090
A male provider	78 (5.2)	66 (4.9)	12(8.0)	
A female provider	825 (55.1)	753 (55.9)	72(48.0)	
No preference	593 (39.6)	527 (39.2)	66(44.0)	
If you had a choice, would you prefer to be attended by:				0.189
A doctor	832 (55.6)	754 (56.0)	78 (52.0)	
A nurse	10 (0.7)	10 (0.7)	0 (0.0)	
A midwife	136 (9.1)	127(9.4)	9 (6.0)	
A combination	365 (24.4)	319(23.7)	46 (30.7)	
No preference	153 (10.2)	136(10.1)	17 (11.3)	

Altogether, 35.9% of the women have reported that they received too little or no information on family planning. The corresponding proportions for the information about breastfeeding, labor, treatment during the index pregnancy, looking after own health, and various tests (blood, urine, etc.) were 30.5%, 25.8%, 13.7%, 11.7%, and 10.0%, respectively. All questions related to the information given to the women were significantly associated with the satisfaction with the antenatal care in crude analysis (Table 3).

Table 3. Bivariate associations between satisfaction with antenatal care and answers to the questions on the information received in antenatal care.

Questions	N (%)	Satisfied, N (%)	Not Satisfied, N (%)	p
Was the information you received about looking after your own health:				<0.001
Not enough	144 (9.6)	95 (7.1)	49 (32.7)	
As much as you wanted	1135 (75.9)	1050 (78.0)	85 (56.7)	
Too much	87 (5.8)	84 (6.2)	3 (2.0)	
No information received	32 (2.1)	24 (1.8)	8 (5.3)	
Don't remember	98 (6.6)	93 (6.9)	5 (3.3)	
Was the information you received about tests (e.g., blood, urine) during this pregnancy:				<0.001
Not enough	92 (6.1)	53 (3.9)	39 (26.0)	
As much as you wanted	1190 (79.5)	1100 (81.7)	90 (60.0)	
Too much	99 (6.6)	96 (7.1)	3 (2.0)	
No information received	58 (3.9)	43 (3.2)	15 (10.0)	
Don't remember	57 (3.8)	54 (4.0)	3 (2.0)	
Was the information you received about any treatment you might need during this pregnancy:				<0.001
Not enough	92 (6.1)	60 (4.5)	32 (21.3)	
As much as you wanted	1098 (73.4)	1016 (75.5)	82 (54.7)	
Too much	73 (4.9)	71 (5.3)	2 (1.3)	
No information received	114 (7.6)	90 (6.7)	24 (16.0)	
Don't remember	119 (8.0)	109 (8.1)	10 (6.7)	
Was the information you received about labor:				<0.001
Not enough	149 (10.0)	112 (8.3)	37 (24.7)	
As much as you wanted	938 (62.7)	877 (65.2)	61 (40.7)	
Too much	101 (6.8)	99 (7.4)	2 (1.3)	
No information received	237 (15.8)	189 (14.0)	48 (32.0)	
Don't remember	71 (4.7)	69 (5.1)	2 (1.3)	
Was the information you received about breastfeeding:				<0.001
Not enough	121 (8.1)	92 (6.8)	29 (19.3)	
As much as you wanted	829 (55.4)	793 (58.9)	36 (24.0)	
Too much	148 (9.9)	141 (10.5)	7 (4.7)	
No information received	334 (22.4)	261 (19.4)	73 (48.7)	
Don't remember	64 (4.3)	59 (4.4)	5 (3.3)	
Was the information you received about family planning:				<0.001
Not enough	84 (5.6)	71 (5.3)	13 (8.7)	
As much as you wanted	728 (48.6)	683 (50.7)	45 (30.0)	
Too much	105 (7.0)	97 (7.2)	8 (5.3)	
No information received	454 (30.3)	374 (27.8)	80 (53.3)	
Don't remember	125 (8.4)	121 (9.0)	4 (2.7)	

In adjusted analysis, the only socio-demographic variable associated with satisfaction with the antenatal care was maternal education—women with secondary or vocational education were more likely to be dissatisfied than women with higher education. Women who were dissatisfied with the care would have preferred more checkups, more time with the antenatal care provider, and shorter intervals between checkups. Moreover, the overall dissatisfaction was associated with the time they had to wait and with either insufficient or no information on looking after own health, tests in the index pregnancy, treatment during this pregnancy, and breastfeeding. Women who had to wait for 60–119 min or did not remember whether they received information on family planning were more likely to be satisfied with the antenatal care than the reference categories (Table 4).

Table 4. Results of multivariable logistic regression analysis.

Questions	aOR	95% CI
How long do you usually have wait at the clinic before being seen by a doctor/nurse/midwife who provides you antenatal care?		
0–59 min	1.00	Reference
60–119 min	0.52	0.28–0.96
120 or more min	1.57	0.77–3.21
Education		
Secondary	1.87	1.07–3.27
Vocational	1.66	1.04–2.63
Higher	1.00	Reference
Was the information you received about looking after your own health		
Not enough	1.82	1.04–3.20
As much as you wanted	1.00	Reference
Too much	0.58	0.15–2.25
No information received	1.13	0.37–3.42
Don't remember	0.69	0.24–1.94
Was the information you received about tests (e.g., blood, urine) during this pregnancy		
Not enough	4.77	2.63–8.68
As much as you wanted	1.00	Reference
Too much	0.55	0.16–1.95
No information received	3.64	1.72–7.73
Don't remember	0.68	0.18–2.59
Was the information you received about any treatment you might need during this pregnancy		
Not enough	2.19	1.17–4.09
As much as you wanted	1.00	Reference
Too much	0.26	0.05–1.36
No information received	1.48	0.78–2.81
Don't remember	0.88	0.38–2.05
Was the information you received about breastfeeding		
Not enough	4.82	2.52–9.25
As much as you wanted	1.00	Reference
Too much	0.97	0.36–2.63
No information received	3.22	1.93–5.38
Don't remember	1.67	0.53–5.38
Was the information you received about family planning		
Not enough	0.78	0.32–1.85
As much as you wanted	1.00	Reference
Too much	1.47	0.54–3.99
No information received	1.42	0.88–2.29
Don't remember	0.22	0.06–0.79
Are you happy about the number of antenatal checkups you have had, or would you have preferred		
More checkups	1.96	1.17–3.28
Fewer checkups	0.97	0.38–2.48
Number of checkups was right	1.00	Reference
Has the time between checkups been		
Too short	0.50	0.21–1.16
Too long	2.28	1.32–3.94
About right	1.00	Reference
Are you happy with the time you normally have to wait?		
No	2.44	1.51–3.96
Yes	1.00	Reference
Do you have enough time with the doctor/nurse/midwife during your checkups, or would you prefer		
A lot more time	1.48	0.84–2.61
A little more time	1.84	1.10–3.07
Time is about right	1.00	Reference

4. Discussion

This is, to the best of our knowledge, the first study on the satisfaction of Kazakhstani women with antenatal services after the new women-oriented antenatal care was introduced in Kazakhstan.

Our findings are generally in line with the results of most of the studies conducted in developing countries which have shown that most of the women are satisfied with antenatal care [25]. However, this proportion is lower than what was reported from the pilot site in Zheskazgan in 2005 [11]. This may be explained by the fact that the pilot study was conducted in close cooperation with international agencies and the local health providers were more enthusiastic about new routines compared with the situation in Semey.

Social variations have been shown to influence the level of satisfaction in some settings [17] but not all [14,26]. Positive associations between satisfaction and maternal age, parity, and education have been observed in several developing settings and were explained by more experience and better utilization of services by older, multiparous, and better educated women [25]. This may also be true for the association between education and satisfaction observed in this study, although no associations with other socio-demographic factors such as age, parity, ethnic background, or income were found.

Promptness of care and time spent with health care provider has been consistently shown to be among the most important factors for satisfaction with antenatal services [25]. Similar to in other studies, women who were dissatisfied with antenatal care reported that they were unhappy with the waiting time, and would have preferred to have more time with the provider, more checkups, and shorter intervals between checkups [14,19,28]. At the same time, women who had to wait between 1 and 2 h were more likely to be satisfied than women who waited for less than an hour in our study. This may be partly explained by the general perception among women that a thorough checkup should take time and long queues can reflect providers' popularity, careful filling out of documentation, etc., thus warranting a qualitative study to explain this unexpected finding. It is interesting that dissatisfied women wished more often to be seen by a combination of different health professionals (30.7% vs. 23.7% for those satisfied). Although the difference did not reach the level of statistical significance, the reasons behind this are worth studying.

Another significant source of dissatisfaction in our study is insufficient information the women receive from their providers about their own health, laboratory tests, treatment, and breastfeeding. Provision of cognitive support has been considered a critical determinant of satisfaction in maternity care in several countries [13,24,26]. While insufficient information in countries with a considerable proportion of foreign providers and high prevalence of illiteracy among women can be attributed to language barriers [14], this is unlikely to be the case in Kazakhstan where virtually everyone speaks Russian and many speak both Russian and Kazakh. The observed high prevalence of either insufficient or even no information on several important aspects related to maternal health should be of concern for the health authorities in Semey.

Our findings should be interpreted with caution taking into account strengths and potential weaknesses of the cross-sectional study design [31]. The relatively large sample size if compared to many similar surveys from developing settings is an advantage that allows detection of more factors associated with the outcome. Consecutive inclusion of all women who delivered in the municipal maternity facilities over the specified period is another strength reducing the probability of sampling bias. It is unlikely that the general level of satisfaction with antenatal services or associations between the satisfaction and selected predictors will vary across seasons in Kazakhstan. Even if so, our study included a part of the cold season and a part of the warm season, reducing the probability of seasonal bias. The questionnaire was previously validated and used in other countries allowing comparability of the findings. Moreover, its Russian and Kazakh versions used in this study were back-translated into English with nearly a perfect match. In addition, they were pretested both on health professionals and on pregnant women. Antenatal care is provided at policlinics while the data on satisfaction with antenatal care were intentionally collected at maternity clinics after delivery to avoid social desirability bias. Policlinics and maternity clinics are two different types of institutions in the Kazakhstani healthcare system, ensuring elimination of social desirability or fear of retaliation. Moreover, this survey was performed by trained interviewers unrelated to medical personnel at the clinics. The participants were assured that the questionnaires were anonymous and the data were treated confidentially by the research team. Thus, fear of retaliation or simple social desirability is very unlikely.

However, the study excluded women with severe complications during delivery, which could have influenced the overall level of satisfaction. Women with unfavorable pregnancy outcomes are less likely to report being satisfied with maternity care [32]. Thus, our estimates of the general satisfaction may be overestimated, although given the fact that we excluded only 5 women, the degree of overestimation is very small. When we repeated our analyses for term pregnancy only, the coefficients changed only marginally and did not influence any of the results. Another limitation is that we studied women's satisfaction in only one town, reducing generalizability of the findings. However, Semey is similar to most middle-sized Kazakhstani towns in terms of socio-economic characteristics of the population and the quality of healthcare, allowing extrapolation of our findings to comparable settings. At the same time, we do not recommend generalization of our results to rural areas where socio-demographic characteristics of the population as well as availability of antenatal care are different from in the urban areas.

5. Conclusions

Most women are satisfied with antenatal care in the study setting. Main sources of dissatisfaction have been identified. While dissatisfaction with the number of visits and longer spacing between them can be solved by better information about safety of these new routines for women without complications, a considerable proportion of women who do not receive sufficient information about various aspects of maternal health should be addressed by training of the health providers in health communication.

Acknowledgments: We thank all of the women who participated in the study. We thank Sonja Myhre from the Norwegian Institute of Public Health for editing the language in the final version of the manuscript.

Author Contributions: Marzhan A. Dauletyarova, Andrej M. Grjibovski, Aidos S. Tlemissov and Yuliya M. Semenova conceived and designed the study; Marzhan A. Dauletyarova, Yuliya M. Semenova, Aidos S. Tlemissov, Galiya Kaylubaeva, Gulshat K. Manabaeva, Bakytkul Toktabayeva, Maryash S. Zhelpakova, Oxana A. Yurkovskaya and Galina Antonova performed the study; Marzhan A. Dauletyarova, Andrej M. Grjibovski, Aidos S. Tlemissov and Yuliya M. Semenova analyzed the data; Marzhan A. Dauletyarova, Andrej M. Grjibovski, Aidos S. Tlemissov, Yuliya M. Semenova, Oxana A. Yurkovskaya, Maryash S. Zhelpakova, Bakytkul Toktabayeva, Gulshat K. Manabaeva and Galiya Kaylubaeva wrote the paper.

Conflicts of Interest: The authors declare no conflict of interest.

References

1. World Health Organization (WHO). *Antenatal Care in Developing Countries. Promises, Achievements and Missed Opportunities. An Analysis of Trends, Levels and Differentials*; WHO: Geneva, Switzerland, 2003.
2. Chalmers, B. Maternity care in the former Soviet Union. *Br. J. Obstet. Gynaecol.* **2005**, *112*, 495–499. [CrossRef] [PubMed]
3. Chalmers, B.; Quliyeva, D. A report of women's birth experiences in Baku, Azerbaijan. *J. Psychosom. Obstet. Gynaecol.* **2004**, *25*, 3–14. [CrossRef] [PubMed]
4. Dennis, L.I.; Flynn, B.C.; Martin, J.B. Characteristics of pregnant women, utilization, and satisfaction with prenatal services in St. Petersburg, Russia. *Public Health Nurs.* **1995**, *12*, 347–377. [CrossRef]
5. Ivanov, L.L.; Flynn, B.C. Utilization and satisfaction with prenatal care services. *West. J. Nurs. Res.* **1999**, *21*, 372–386. [CrossRef] [PubMed]
6. Kamiya, Y. Women's autonomy and reproductive health care utilisation: Empirical evidence from Tajikistan. *Health Policy* **2011**, *102*, 304–313. [CrossRef] [PubMed]
7. Fan, L.; Habibov, N.N. Determinants of accessibility and affordability of health care in post-socialist Tajikistan: Evidence and policy options. *Glob. Public Health* **2009**, *4*, 561–574. [CrossRef] [PubMed]

8.   Wiegers, T.A.; Boerma, W.G.; de Haan, O. Maternity care and birth preparedness in rural Kyrgyzstan and Tajikistan. *Sex. Reprod. Healthc.* **2010**, *1*, 189–194. [CrossRef] [PubMed]

9.   Falkingham, J. Inequality and changes in women's use of maternal health-care services in Tajikistan. *Stud. Fam. Plan.* **2003**, *34*, 32–43. [CrossRef]

10.   Smailov, A.A. *Multiple Indicator Cluster Survey (MICS) in the Republic of Kazakhstan 2010–2011. Monitoring the Situation of Children and Women*; Statistics Committee of the Ministry of National Economy of the Republic of Kazakhstan: Astana, Kazakhstan, 2012.

11.   Anonymous. *Introducing International Approaches to Safe Motherhood in Zheskazgan: Results of a Pilot Project in Kazakhstan*; United States Agency for International Development: Almaty, Kazakhstan, 2005.

12.   World Health Organization. Health for All Database. Available online: http://data.euro.who.int/hfadb (accessed on 11 September 2015).

13.   Dauletyarova, M.; Semenova, Y.; Kaylubaeva, G.; Manabaeva, G.; Khismetova, Z.; Akilzhanova, Z.; Tussupkaliev, A.; Orazgaliyeva, Z. Are women of East Kazakhstan satisfied with the quality of maternity care? Implementing the WHO tool to assess the quality of hospital services. *Ir. J. Public Health* **2016**, *45*, 729–738.

14.   Ghobashi, M.; Khandekar, R. Satisfaction among Expectant Mothers with Antenatal Care Services in the Musandam Region of Oman. *Sult. Qaboos Univ. Med. J.* **2008**, *8*, 325–332.

15.   Richard, L.; Séguin, L.; Champagne, F.; Therrien, R. Determinants of satisfaction with medical prenatal care in Quebec women. *Can. J. Public Health* **1992**, *83*, 66–70. [PubMed]

16.   Fawole, A.O.; Okunlola, M.A.; Adekunle, A.O. Clients' perceptions of the quality of antenatal care. *J. Natl. Med. Assoc.* **2008**, *100*, 1052–1058. [CrossRef]

17.   Esimai, O.A.; Omoniyi-Esan, G.O. Wait time and service satisfaction at Antenatal Clinic, Obafemi Awolowo University Ile-Ife. *East Afr. J. Public Health* **2009**, *6*, 309–311. [PubMed]

18.   Hundley, V.; Rennie, A.M.; Fitzmaurice, A.; Graham, W.; van Teijlingen, E.; Penney, G. A national survey of women's views of their maternity care in Scotland. *Midwifery* **2000**, *16*, 303–313. [CrossRef] [PubMed]

19.   Langer, A.; Villar, J.; Romero, M.; Nigenda, G.; Piaggio, G.; Kuchaisit, C.; Rojas, G.; Al-Osimi, M.; Belizán, J.; Farnot, U.; et al. Are women and providers satisfied with antenatal care? Views on a standard and a simplified, evidence-based model of care in four developing countries. *BMC Women's Health* **2002**, *2*, 7. [CrossRef] [PubMed]

20.   Sikorski, J.; Wilson, J.; Clement, S.; Das, S.; Smeeton, N. A randomised controlled trial comparing two schedules of antenatal visits: The antenatal care project. *Br. Med. J.* **1996**, *312*, 546–553. [CrossRef]

21.   Nigenda, G.; Langer, A.; Kuchaisit, C.; Romero, M.; Rojas, G.; Al-Osimy, M.; Villar, J.; Garcia, J.; Al-Mazrou, Y.; Ba'aqeel, H.; et al. Womens' opinions on antenatal care in developing countries: Results of a study in Cuba, Thailand, Saudi Arabia and Argentina. *BMC Public Health* **2003**, *3*, 17. [CrossRef] [PubMed]

22.   Langer, A.; Nigenda, G.; Romero, M.; Rojas, G.; Kuchaisit, C.; al-Osimi, M.; Orozco, E. Conceptual bases and methodology for the evaluation of women's and providers' perception of the quality of antenatal care in the WHO Antenatal Care Randomised Controlled Trial. *Paediatr. Perinat. Epidemiol.* **1998**, *12* (Suppl. 2), 98–115. [CrossRef]

23.   Clement, S.; Candy, B.; Sikorski, J.; Wilson, J.; Smeeton, N. Does reducing the frequency of routine antenatal visits have long term effects? Follow up of participants in a randomised controlled trial. *Br. J. Obstet. Gynaecol.* **1999**, *106*, 367–370. [CrossRef] [PubMed]

24.   Clement, S.; Sikorski, J.; Wilson, J.; Das, S.; Smeeton, N. Women's satisfaction with traditional and reduced antenatal visit schedules. *Midwifery* **1996**, *12*, 120–128. [CrossRef]

25.   Srivastava, A.; Avan, B.I.; Rajbangshi, P.; Bhattacharyya, S. Determinants of women's satisfaction with maternal health care: A review of literature from developing countries. *BMC Pregnancy Childbirth* **2015**, *15*, 97. [CrossRef] [PubMed]

26.   Craig, B.J.; Kabylbekova, Z. Culture and Maternity Care in Kazakhstan: What New Mothers Expected. *Health Care Women Int.* **2015**, *36*, 41–56. [CrossRef] [PubMed]

27.   Oladapo, O.T.; Osiberu, M.O. Do sociodemographic characteristics of pregnant women determine their perception of antenatal care quality? *Matern. Child J.* **2009**, *13*, 505–511. [CrossRef] [PubMed]

28.   Das, P.; Basu, M.; Tikadar, T.; Biswas, G.; Mridha, P.; Pal, R. Client satisfaction on maternal and child health services in rural Bengal. *Indian J. Community Med.* **2010**, *35*, 478–481. [PubMed]

29.   Grjibovski, A.M. Confidence intervals for proportions. *Ekol. Cheloveka* **2008**, *6*, 57–60.

30. Field, A. *Discovering Statistics Using IBM SPSS Statistics*, 2nd ed.; SAGE Publications: Thousand Oaks, CA, USA, 2005.
31. Kholmatova, K.K.; Grjibovski, A.M. Cross-sectional studies: Planning, sample size and data analysis. *Ekol. Cheloveka* **2016**, *2*, 49–56.
32. Cham, M.; Sundby, J.; Vangen, S. Availability and quality of emergency obstetric care in Gambia's main referral hospital: Women-users' testimonies. *Reprod. Health* **2009**, *6*, 5. [CrossRef] [PubMed]

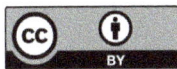

© 2018 by the authors. Licensee MDPI, Basel, Switzerland. This article is an open access article distributed under the terms and conditions of the Creative Commons Attribution (CC BY) license (http://creativecommons.org/licenses/by/4.0/).

International Journal of
*Environmental Research
and Public Health*

MDPI

Article

"I Was Relieved to Know That My Baby Was Safe": Women's Attitudes and Perceptions on Using a New Electronic Fetal Heart Rate Monitor during Labor in Tanzania

Sara Rivenes Lafontan [1,*]**, Johanne Sundby** [1]**, Hege L. Ersdal** [2]**, Muzdalifat Abeid** [3]**, Hussein L. Kidanto** [4] **and Columba K. Mbekenga** [5]

[1] Institute of Health and Society, Faculty of Medicine, University of Oslo, Forskningsveien 3A, 0373 Oslo, Norway; johanne.sundby@medisin.uio.no
[2] Department of Anesthesiology and Intensive Care, University of Stavanger, 4036 Stavanger, Norway; hege.ersdal@safer.net
[3] Temeke Regional Referral Hospital, Dar es Salaam, Tanzania; amuzdalifat29@gmail.com
[4] Ministry of Health Community Development Gender Elderly and Children, Dodoma, Tanzania; hkidanto@gmail.com
[5] School of Nursing and Midwifery, Aga Khan University, Dar es Salaam, Tanzania; kokumbekenga@gmail.com
*   Correspondence: s.r.lafontan@medisin.uio.no; Tel.: +47-2285-0550

Received: 15 December 2017; Accepted: 7 February 2018; Published: 9 February 2018

Abstract: To increase labor monitoring and prevent neonatal morbidity and mortality, a new wireless, strap-on electronic fetal heart rate monitor called Moyo was introduced in Tanzania in 2016. As part of the ongoing evaluation of the introduction of the monitor, the aim of this study was to explore the attitudes and perceptions of women who had worn the monitor continuously during their most recent delivery and perceptions about how it affected care. This knowledge is important to identify barriers towards adaptation in order to introduce new technology more effectively. We carried out 20 semi-structured individual interviews post-labor at two hospitals in Tanzania. A thematic content analysis was used to analyze the data. Our results indicated that the use of the monitor positively affected the women's birth experience. It provided much-needed reassurance about the wellbeing of the child. The women considered that wearing Moyo improved care due to an increase in communication and attention from birth attendants. However, the women did not fully understand the purpose and function of the device and overestimated its capabilities. This highlights the need to improve how and when information is conveyed to women in labor.

Keywords: Tanzania; low-resource setting; labor care; laboring women's attitudes; (electronic) fetal heart rate monitoring; labor monitoring; health literacy; informed consent; Moyo; wireless fetal heart rate monitor

---

1. Introduction

While there have been global improvements in child survival, perinatal mortality remains nearly unchanged [1]. Each year, as many as 2 million babies die during labor (fresh stillbirths) [2–5] and almost 3 million newborn babies die within their first month of life (neonatal deaths). The global target for reducing neonatal mortality as stated by the Sustainable Development Goal 3.2 aims to reduce neonatal mortality to 12 per 1000 live births by 2030 [6]. The countries in the world with the highest neonatal mortality are located in South Asia and Sub-Saharan Africa [7]. While Tanzania has made great improvements in reducing neonatal mortality, 27% of the estimated 8000 newborn deaths occurring each year in the country are caused by birth asphyxia [7]. Birth asphyxia can be detected through regular fetal heart rate monitoring (FHRM). The most common way to monitor FHR is by using a Pinard fetoscope. However, in low-income settings where there is a lack of skilled birth attendants, such monitoring is often not done according to guidelines [8], partly due to time constraints [9]. FHRM has also been found to be suboptimal as the partogram used for monitoring and documenting the progress of labor through regular FHRM and maternal assessment is considered to be a complex tool [10]. While it provides guidance for obstetric interventions based on the progress of labor, it is often under-utilized or incorrectly completed [11,12].

To improve FHRM, a new strap-on automatic fetal heart rate monitor, Moyo, was developed by Laerdal Global Health (see Appendix A). It helps detect fetal heart rate and alerts the skilled birth attendant in an effort to ensure timely obstetrical actions and prevent birth asphyxia and fresh stillbirths. Acceptance by users is essential for the success of technological devices [8,13]. While investigated in high-income countries, there is limited knowledge about laboring women's views about new technological devices used in maternal care in low-resource settings. We believe it is important to bring forward their perspectives in an effort to improve care. This knowledge is important to identify potential barriers towards adaptation in order to introduce new technology more effectively and ensure long-term use. Through a review of literature, we were unable to identify other studies that investigated laboring women's attitudes and perceptions about a wireless strap-on electronic fetal heart rate monitor in low-resource settings. Research is therefore needed as new technological devices are increasingly introduced in maternal care in low-resource settings. The objective of this present study is to explore the attitudes and perceptions of mothers who wore Moyo during their most recent delivery about the device and its effects on the care they received.

This study is part of the ongoing evaluation of the introduction of Moyo and was conducted in parallel with the quantitative Safer Births Moyo studies in Dar es Salaam. At a tertiary health facility in the city, a 2-arm randomized control study testing the use of Moyo versus a hand-held Doppler for fetal heart rate monitoring was conducted. At a municipal referral hospital, a descriptive study evaluating the use of Moyo and its effects on timely obstetrical actions/referrals and perinatal outcome was carried out.

2. Materials and Methods

2.1. Study Design and Data Collection

As the current study aimed to explore the attitudes and perceptions of laboring women, a qualitative approach was chosen [14]. In order to capture individual experiences, a total of 20 semi-structured individual interviews were carried out [15], ten (10) at each study site. An interview guide was used which included open-ended questions about the information received about the device, opinions about wearing it, and the care received while wearing the device. When necessary, follow-up questions were asked for elaborations or clarifications. Each interview ended by asking the participant if she had any questions for the interviewer. Interviews at both hospitals were conducted in Kiswahili by a research assistant who was a teacher in midwifery with experience in conducting qualitative research. The first author (Sara Rivenes Lafontan) was present during all interviews. Data collection continued until saturation and no new themes arose [15]. Additional interviews were consequently carried out at both study sites in an effort to validate findings with new respondents. This process aims to verify the collected data in order to increase the validity of the findings and is often referred to as respondent validation or member checking [15]. These interviews were part of the total number of interviews carried out. The interviews were conducted 12–24 h post labor at different private locations inside both hospitals to ensure privacy, and lasted 20–25 min. The data collection took place from January to March 2017.

2.2. Recruitment of Participants and Ethics

Twenty mothers were recruited to participate in the study and all participants were interviewed once. Recruitment was done through convenience sampling [15]. The mothers were approached before discharge from the post-natal ward and informed about the study by two members of the research team at both hospitals. All the women who were asked to participate in the study accepted. The recruitment was conducted by the Tanzanian research assistant with assistance from nursing staff at the maternity wards. The inclusion criteria to participate in the study were that Moyo had been used during the most recent delivery, that there had been a positive fetal outcome, and that the women were multiparous.

The study was conducted according to the Declaration of Helsinki [16]. All participants received oral and written information about the purpose of the study before giving their written consent to participate. The Safer Births studies are approved by the Norwegian Regional Ethics Committee (REK Vest; Ref: 2013/110/REK vest) and the Tanzanian National Institute for Medical Research (Ref: NIMR/HQ/R.8a/Vol.IX/388). The first author obtained a research permit to carry out the study from the Tanzania Commission for Science and Technology, COSTECH, (No. 2016-396-NA-2016-277). The study obtained ethical approval from all relevant entities, both at the institutions where the study was carried out and at the local government.

2.3. Study Setting

The study was carried out at two hospitals in Dar es Salaam, Tanzania. Hospital 1 is a tertiary referral hospital with 10,000 annual deliveries. It receives patients referred from both public and private practice and also serves paying private patients. The obstetric department is staffed with a number of obstetric and gynecologic (Ob-Gyn) specialists, resident doctors, intern doctors, and nurses/midwives. The labor ward includes 19 beds and five birth attendants per shift. Hospital 2 is a municipal referral hospital receiving patients from health centers and peripheral hospitals in a primarily high-density area of Dar es Salaam. There are two Ob-Gyn specialists per day working in the obstetrics department in addition to medical doctors, intern doctors, and nurses/midwives. The hospital has approximately 17,000 annual deliveries, between 40 and 50 each day. The labor ward has 12 beds and five birth attendants during the day. Women at the two facilities were monitored using a Pinard prior to the introduction of Moyo (as a trial). Both facilities have the capacity to perform what is described as comprehensive emergency obstetric and newborn care signal functions [17].

2.4. Data Analysis

The interviews were recorded and transcribed verbatim by a transcriber who was trained by the first author (Sara Rivenes Lafontan) and who had previous experience transcribing qualitative interviews in Kiswahili. The transcripts were translated into English by a native speaker fluent in both Kiswahili and English and familiar with the study context. Both transcripts and translated versions of the interviews were verified by members of the research team. The translated interviews were read and re-read to deepen the familiarity with the content. Data organization was undertaken using the software package NVivo 11 (QSR International Pty Ltd., Melbourne, Australia). The data was analyzed using qualitative content analysis which is considered suitable for descriptive research questions [18]. During this stepwise process, the material was systematically divided into codes and categories as described by Graneheim and Lundman [19,20]. Transcripts were analyzed line by line and assigned to relevant codes. A coding list was generated and codes were subsequently merged into categories; see Table 1 below for an example of the coding process. Throughout this process, emphasis was on keeping the original wording of the mothers participating in the study. Condensed meaning units, codes, and categories were discussed and agreed upon among the authors.

Table 1. Example of the analysis process.

Translated Transcribed Interview	Code	Category
I: Okay, great, so can you tell us if this device changed your birth experience compared to your previous deliveries where devices like Pinard were used? R: Yes, I saw the difference because this device allowed the nurse to be closer as opposed to previously where they'd walk around and monitor from afar, they would come to me more often too.	Feels that she received closer and more frequent attention from the nurse compared to previous deliveries due to the device.	Receiving close care [1]

[1] The category was formed by several codes.

3. Results

3.1. Demographic Characteristics

The age range of participants was 23–43 years, median age 32 years. A summary of participant characteristics by age group, occupation, and number of children is presented in Table 2 below.

Table 2. Demographic description of participants by age group, occupation, and number of children.

Variable	Sub-Groups	*n* (20)	%
Age	20–29	6	30
	30–40	13	65
	above 40	1	5
Occupation	Run a small business	7	35
	Maid	1	5
	Teacher	2	10
	Stay at home	5	25
	Farmer	2	10
	Nurse	1	5
	Entrepreneur	1	5
	Business woman	1	5
Number of children	1		
	2	6	30
	3	4	20
	4	8	40
	above 4	1	5

3.2. Categories

The attitudes and perceptions of the women participating in the study towards using the device and their perceptions about how the use affected care were divided into four categories: understanding Moyo's purpose and functions, feeling the device had a positive effect on the delivery, receiving close care, and feeling good knowing the baby was safe. An additional category was developed to capture the women's suggestions for how the introduction of Moyo could be improved.

3.2.1. Understanding Moyo's Purpose and Functions

Half of the participants at Hospital 2 and one participant at Hospital 1 responded that they had not been informed about the purpose of the device and its main functions when it was put on them. All but one of the participants who responded that they had not been informed had asked the health care provider what it was or understood it themselves. This was the only category where there was a clear difference in the responses at the two study sites. Of those who reported that they were informed, the information received and/or retained by the participants seemed to be related to the purpose of the device and less about its functions; they knew that Moyo measured fetal heart rate (purpose), but were unaware of the meaning of the colors on the display and sounds coming from the monitor (functions). None of the participants seemed to have fully understood the functions of the device, including the alarm function. One woman was unable to see the monitor because it was hung on the IV drip stand with the display away from her:

> *I would like if they could turn the device around so I am able to see and know what's going on, also if they could give us more information about the meaning of colors and what to do if anything ever happens.*

> Hospital 1#3

As an explanation for why they did not know certain functions of Moyo or the purpose of the device, six women said that they were unable to absorb information or ask questions about Moyo due to labor pains. One participant indicated that while she had been informed about what the device measured, she had not been informed about its functions but she trusted the health care providers to take the appropriate action if needed. Those who said they had not received information about the purpose of the device did not express more negative attitudes towards the device or about wearing it. However, they more frequently attributed functions to the device; one woman who reported that she had not been initially informed suggested it might be a form of lucky charm since it was worn around her neck. Another thought it was a clock because she saw numbers on the monitor's display. There was also a tendency by some to overestimate the diagnostic power of the device; one woman said she thought that fetal abnormalities would be detected faster when the device was used. Some of the participants also mentioned that they believed the device helped the baby breathe and helped the baby overall to ensure a safe delivery.

One woman at Hospital 2, who also responded that she had not received information, explained that the woman lying in the bed next to her had said that if Moyo did not make a sound it meant that the fetus was dead. Another also expressed fear of the consequences of the device not making a sound:

> *In my mind I was thinking maybe if the device did not produce any sound my baby was no longer alive. So from time to time I pulled the straps of the device and waited for the sound.*

> Hospital 2#20

3.2.2. Feeling the Device Had a Positive Effect on the Delivery

All participants in the study delivered vaginally and on term without major complications during their most recent delivery. The women expressed that wearing the device had positive effects during the delivery. Three of the participants at Hospital 2 mentioned that Moyo helped the labor progress due to the belt which some said held the abdomen up, while another said helped the baby progress through the birth canal:

> *Previously when pushing the baby after some time the baby returned inside the womb and I had to push again and again. But this time with the device when pushing the baby did not return inside because there were no room for returning, the device had occupied the remaining space.*

> Hospital 2#16

Despite it being a new device, none of the participants expressed any doubt about the accuracy or safety of the device. For some of the women, the use of Moyo seemed to be linked with medical advancement and improvements in care which translated into an easier delivery for the women:

> *A high number of women lost their babies but now when the labor pains start when you attempt to push, the baby arrives with little hustle not like in the past when you would be in labor for six to eight hours.*

> Hospital 1#7

None of the participants said the device was painful to wear compared to the Pinard which some said was painful when it was pressed on the abdomen. Some of the women also expressed feeling that Moyo had given them strength and energy; they had felt less tired and Moyo gave them the strength to push during contractions. There were some conflicting opinions about the effect of Moyo on labor pains. Some participants wondered if wearing Moyo resulted in more labor pain as the pain had become more intense when Moyo was put on. One mother felt that Moyo had contributed to less labor pain. The issue of labor pain and its effects was raised by the mothers and was not part of the interview guide.

3.2.3. Feeling Good Knowing the Baby Was Safe

Several of the mothers at both study sites reported previous negative experiences in childbirth, some having lost a child. Many explained being worried about the wellbeing of the baby and receiving limited information about the progress of the baby during previous deliveries:

> *I lost a child 2 years ago—they found out that one of the babies I carried died and I only found out after I gave birth to the other baby.*

Hospital 2#13

This was compared to the feeling of reassurance about the wellbeing of their unborn child when Moyo was used. The continuous signs from the monitor that the baby was doing well, and being able to hear the heartbeats from the monitor and see the FHR marked on the display enabled the women to experience for themselves that the baby was doing well. One woman, when asked what was different during this delivery compared to previous ones, said:

> *I: Did you feel anything different?*
> *R: Yes, I felt the difference, the difference is this time I could see how my baby was progressing while I was going through labor, the device gave me hope that the baby was ok.*

Hospital 1#9

The main focus for the women interviewed was how Moyo positively affected their unborn child and not about how the women themselves felt about wearing the device. Questions about particular features of the device were often answered with the benefits of using the device for the fetus. When asked what it felt like to wear Moyo during the delivery, one woman simply responded:

> *I was relieved to know that my baby was safe.*

Hospital 2#7

3.2.4. Receiving Close Care

The use of the device seemed to increase the sense of receiving care and being monitored for many of the women in the study. Some of the participants said they felt they had received closer follow-up from the health care provider compared to previous deliveries and said that even if the nurse/midwife was not by the bedside, she was monitoring the progress of the delivery from afar:

> *Respondent: even though the midwife was away she was able to hear.*
> *Interviewer: she listening when away?*
> *Respondent: Yes.*

Hospital 2#7

When comparing Moyo to the Pinard, the increased monitoring was something that was pointed out by some of the women:

> *I think there's more care and attention given when Moyo device was used, they'd attach it from the beginning until you give birth and they'd monitor it in between whereas with Pinard, they'd only monitor once in a while—when you are first admitted and when you are giving birth.*

Hospital 1#8

Moreover, two participants said that they felt they had received more attention from the health care provider when Moyo was used. One of these said that despite receiving less attention, she felt reassured about the progress of her child because she could see it on the device. It could seem as though the use of Moyo gave the health care providers more reason to attend to the mother if only to check on the device. Participants explained how the midwives came to look at the display of the device and left again without taking any other measurements or observations.

When Moyo was used, the mothers felt more actively engaged in the labor monitoring process which they also expressed as positive. Several respondents described how the monitoring of the fetus became a shared responsibility between the mother and the health care providers because the mother could follow the fetal heart rate. One participant said she felt there was an increased collaboration between her, the doctor, and the midwife.

> I: So how did you feel when you saw that your baby was ok?
>
> R: I felt more confident... there was also a lot of cooperation around, compared to the first device (Pinard).
>
> I: Why was there no cooperation when the first device was used?
>
> R: Because only a doctor/nurse could hear.

Hospital 2#11

3.2.5. Suggestions for Improvements

None of the participants in the study had suggestions for how the functions and characteristics of the device could be improved. However, it was suggested that Moyo should be introduced during ante-natal care (ANC) visits in order for the mothers to receive adequate information and have time to familiarize themselves with the device before arriving at the labor ward.

> I would suggest that the patient is educated about the device before coming into the labor ward, we are often in so much pain when we enter the (labor) ward, so it's not easy to listen and take everything in, some may refuse to wear the device because they are worried or in doubt and don't want to add more pain, so it's best that patients are told about the device before they enter the ward.

Hospital 1#8

Others said that their only suggestion was that Moyo should be available to as many women as possible during labor. It was explained that it would benefit both women and their babies, making the childbirth easier for the women.

4. Discussion

In the present study, we explored the attitudes and perceptions of women using a new electronic fetal heart rate monitor during labor. Our results indicate that the use of the monitor positively affected the women's birth experience by providing much-needed reassurance about the wellbeing of the child. The mothers also believed that the care had improved due to a perceived increase in communication and attention from the health care providers, but also to what the women described as being "monitored from afar".

Expressing that they were being monitored while the health care provider was away suggests that the women felt monitored due to the fact that they were wearing the device. As such, wearing the device became an extended part of the care provided by the birth attendant. Central to perceptions about care is the presence of the provider and by wearing the device the women expressed increased satisfaction with the care received [21]. However, it has been found that women are positive towards any intervention received during ANC or labor, regardless of the efficacy of the intervention [22]. The fact that many expressed that they felt care improved with the use of Moyo could also have to do with possible neglect experienced in the past [23]. Expressed satisfaction with the care received could also be an indication of low expectations, or not knowing what to expect [24,25]. Often, during labor and delivery, women with low socio-economic status in overburdened public facilities are seemingly quite powerless, passive, and poorly informed, and have low expectations about care and information [26,27]. One could also argue that it might be difficult for the women to judge the quality of care without having experienced good care in the past. Several of the women in the study expressed receiving limited information and labor monitoring during previous deliveries, which could be another reason why the perceptions about care were mainly positive. Studies indicate that receiving medicines or items such as bed nets is described by women as good care while not receiving information from health care providers was not associated with poor care [24].

The reported lack of information by some of the participants about the purpose and functions of Moyo seemed to generate misconceptions and an overestimation of the capabilities of the device. The device was considered by some as almost magical in its abilities and some participants believed that Moyo not only detected but also solved problems by helping the baby to breathe or giving the mother the strength to push during delivery. This finding is similar to a qualitative study about the use of ultrasound in antenatal care in Botswana [28]. The women who reported that they were not informed more frequently reported attributions and an overestimation of the capabilities the device. This indicates an unmet need for information about Moyo and draws on models of health literacy and informed consent. These concepts imply that the patient receives and understands information about purpose, limitations, and procedure and the choice to accept or decline prior to a medical procedure [23]. To increase people's health literacy is an international priority as low health literacy is linked to increased morbidity and mortality [29]. Health literacy is also a critical component of empowerment as limited health literacy reduces autonomy in self-care and decision-making [30].

For the women in our study, the use of Moyo seemed to have strengthened their position during the delivery and the device became a tool of empowerment. In low-income settings, women are perceived as having less access to essential resources and less autonomy and decision-making power compared to men according to studies [31]. Each year, roughly a third of maternal deaths worldwide are directly related to inadequate care during pregnancy [32]. Conversely, empowered women have lower infant mortality and better overall health [31,33]. By wearing the device and monitoring the FHR, the women took on a more active role as they themselves were part of the important task of monitoring the progress of their baby. The combined effect of knowing the status of their unborn child and what they perceived as increased attention from the health care providers created a feeling of confidence, particularly among the participants in the study with the lowest socio-economic status. This contribution to the empowerment of the women in the study is an aspect of technology diffusion in low-income settings that we believe should be investigated further.

To measure FHR, many of the women in the current study preferred Moyo compared to the Pinard fetoscope and did not express concern about Moyo being a new device. It is argued that women have more confidence in information produced by technological devices rather than in their own bodily sensations as technology is often associated with experts and valued over local practices and the intervention-free birth which is perceived as "risky" [28,34,35]. This phenomenon is described as Gizmo idolatry, defined as *the willingness to accept, in fact to prefer, unproven, technologically-oriented medical measures* and that machinery is considered more valuable than a "low-tech" approach [36]. This attitude could explain why none of the participants expressed any fears about the potential harm of using the device which was a surprising finding and contrary to previous studies on the use of ultrasound [23,28].

Many of the respondents expressed a sense of relief knowing that their child was doing well when using Moyo. FHRM seemed to be considered a test to find out if everything was okay, compared to a confirmation that it was. This finding is similar to other studies in Sub-Saharan Africa investigating attitudes toward the use of ultrasound during pregnancy [37]. The anxieties of childbirth, particularly pertaining to uncertainties about the wellbeing of the unborn child, had been largely ignored by health providers during previous deliveries. The need for reassurance due to the risks involved in pregnancy and childbirth for mothers in low-resource settings is closely linked to the need for information about the labor progress. The fact that some of the women who said they had not been informed either guessed or asked the health care provider about the purpose of the device also indicates a need for control over the labor process, not solely relying on the expertise of the health care providers. Studies from Tanzania indicate that women during ANC and labor receive inadequate information about the status of the fetus and indications, process, and results of medical interventions [23,38]. However, it is argued that most patients are unable to recall information provided to them [39]. As mentioned by some of the women, labor pain makes it difficult to absorb information and the women would most likely have been more susceptible to retaining information provided at an earlier stage of the labor when they were in less pain.

Strengths and Limitations

Several steps were taken to increase the validity of the study findings and ensure trustworthiness [20,40,41]. In an effort to increase credibility by shedding light on the research question from different angles, participants in the study varied in socio-economic background, occupation and age. As interviews were conducted in Kiswahili and translated to English, there was a risk that meaning might be lost during the translation process. Translations were therefore verified by members of the research team and the findings were validated with new participants after saturation was reached, in an effort to ensure that concepts were accurately captured. During the data collection, analysis codes were shared, discussed, and agreed upon among authors. The research team was multi-professional with both Tanzanian and Norwegian members, which facilitated interpretation of the data from different angles in order to capture diverse perspectives on the findings. Qualitative findings cannot be generalized due to small and demographically non-representative sample size; however, by describing in detail the context and characteristics of the participants in the current study, we allow the reader to make an informed decision about the transferability of study findings to other contexts [41]. While the women in the study seemed at ease during the interview, they might have felt uncomfortable saying anything negative about the care due to fears of repercussions as they were still admitted to the hospital. A suggestion for future studies is therefore to broaden the group of participants and to interview participants outside of the health care facilities. The women in the current study did not report experiencing severe complications during the most recent delivery and often described it as faster or less painful than previous deliveries. Overall, women with uncomplicated deliveries without unexpected levels of pain and duration of the labor report higher levels of satisfaction with care compared to those who do experience complications. This might be one of the reasons the responses were largely positive, both about the device and about the care received [21,42,43].

5. Conclusions

This study provides an understanding of how the use of a new electronic fetal heart rate monitor had a positive effect on the birth experience of the women in our study. This was largely due to an increased knowledge about the wellbeing of the unborn child and a perceived improvement in care. The study highlights the unacknowledged anxiety of childbirth which should be addressed by both health care providers and policy makers. A lack of understanding of the basic functions and purpose of the device raises the issue of informed consent and health literacy and the need to improve how and when information is conveyed to women in labor. We recommend that information about new devices used in the labor ward is included in the information provided to pregnant women during ante natal care and/or provided in the early stages of labor. This information should also include limitations of a technological device to avoid overestimation of the diagnostic power.

Acknowledgments: The authors wish to thank the women who participated in the study as well as staff and administration at the two hospitals where the data was collected. The study was supported by the Laerdal Foundation and the Research Council of Norway through the Global Health and Vaccination Program (GLOBVAC), project number 228203. The founding sponsors had no role in the design of the study; in the collection, analyses, or interpretation of data; in the writing of the manuscript, and in the decision to publish the results.

Author Contributions: Sara Rivenes Lafontan formulated the study design, carried out the data collection and analysis and drafted the paper. Johanne Sundby, Hege L. Ersdal, Columba K. Mbekenga contributed substantially to the design, data collection and analysis and critically revised the paper draft. Muzdalifat Abeid and Hussein L. Kidanto participated substantially in the acquisition of data and in critically revising the paper draft. All authors read and approved the final manuscript.

Conflicts of Interest: The authors declare no conflict of interest. The founding sponsors had no role in the design of the study; in the collection, analyses, or interpretation of data; in the writing of the manuscript, and in the decision to publish the results.

Appendix

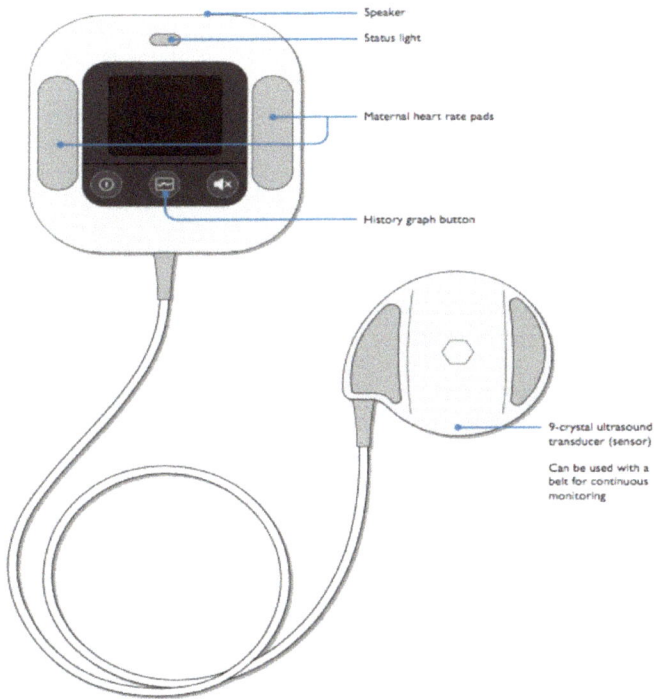

Figure A1. The Fetal Heart Rate (FHR) monitor, Moyo (Laerdal Global Health).

References

1. Wang, H.; Liddell, C.A.; Coates, M.M.; Mooney, M.D.; Levitz, C.E.; Schumacher, A.E.; Apfel, H.; Iannarone, M.; Phillips, B.; Lofgren, K.T.; et al. Global, regional, and national levels of neonatal, infant, and under-5 mortality during 1990–2013: A systematic analysis for the global burden of disease study 2013. *Lancet* **2014**, *384*, 957–979. [CrossRef]
2. Ersdal, H.L.; Mduma, E.; Svensen, E.; Perlman, J. Birth asphyxia: A major cause of early neonatal mortality in a Tanzanian rural hospital. *Pediatrics* **2012**, *129*, e1238–e1243. [CrossRef] [PubMed]
3. Lawn, J.; Shibuya, K.; Stein, C. No cry at birth: Global estimates of intrapartum stillbirths and intrapartum-related neonatal deaths. *Bull. World Health Organ.* **2005**, *83*, 409–417. [PubMed]
4. Lawn, J.E.; Kinney, M.; Lee, A.C.; Chopra, M.; Donnay, F.; Paul, V.K.; Bhutta, Z.A.; Bateman, M.; Darmstadt, G.L. Reducing intrapartum-related deaths and disability: Can the health system deliver? *Int. J. Gynaecol. Obstet.* **2009**, *107* (Suppl. 1), S123–S140. [CrossRef] [PubMed]

5. Cousens, S.; Blencowe, H.; Stanton, C.; Chou, D.; Ahmed, S.; Steinhardt, L.; Creanga, A.A.; Tuncalp, O.; Balsara, Z.P.; Gupta, S.; et al. National, regional, and worldwide estimates of stillbirth rates in 2009 with trends since 1995: A systematic analysis. *Lancet* **2011**, *377*, 1319–1330. [CrossRef]
6. Kumar, S.; Kumar, N.; Vivekadhish, S. Millennium Development Goals (MDGs) to Sustainable Sevelopment Goals (SDGs): Addressing unfinished agenda and strengthening sustainable development and partnership. *Indian J. Community Med.* **2016**, *41*, 1–4. [CrossRef] [PubMed]
7. United Nations Inter-agency Group for Child Mortality. *Levels and Trends in Child Mortality Report 2017*; United Nations International Children's Emergency Fund: New York, NY, USA, 2017.
8. Kidanto, H.L.; Mogren, I.; van Roosmalen, J.; Thomas, A.N.; Massawe, S.N.; Nystrom, L.; Lindmark, G. Introduction of a qualitative perinatal audit at muhimbili national hospital, Dar es Salaam, Tanzania. *BMC Pregnancy Childbirth* **2009**, *9*, 45. [CrossRef] [PubMed]
9. Lewis, D.; Downe, S.; Panel, F.I.F.M.E.C. Figo consensus guidelines on intrapartum fetal monitoring: Intermittent auscultation. *Int. J. Gynaecol. Obstet.* **2015**, *131*, 9–12. [CrossRef] [PubMed]
10. World Health Organization. *World Health Organization Partograph in Management of Labour, World Health Organization Maternal Health and Safe Motherhood Programme*; World Health Organization: Geneva, Switzerland, 1994.
11. Wyatt, J. Appropriate medical technology for perinatal care in low-resource countries. *Ann. Trop. Paediatr.* **2008**, *28*, 243–251. [CrossRef] [PubMed]
12. Wrammert, J.; Clark, R.B.; Ewald, U.; Målqvist, M. Inadequate fetal heart rate monitoring and poor use of partogram associated with intrapartum stillbirth: A case-referent study in Nepal. *BMC Pregnancy Childbirth* **2016**, *16*, 233.
13. Holden, R.J.; Karsh, B.T. The technology acceptance model: Its past and its future in health care. *J. Biomed. Inf.* **2010**, *43*, 159–172. [CrossRef] [PubMed]
14. Moen, K.; Middelthon, A.-L. Qualitative research methods. In *Research in Medical and Biological Sciences: From Planning and Preparation to Grant Application and Publication*; Laake, P., Breien Benestad, H., Reino Olsen, B., Eds.; Academic Press: London, UK, 2015; pp. 321–378.
15. Green, J.; Thorogood, N. *Qualitative Methods for Health Research*, 2nd ed.; SAGE: London, UK, 2009.
16. Rickham, P.P. Human experimentation. Code of ethics of the world medical association, Declaration of Helsinki. *Br. Med. J.* **1964**, *2*, 177. [PubMed]
17. Freedman, L.P.; Graham, W.J.; Brazier, E.; Smith, J.M.; Ensor, T.; Fauveau, V.; Themmen, E.; Currie, S.; Agarwal, K. Practical lessons from global safe motherhood initiatives: Time for a new focus on implementation. *Lancet* **2007**, *370*, 1383–1391. [CrossRef]
18. Schreier, M. *Qualitative Content Analysis in Practice: Margrit Schreier*; SAGE: London, UK, 2012.
19. Graneheim, U.H.; Lindgren, B.M.; Lundman, B. Methodological challenges in qualitative content analysis: A discussion paper. *Nurse Educ. Today* **2017**, *56*, 29–34. [CrossRef] [PubMed]
20. Graneheim, U.H.; Lundman, B. Qualitative content analysis in nursing research: Concepts, procedures and measures to achieve trustworthiness. *Nurse Educ. Today* **2004**, *24*, 105–112. [CrossRef] [PubMed]
21. Tesfaye, R.; Worku, A.; Godana, W.; Lindtjorn, B. Client satisfaction with delivery care service and associated factors in the public health facilities of Gamo Gofa zone, Southwest Ethiopia: In a resource limited setting. *Obstet. Gynecol. Int.* **2016**, *2016*, 5798068. [CrossRef] [PubMed]
22. Mbaruku, G.; Msambichaka, B.; Galea, S.; Rockers, P.C.; Kruk, M.E. Dissatisfaction with traditional birth attendants in rural Tanzania. *Int. J. Gynaecol. Obstet.* **2009**, *107*, 8–11. [CrossRef] [PubMed]
23. Stal, K.B.; Pallangyo, P.; van Elteren, M.; van den Akker, T.; van Roosmalen, J.; Nyamtema, A. Women's perceptions of the quality of emergency obstetric care in a referral hospital in rural Tanzania. *Trop. Med. Int. Health* **2015**, *20*, 934–940. [CrossRef] [PubMed]
24. Kumbani, L.C.; Chirwa, E.; Malata, A.; Odland, J.O.; Bjune, G. Do Malawian women critically assess the quality of care? A qualitative study on women's perceptions of perinatal care at a district hospital in Malawi. *Reprod. Health* **2012**, *9*, 30. [CrossRef] [PubMed]
25. Solnes Miltenburg, A.; Lambermon, F.; Hamelink, C.; Meguid, T. Maternity care and human rights: What do women think? *BMC Int. Health Hum. Rights* **2016**, *16*, 17. [CrossRef] [PubMed]
26. Thaddeus, S.; Maine, D. Too far to walk: Maternal mortality in context. *Soc. Sci. Med.* **1994**, *38*, 1091–1110. [CrossRef]

27. Gabrysch, S.; Campbell, O.M. Still too far to walk: Literature review of the determinants of delivery service use. *BMC Pregnancy Childbirth* **2009**, *9*, 34. [CrossRef] [PubMed]
28. Tautz, S.; Jahn, A.; Molokomme, I.; Gorgen, R. Between fear and relief: How rural pregnant women experience foetal ultrasound in a Botswana district hospital. *Soc. Sci. Med.* **2000**, *50*, 689–701. [CrossRef]
29. Raynor, D.K. Health literacy. *BMJ* **2012**, *344*, e2188. [CrossRef] [PubMed]
30. Osman, H.M.; Egal, J.A.; Kiruja, J.; Osman, F.; Byrskog, U.; Erlandsson, K. Women's experiences of stillbirth in somaliland: A phenomenological description. *Sex Reprod. Health* **2017**, *11*, 107–111. [CrossRef] [PubMed]
31. Lailulo, Y.A.; Susuman, A.S.; Blignaut, R. Correlates of gender characteristics, health and empowerment of women in ethiopia. *BMC Womens Health* **2015**, *15*, 116. [CrossRef] [PubMed]
32. Jennings, L.; Na, M.; Cherewick, M.; Hindin, M.; Mullany, B.; Ahmed, S. Women's empowerment and male involvement in antenatal care: Analyses of demographic and health surveys (DHS) in selected African countries. *BMC Pregnancy Childbirth* **2014**, *14*, 297. [CrossRef] [PubMed]
33. Adhikari, R.; Sawangdee, Y. Influence of women's autonomy on infant mortality in Nepal. *Reprod. Health* **2011**, *8*, 7. [CrossRef] [PubMed]
34. Georges, E. Fetal ultrasound imaging and the production of authoritative knowledge in Greece. *Med. Anthropol. Q.* **1996**, *10*, 157–175. [CrossRef] [PubMed]
35. Newnham, E.C.; McKellar, L.V.; Pincombe, J.I. Documenting risk: A comparison of policy and information pamphlets for using epidural or water in labour. *Women Birth* **2015**, *28*, 221–227. [CrossRef] [PubMed]
36. Leff, B.; Finucane, T.E. Gizmo idolatry. *JAMA* **2008**, *299*, 1830–1832. [CrossRef] [PubMed]
37. Oluoch, D.A.; Mwangome, N.; Kemp, B.; Seale, A.C.; Koech, A.; Papageorghiou, A.T.; Berkley, J.A.; Kennedy, S.H.; Jones, C.O. "You cannot know if it's a baby or not a baby": Uptake, provision and perceptions of antenatal care and routine antenatal ultrasound scanning in rural Kenya. *BMC Pregnancy Childbirth* **2015**, *15*, 127. [CrossRef] [PubMed]
38. Tancred, T.; Schellenberg, J.; Marchant, T. Using mixed methods to evaluate perceived quality of care in Southern Tanzania. *Int. J. Qual. Health Care* **2016**, *28*, 233–239. [CrossRef] [PubMed]
39. Shekelle, P.G.; Wachter, R.M.; Pronovost, P.J.; Schoelles, K.; McDonald, K.M.; Dy, S.M.; Shojania, K.; Reston, J.; Berger, Z.; Johnsen, B.; et al. Making health care safer II: An updated critical analysis of the evidence for patient safety practices. *Evid. Rep. Technol. Assess. (Full Rep.)* **2013**, *211*, 1–945.
40. Maxwell, J.A. *Qualitative Research Design: An Interactive Approach*; SAGE: London, UK, 2013; Volume 41.
41. Dahlgren, L.; Emmelin, M.; Winkvist, A. *Qualitative Methodology for International Public Health*; Umeå International School of Public Health: Umeå, Sweden, 2007.
42. Henriksen, L.; Grimsrud, E.; Schei, B.; Lukasse, M.; Bidens Study, G. Factors related to a negative birth experience–A mixed methods study. *Midwifery* **2017**, *51*, 33–39. [CrossRef] [PubMed]
43. Bitew, K.; Ayichiluhm, M.; Yimam, K. Maternal satisfaction on delivery service and its associated factors among mothers who gave birth in public health facilities of Debre Markos town, northwest Ethiopia. *BioMed Res. Int.* **2015**, *2015*, 460767. [CrossRef] [PubMed]

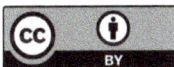

© 2018 by the authors. Licensee MDPI, Basel, Switzerland. This article is an open access article distributed under the terms and conditions of the Creative Commons Attribution (CC BY) license (http://creativecommons.org/licenses/by/4.0/).

International Journal of
*Environmental Research
and Public Health*

MDPI

Article

Adverse Pregnancy Outcomes among Adolescents in Northwest Russia: A Population Registry-Based Study

Anna A. Usynina [1,2,*], Vitaly Postoev [3], Jon Øyvind Odland [1] and Andrej M. Grjibovski [4,5]

[1] Department of Community Medicine, Faculty of Health Sciences, UiT The Arctic University of Norway, 9037 Tromsø, Norway; jon.oyvind.odland@uit.no
[2] Department of Neonatology and Perinatology, Northern State Medical University, 51 Troitsky Ave., Arkhangelsk 163000, Russia
[3] Department of Public Health, Health Care and Social Work, Northern State Medical University, 51 Troitsky Ave., Arkhangelsk 163000, Russia; vipostoev@yandex.ru
[4] Central Scientific Research Laboratory, Northern State Medical University, 51 Troitsky Ave., Arkhangelsk 163000, Russia; andrej.grjibovski@gmail.com
[5] Department of Public Health and Healthcare, Hygiene and Bioethics, North-Eastern Federal University, 58 Belinsky Str., Yakutsk 677000, Russia
* Correspondence: perinat@mail.ru; Tel.: +7-921-245-1078

Received: 14 December 2017; Accepted: 30 January 2018; Published: 3 February 2018

Abstract: This study aimed to assess whether adolescents have an increased risk of adverse pregnancy outcomes (APO) compared to adult women. We used data on 43,327 births from the population-based Arkhangelsk County Birth Registry, Northwest Russia, for 2012–2014. The perinatal outcomes included stillbirth, preterm birth (<37 and <32 weeks), low and very low birthweight, 5 min Apgar score <7 and <4, perinatal infections, and the need for neonatal transfer to a higher-level hospital. Multivariable logistic regression was applied to assess the associations between age and APO. Altogether, 4.7% of deliveries occurred in adolescents. Both folic acid intake and multivitamin intake during pregnancy were more prevalent in adults. Adolescents were more likely to be underweight, to smoke, and to have infections of the kidney and the genital tract compared to adult women. Compared to adults, adolescents were at lower risk of low birthweight, a 5 min Apgar score <7, and need for neonatal transfer. Adolescents had no increased risk of other APO studied in the adjusted analysis, suggesting that a constellation of other factors, but not young age per se, is associated with APO in the study setting.

Keywords: Apgar score; birth registry; low birthweight; preterm birth; Russia; stillbirth; adolescent pregnancy; very low birthweight

1. Introduction

Pregnancy in adolescents continues to be an important public health challenge worldwide. Approximately 11% of all births occur among 15–19-year-olds [1]. In 2014, the global birth rate in 15–19 years old adolescents was 49 per 1000 women [2]. In 2015, women aged 15–19 years gave birth to 229,715 infants in the United States [3]. The adolescent pregnancy rate in the US remains the highest among the western high-income countries and comprises 57 pregnancies per 1000 women aged 15–19 years [4]. In Europe, the pregnancy rates in adolescents aged 18 and less years vary from less than 2.0 per 1000 women aged 15–17 years in Denmark, Netherland, Finland, and Sweden to 35.5 and 29.2 per 1000 in Bulgaria and Romania, respectively [5]. In low-income countries, the adolescent pregnancy rate is several times higher; in Niger, for example, every fifth pregnancy occurs in 15–19-years-old women [6].

Different factors contribute to adverse pregnancy outcomes (APO). Maternal cigarette smoking [7,8], alcohol drinking [9], and drug use [8] during pregnancy increase the risk of stillbirth. Compared to healthy women, pregnant women with infections of the urinary [10,11] and genital tract [12] are at higher risk of preterm birth. Poor antenatal care [13] and maternal infections [14] are associated with early-onset infections in newborns. An antepartum urinary tract infection is an established risk factor of low birthweight (LBW), small for gestational age (GA), and perinatal death among babies born to women aged 20–29 years [11].

Earlier studies have shown that, compared to adult women, pregnant adolescents have a higher prevalence of smoking [15–17] and age-inappropriate education [18]. Young women are more likely to be underweight [15,19,20] and have inadequate antenatal care [15,17,18,20–22]. Mothers aged 16–19 years have a higher prevalence of recreational drug use and smoking compared with women aged 20–24 years [19]. The adolescents are more likely to initiate antenatal care later [22] and to have urinary tract infections [16,23]. Women aged <25 years are less likely to use dietary supplements compared to older women [24].

The results of studies on the associations between maternal age and pregnancy outcomes in young women are controversial. Numerous studies have reported that adolescent pregnancy is associated with preterm birth [17–22,25–27], neonatal mortality [17], combined perinatal and neonatal mortality [27], stillbirth [21], low Apgar score [17,22], LBW or very LBW (VLBW) [17,18,20,22,25], small for GA [18,20] or intrauterine growth restriction [21], as well as neonatal intensive care unit (NICU) admission [22]. Other studies have not found an increased risk for perinatal [15,22] and neonatal [17,20] mortality, as well as small for GA [26,27]. This heterogeneity in the results can be at least partly explained by the use of different definitions of adolescent pregnancy, the study of different age groups, and the use of different variables for adjustment that makes the comparison and interpretation of the results complicated [28], warranting further research.

In Russia, the adolescent pregnancy rates have been decreasing over the last decades. The annual number of births per 1000 women aged 15–19 comprised 55.0, 44.8, 27.4, and 21.5 in 1990, 1995, 2000, and 2016, respectively [29]. Abortions before 12 weeks are free in Russia. In 2014, four percent of the total number of legal abortions were among adolescents aged 15–19 years [30]. Data on the prevalence of illegal abortions in adolescents is not available.

Available data on adolescent pregnancy in Northwest Russia are scarce. Arkhangelsk County is partially located in the Arctic zone of Russia. In 2016, Arkhangelsk County had a total area of 413,100 km^2 and a population exceeding 1.1 million [30]. People aged 15–29 years comprised 284,000 (23.4%) of the population [31]. In 2004, Grjibovski et al. [32] demonstrated that infants born to 15–19-year-olds were lighter at birth and more likely to have LBW compared to babies born to older women. From 2011 to 2013, the prevalence of pelvic inflammatory diseases in 15–17-years-old girls increased by 40%, corresponding to 84.8 per 1000 girls of that age. In 2013, salpingitis and oophoritis were revealed in 1.2% of female adolescents aged 15–17 years. As many as 1.7% of 10–14-years-old girls experienced menstrual cycle disorders [33]. In the Russian Arctic zone, 12.6% of current and former smokers began to smoke before 15 years of age [34]. Women younger than 20 years comprised 12.8% of all women who smoked before or during pregnancy [35].

At present, no study has assessed the perinatal outcomes in adolescent pregnancies in Northwest Russia using large population-based samples. The aim of this study was to assess whether adolescent pregnancy is associated with selected APO in Northwest Russia.

2. Materials and Methods

2.1. Study Population and Design

This study is a retrospective registry-based study with data from the Arkhangelsk County Birth Registry (ACBR), Northwest Russia. A detailed description of the ACBR was published earlier [36]. The ACBR includes data on virtually all live- and stillbirths from 22 weeks of gestation in Arkhangelsk

County from 1 January 2012. The coverage of the ACBR is 99.6%. The identity of information in medical documents, registration forms, as well as in electronic databases was approved by quality controls [36]. The ACBR contains maternal sociodemographic, lifestyle, and behavior information, data about the mother's health before and during the pregnancy in consideration, information about the delivery and the newborn's health. To the date, the ACBR is a systematic data collection in medical documents. Standard paper registration forms are used. The data are collected at delivery units after the birth of the child before his discharge and transfer from the hospital, or before the woman's discharge in stillbirth or the baby's death. Midwives and nurses or other health workers are responsible for data registration. They use both data on antenatal care and data on pregnancy outcomes documented in medical records. No additional interviews with postpartum women are used. All records from paper-based registration forms are then transferred to a depersonified electronic database [36].

For the purpose of this study, we used quality assured data on all live- and stillbirths recorded in the ACBR between 1 January 2012 and 31 December 2014 (*n* = 43,327). The number of births included in the prevalence analyses of each of the studied maternal characteristics varied, as we excluded births with missing information. To perform the prevalence analyses of APO, we excluded multiple births (*n* = 494), births prior to 22 and after 45 completed weeks of gestation (*n* = 1), and births with unknown GA at delivery (*n* = 200). Births with missing information on each of the studied maternal medical and behavior characteristics, as well as potential confounders were excluded from the study population when we performed logistic regression analyses. The number of excluded births varied, as we used several logistic models for each APO when used as the dependent variable.

GA was assessed by obstetricians and recorded in medical documents as well as in the birth registry. The assessment of GA was primarily based on first ultrasound data. In women with missed data of ultrasound examination, the data of the last menstrual period were used. Preterm births were defined as those that occurred before 37 completed weeks [37]. We used the World Health Organization's definition of adolescent pregnancy, that is pregnancy in a woman aged 10–19 years [38]. In this study, we defined the age of the woman as her age at the time of the baby's delivery. Women aged ≥20 years were considered as adults.

2.2. Outcome Variables

We used each of the studied pregnancy outcome (stillbirth, preterm birth <37 weeks, preterm birth <32 weeks, LBW, VLBW, neonatal transfer to higher-level hospital, infections specific to the perinatal period, as well as the 5 min Apgar score less than 7 and 4) as a dichotomous dependent variable. LBW and VLBW were defined as birthweight <2500 g and <1500 g, respectively [37]. We treated the variable "infections specific to the perinatal period" as a dichotomous variable that corresponded to the information on this particular issue recorded by the check-box method in the ACBR registration forms.

2.3. Independent Variables

In this study, the timing of the first antenatal visit, maternal smoking in pregnancy, body mass index (BMI), multivitamin and folic acid intake in pregnancy, evidence of alcohol and drug abuse, as well as infections of the kidney and the genital tract in pregnancy were used as independent variables. The first antenatal visit at 12 and more weeks of gestation was defined as late antenatal visit. Maternal education was classified as none or primary [class 1–9], secondary [class 10–11], vocational school, and higher. We calculated the BMI by dividing the weight (kg) by the height squared (m^2). The maternal BMI at the first antenatal visit were categorized into three groups: underweight (BMI < 18.5 kg/m^2), normal weight (BMI = 18.5–24.9 kg/m^2) (reference group), and overweight and obese (BMI ≥ 25.0 kg/m^2) [39]. The mothers were categorized as smokers and nonsmokers according to their smoking status during pregnancy. Evidence of maternal alcohol abuse in pregnancy was recorded as "no" or "yes". The same was done for the variable "evidence of maternal drug abuse in pregnancy". Nonsmokers and those who had no evidence of either alcohol or drug abuse served as reference groups. "Infections of kidney in pregnancy" and "Infections of the genital tract in pregnancy" were recorded as "no" or "yes". We used information on International Statistical Classification of Diseases and Related Health Problems 10th revision (ICD-10) codes O23.0 and O23.5 in the ACBR for "Infections of kidney in pregnancy" and "Infections of the genital tract in pregnancy", respectively. In registration forms, information on ICD-10 codes O23.0 and O23.5 was recorded by the check-box method. We categorized parity as primipara (reference group) and para.

2.4. Data Analysis

Chi-squared tests were employed to compare the distribution of the selected medical and behavior characteristics between adolescents and adult women. Multivariable logistic regression was applied to assess independent associations between adolescent age and the outcomes adjusted for potential confounders. As all studied APO are rare, odds ratios (ORs) were used as proxy estimates for relative risks. In multivariable analyses, we adjusted for maternal education, smoking, BMI, year of delivery, multivitamin and folic acid intake, infections of the kidney and the genital tract in pregnancy, and timing of the first antenatal visit. Associations between maternal age and LBW and between maternal age and VLBW were also adjusted for preterm birth. The statistical analyses were performed using IBM SPSS Statistics for Macintosh, Version 24.0. (IBM Corp, Armonk, NY, USA).

2.5. Ethics Approval

The Ethical Committee of the Northern State Medical University (Arkhangelsk, Russia) approved this study (Protocol 01/02-17). The ethical approval was also obtained from the Regional Committee for Medical and Health Research Ethics in Northern Norway (2013/2300/REK Nord).

3. Results

Out of a total of 43,327 births, 2033 (4.7%) were from adolescents.

3.1. Prevalence of Medical and Behavior Characteristics in Adolescents and Adult Women

Compared with adults, adolescents were more likely to be underweight, primipara, to smoke, to have infections of the kidney and the genital tract, and less likely to take folic acid and multivitamins during pregnancy (Table 1). Young women were 2.4 times as likely as adults to initiate antenatal care after 12 weeks of gestation. There were no significant differences between the groups in the prevalence of alcohol or drug abuse.

Table 1. Bivariate analyses of maternal medical and behavior characteristics, according to mothers' age, the ACBR, Russia, 2012–2014.

Maternal Characteristics	*n* Without Missing Information	Adolescents *n* (%)	Adult Women *n* (%)	*p*-Value *
Late antenatal visit	42,855	614 (30.7)	5148 (12.6)	<0.001
BMI, kg/m^2	42,751			<0.001
<18.5		219 (11.0)	2604 (6.4)	
18.5–24.9		1465 (73.3)	25,985 (63.8)	
≥25		314 (15.7)	12,164 (29.8)	
Smoking	39,888	604 (31.6)	5875 (15.5)	<0.001
Evidence of alcohol abuse	43,318	7 (0.3)	171 (0.4)	0.631
Evidence of drug abuse	43,320	0 (0.0)	14 (0.0)	0.406
Folic acid intake	43,191	866 (42.9)	22,117 (53.7)	<0.001
Multivitamin intake	43,192	961 (47.6)	22,332 (54.2)	<0.001
Infections of kidney in pregnancy [1]	43,327	762 (37.5)	13,980 (33.9)	0.001
Infections of the genital tract in pregnancy [2]	43,327	495 (24.3)	6600 (16.0)	<0.001
Parity (para)	39,249	160 (8.9)	21,553 (57.6)	<0.001

ACBR: Arkhangelsk County Birth Registry; *n*: number; BMI: body mass index. * *p* for chi-squared tests.
[1] ICD-10 code O23.0; [2] ICD-10 code O23.5.

3.2. Prevalence of Pregnancy Outcomes in Adolescent and Adult Women

Compared to infants born to adult women, the infants of adolescents were more likely to have LBW and required more frequent transfer to a higher-level hospital (Table 2). We did not find differences in the proportions of other studied APO between the groups of adolescents and adults.

Table 2. Bivariate analyses of adverse pregnancy outcomes, according to mothers' age, the ACBR, Russia, 2012–2014.

Perinatal Outcomes	n Without Missing Information	Adolescents n (%)	Adult Women n (%)	p-Value *
Stillbirth	42,757	18 (0.9%)	279 (0.7%)	0.278
Preterm birth (<37 weeks)	42,633	23 (1.1%)	530 (1.3%)	0.540
Preterm birth (<32 weeks)	42,633	140 (7.0%)	2452 (6.0%)	0.085
Neonatal transfer to a higher-level hospital	42,831	227 (11.2%)	4012 (9.8%)	0.042
Low birthweight	42,824	133 (6.6%)	2158 (5.8%)	0.012
Very low birthweight	42,824	18 (0.9%)	413 (1.0%)	0.589
Perinatal infections in infants	42,833	5 (0.2%)	43 (0.1%)	0.063
The 5 min Apgar score <7	42,425	36 (1.8%)	778 (1.9%)	0.694
The 5 min Apgar score <4	42,425	14 (0.7%)	232 (0.6%)	0.467

ACBR: Arkhangelsk County Birth Registry; *n*: number. * *p* for chi-squared tests.

3.3. Association between Maternal Age and APO

Only the variables that were significantly associated with outcomes in the bivariate analyses (Table 2) were included in the multivariable models (Table 3). In the bivariate analysis, the risk of neonatal transfer to a higher-level hospital was 16% higher in adolescents compared to adult women (Table 3). The young maternal age was associated with an increased risk of LBW. After adjusting for confounding factors, we found associations between young maternal age and decreased risk of neonatal transfer, LBW, and a 5 min Apgar score <7.

Table 3. The crude and adjusted odds ratios for adverse pregnancy outcomes in adolescents, the ACBR, Russia, 2012–2014.

Perinatal Outcomes	n (n₁)	Unadjusted ORs	95% CI	Adjusted * ORs	95% CI
Stillbirth	35,066 (232)	1.30	0.81, 2.10	0.88	0.49, 1.58
Preterm birth (<37 weeks)	35,110 (2095)	1.17	0.98, 1.39	0.94	0.76, 1.17
Preterm birth (<32 weeks)	35,110 (438)	0.88	0.58, 1.34	0.66	0.39, 1.11
Neonatal transfer to a higher-level hospital	35,110 (3412)	1.16	1.01, 1.34	0.81	0.68, 0.96
Low birthweight	35,104 (1872)	1.26	1.05, 1.51	0.72 **	0.55, 0.95
Very low birthweight	35,104 (348)	0.88	0.55, 1.41	0.58 **	0.30, 1.09
Perinatal infections in infants	35,224 (40)	2.35	0.93, 5.93	3.05	0.92, 10.12
The 5 min Apgar score <7	34,799 (640)	0.94	0.67, 1.31	0.55	0.37, 0.84
The 5 min Apgar score <4	34,799 (184)	1.22	0.71, 2.10	0.64	0.33, 1.27

ACBR: Arkhangelsk County Birth Registry; *n*: number of births included in the final regression model; *n₁*: number of studied outcomes in the final regression model; ORs: odds ratio; CI: confidence intervals. * Adjusted for maternal body mass index, education, smoking, year of delivery, multivitamin and folic acid intake, infections of the kidney and the genital tract in pregnancy, timing of the first antenatal visit, parity; ** Adjusted for all variables and potential confounders listed above and preterm birth (<37 weeks of gestation).

4. Discussion

Adolescents had no increased risk of any studied APO. After adjustment for potential confounders, adolescents' infants were less likely to have LBW, a 5 min Apgar score <7, and to need neonatal transfer compared to babies of adult women.

4.1. Prevalence of Maternal Medical and Behavior Characteristics and Birth Outcomes

In this population-based study, 4.7% of births occurred to women younger than 20 years old. Lewis et al. [16] demonstrated that 11% of births in Western Australia were to young women aged 12–18 years. Chen et al. [17] also showed a higher prevalence of births (8.75%) in women <20 years in the United States. The increase of the quality of individual contraceptive counseling and contraceptive knowledge in Russian youth [40] could partly explain our findings on birth prevalence among adolescents. After 1995, the Government of the Russia reduced the benefits to young families, which could also contribute to a postponed parenthood. The postponement of the first birth was attributed to the absence of supportive family policies and economic uncertainty [41].

In our study, the use of 25–29 as a control group was not possible because of the low number of APO that caused a failure of the models to converge. Lewis et al. [16] also treated adults as a whole group to compare pregnancy outcomes between adolescents and adult women. Shrim et al. (2011) [27] compared APO between adolescents and 20–39-years-old women.

Our finding that adolescents were more likely to initiate antenatal care late compared to adult women is supported by the literature [22]. However, direct comparisons of studies are complicated, as the definition of appropriate antenatal care varies. Some studies, like the current one, register GA at the first antenatal visit [25,42] or the number of visits during pregnancy [22,43], while others use more complicated characteristics of antenatal care adequacy that include both the timing and the number of antenatal visits [17,18,20,21] and the infant's birthweight [15]. The combination of several approaches in one study [22,42] as well as unspecified variables such as "regular visits" [44] have also been reported. Minjares-Granillo et al. (2016) [42] demonstrated a two-week difference in the timing of the first antenatal visit between adolescents and other women, but the results were not statistically significant. Irrespectively of the definition of antenatal care adequacy, the researches mostly demonstrate less adequate care in adolescents compared with adult women [15,17,18,20–22,43,44]. In contrast, de Vienne et al. (2009) [45] reported no difference between younger and older women in the studied age groups among 14–30-year-olds.

In our study, the adolescents were more likely to be underweight as well as less likely to be overweight. Earlier studies have consistently shown a higher prevalence of underweight adolescents compared with young adults [15,19]. The prevalence of overweight among adolescents was half of that observed in adults. Torvie et al. (2009) [20] also reported that adolescents had a lower prevalence of overweight compared with women aged 20–24 years.

In our study, twice as many adolescents were smokers compared with adults. We treated adolescents as a whole group, and our findings are consistent with those of the previously published studies of Salihu et al. [15] and Lewis et al. [16]. Chen et al. [17] and Torvie et al. [20], who categorized adolescents in several age groups, specified that the youngest mothers (10–15 and 11–14 years in Chen et al. [17] and Torvie et al. [20], respectively) had a lower prevalence of smoking compared to "older adolescents". In our study, 3439 (8%) births had no data on smoking, but the proportions of adolescents among those with missing and recorded information on smoking was only 3.5% and 4.8%, respectively.

We did not find any difference in the prevalence of alcohol abuse between adolescents and adult women. This is consistent with other researchers' results [15,17,19,42]. Salas-Wright et al. (2015) [46] reported that, compared to their non-pregnant counterparts, pregnant adolescents in the United States were 1.4 and 1.7 times more likely to use alcohol and to have alcohol use disorders, respectively.

In our study, there were no adolescents with recorded drug abuse. Kawakita et al. (2016) [19] specified that older adolescents (aged 15–19 years) are 1.5 times more likely to be addicted to drugs compared to adults. Salas-Wright et al. (2015) [46] showed that the rate of use of any substances in pregnant adolescents remained 60% higher than in non-pregnant adolescents after adjusting for other studied characteristics, and that young adolescents (12–14 years old) had even a higher rate of substance use compared to older adolescents aged 15–17 years. We did not compare pregnant and non-pregnant adolescents in this study. The ACBR contains information only about pregnant women. Moreover, the information is based on medical records which in turn contains information collected in part as self-reports.

We found a significantly lower prevalence of folic acid and multivitamin intake in pregnant adolescents compared with adults. These results are consistent with those reported by Branum et al. (2013) [24] who demonstrated a 2.5 times lower prevalence of supplement use among pregnant women aged <25 years compared with older women. Kirbas et al. (2016) [22] reported a lower prevalence of both preconception and prenatal folic acid supplementation in adolescents compared with healthy pregnant women aged 20–34 years. However, two previous studies did not reveal a significant difference in folic acid intake between pregnant adolescents and adults [42,47]. The proportion of missing data was relatively small: 135 (0.3%) and 136 (0.3%) births with missing data on multivitamin and folic acid supplementation, respectively. Compared to adults, the proportion of adolescents was higher among those with missing data for both folic acid (9.4%) and multivitamin (9.6%) intake. Because of the small total number of missing data in these two variables, the final results were unlikely to be affected.

Our finding of a high prevalence of kidney infections in pregnant adolescents (37.5% vs. 33.9% in adults) is consistent with other studies. Vettore et al. (2013) [23] reported that among pregnant women with urinary tract infections the proportion of women aged <20 years (28.4%) was 40% higher than that of women without this health problem. Lewis et al. (2009) [16] also demonstrated that mothers aged 17–18 years experienced a 2.6 times greater risk of urinary tract infection compared to adults. Salihu et al. (2011) [15] reported that the prevalence of renal diseases during the second pregnancy in women aged 10–19 years was higher compared to 20–24-year-olds. The researchers did not specify the variable they used, so we could only suspect that they supposed kidney infections too.

We found that the prevalence of genital tract infections in adolescents was 50% higher than in adult women. Carter et al. (2011) [48] demonstrated a twice as high proportion of mothers aged <20 years among those who had genital tract infections compared with healthy women. Similarly, the proportions of adolescents (<20 years) with and without genital tract infections among women who gave birth to infants with birth defects were 19.2% and 9.5%, respectively. Chokephaibulkit et al. (1997) [49] demonstrated that 11.2% of pregnant women aged <19 years were infected with *Chlamydia trachomatis*. In contrast to our study, the authors did not investigate older age women. At the same time, we had no information on specific infections to compare our data with those cited above. In our study, the data on both the genital tract and kidney infections were based on medical records that may have a lower risk of misclassification and underreporting compared with self-reports. Since the prevalence of kidney and genital tract infections in our study is relatively high, we are not able to exclude an overdiagnosis in the ACBR records. Carter et al. [48] indicated that, in their study, some mothers might have misreported genital tract infections as urinary tract infections and, in addition, declared only symptomatic diseases, which could lead to a lower prevalence of reported infections.

In the prevalence analyses of APO, we found that, compared to adult women, only neonatal transfer to a higher-level hospital and LBW were significantly higher in adolescents' infants. Our results are consistent with those of previous studies. Chen et al. (2007) [17] and Torvie et al. (2015) [20] demonstrated that the rate of LBW consistently increased with the decreasing mothers' age and was the highest among babies born to women aged <15 years. Fayed et al. (2017) [44] demonstrated similar results. Malabarey et al. (2012) [21] also reported a 1.5 times significant difference in LBW proportions between those aged younger than 15 years and those aged 15 years and older. Lewis et al. (2009) [16] found a significant difference in LBW prevalence among adolescents and adult women (24% and 19%, respectively) but did not confirm the difference in the NICU admission prevalence between the studied groups. In addition, the abovementioned study did not show a difference in the prevalence of either NICU admission or LBW between 12–16 and 17–18-year-olds. Shrim et al. (2011) [27] reported a twice as high prevalence of NICU admission in infants born to mothers aged <20 years compared with those born to 20–39-year-olds. As we did not specify how many babies transferred from the delivery units to a higher-level hospital were admitted directly to an NICU, we only could speculate that the proportion of those admitted to an NICU might be higher in adolescents' newborns compared with older mothers' babies. In Arkhangelsk County, most severe ill newborns are transported to the NICU at the high-level Regional Children Hospital. Babies with more stable health conditions can be transported to the Pediatric Departments of this or other hospitals. Information about the exact Department where the newborns were transported is partly available in the ACBR.

Although some studies have reported a higher prevalence of stillbirth [16], LBW [50] and VLBW [17], preterm birth <37 [17,19,44] and <32 weeks [17] of gestation, as well as low 5 min Apgar score [16,17,28] in adolescents compared to adult women, we did not identify significant differences of these birth outcomes between the studied age groups. Contrary to studies of other authors, we have not found any difference among adolescents and adult women in APO.

4.2. Risk of APO

We have found that the risk of the most studied APO was similar in adolescents and adult women. In this study, adolescents were at a lower risk of LBW, the 5 min Apgar score <7, and need for neonatal transfer compared with adults. The association of adolescence with APO continues to be a subject of controversy. Our findings are in line with the results of other researchers who have demonstrated no association of maternal young age and stillbirth [15,26,28], VLBW [19], preterm birth [45], or preterm birth at GA < 28 weeks [19]. In our study, the risk of LBW was lower in adolescents compared to adults, which is in contrast with earlier studies [19,45]. Previous studies have not found an increased risk of admission to an NICU [45], or a low Apgar score [19,26,28] in infants born to adolescent women compared to adult women's babies. In our study, we have found a decreased risk of the 5 min Apgar score <7 and of the need for neonatal transfer in adolescents compared to adults. We have not found an increased risk of perinatal infections in infants, consistent with the results of Kawakita et al. (2016) [19] who reported that the young maternal age treated in age groups was not associated with neonatal pneumonia, sepsis, and meningitis.

We suggest that early and late adolescence might entail different risks for APO. The stratification by maternal age and the assessment of risk for APO in age groups demonstrate reliable relationships between maternal age and perinatal outcomes. As seen in other studies, the youngest mothers had a higher risk of LBW [25,43,51], preterm birth [19,25,26], stillbirth [45], and low Apgar score [43] compared to older adolescents. Socioeconomic disadvantages for the adolescents are more likely in early age. In this study, we treated adolescents without age grouping, which should be done in the future studies.

In contrast with the findings of Fraser et al. (1995) [18], some studies [42,51,52] have demonstrated that the socioeconomic status has an impact on the relationship between maternal age and APO. We did not include any economic variables in the multivariable regression models studying the risk of adolescent pregnancy outcomes, because of the limitations of the ACBR database. However, we demonstrated a higher prevalence of smoking, underweight, and late onset of antenatal care in adolescents compared to adults (Table 1). We have found that the inclusion of smoking, underweight, late onset of antenatal care, education, and other potential confounders in all logistic models attenuated the odds of all studied APO, except for perinatal infections in the infants (Table 3). The adjusted odds became significant for LBW, the 5 min Apgar score <7, and the need for neonatal transfer, suggesting confounding effects of the sociodemographic factors.

4.3. Strength and Limitations

The strength of this study is a large and validated database. Since the ACBR covers 99.6% of all births that took place in Arkhangelsk County in 2012–2014 [36], the results of our study can be generalized to the entire population of adolescents in Northwest Russia. In addition, the regions in Northwest Russia are similar in their population structure.

In the ACBR, data on smoking, alcohol, and drug abuse during pregnancy were collected from medical records. This attenuates the risk of an under-report bias, but is not able to completely exclude an information bias, as the medical records contain information originally based in part on self-reports. In our study, the proportion of missing information in all studied variables was the smallest in adolescent mothers (data not shown), which could be considered as an advantage. It is likely that the exclusion of the births with missing data on all studied variables did not affect the present study results because of the large sample size.

The finding of a high prevalence of smoking as well as of kidney and genital tract infections in pregnant adolescents compared to the adults could be considered as one additional advantage for health care providers' and government efforts aimed at the discovery of the risk population.

We did not include data on maternal reproductive history, pre-pregnancy diseases, and complications of pregnancy as potential confounders in the logistic regression analyses, which may be considered as a limitation of this study. However, we adjusted our models for those confounders referring to the association of young maternal age and APO.

5. Conclusions

In this study, adolescents gave birth to 4.7% of all infants recorded in the ACBR in 2012–2014. Compared to adults, women aged ≤19 years were more likely to be underweight, to smoke, to miss folic acid and multivitamin intake, and to have kidney and genital tract infections. We did not identify an increased risk of the studied APO in adolescents compared to adults and suppose that factors apart from young maternal age contribute more to APO. We found a lower risk of LBW, the 5 min Apgar score <7, and the need for neonatal transfer in adolescents' infants. The results of this study may be useful in generating and implementing prevention and intervention strategies in Northwest Russia. Our findings may be also a benefit for doctors and midwives planning their work when dealing with pregnant adolescents. Particular efforts should be undertaken in order to increase the multivitamin and folic acid supplementation rate in pregnant adolescents as well as to provide more effective measures to prevent genital tract infections and promote a healthy life style in adolescents.

Acknowledgments: We acknowledge the staff of the Medical Analytical and Informational Centre, Arkhangelsk, Russia for providing the data for this study.

Author Contributions: Anna A. Usynina, Vitaly Postoev, and Jon Øyvind Odland conceived the idea of the study; all authors contributed to the design; Vitaly Postoev analyzed the data; Anna A. Usynina and Vitaly Postoev wrote the paper; Anna A. Usynina, Vitaly Postoev, and Andrej M. Grjibovski contributed to the discussion of the results; Jon Øyvind Odland and Andrej M. Grjibovski supervised the study.

Conflicts of Interest: The authors declare no conflict of interest.

References

1. WHO. *Early Marriages, Adolescent and Young Pregnancies. A 65/13*; WHO: Geneva, Switzerland, 2012.
2. WHO. Adolescent Pregnancy. Available online: http://www.who.int/mediacentre/factsheets/fs364/en/ (accessed on 28 November 2017).
3. Martin, J.A.; Hamilton, B.E.; Osterman, M.J.K.; Driscoll, A.K.; Mathews, T.J. *Births: Final Data for 2015*; National Vital Statistics Report; National Center for Health Statistics: Hyattsville, MD, USA, 2017; p. 70.
4. Sedgh, G.; Finer, L.B.; Bankole, A.; Eilers, M.A.; Singh, S. Adolescent Pregnancy, Birth, and Abortion Rates across Countries: Levels and Recent Trends. *J. Adolesc. Health* **2015**, *56*, 223–230. [CrossRef] [PubMed]
5. Office for National Statistics. Available online: https://www.ons.gov.uk/ (accessed on 29 November 2017).
6. WHO; UNICEF. *Accountability for Maternal, Newborn and Child Health. The 2013 Update*; WHO: Geneva, Switzerland, 2013; Available online: http://www.who.int/woman_child_accountability/ierg/reports/Countdown_Accountability_2013Report.pdf (accessed on 26 November 2017).

7. Bjørnholt, S.M.; Leite, M.; Albieri, V.; Kjaer, S.K.; Jensen, A. Maternal smoking during pregnancy and risk of stillbirth: Results from a nationwide Danish register-based cohort study. *Acta Obstet. Gynecol. Scand.* **2016**, *95*, 1305–1312. [CrossRef] [PubMed]

8. Varner, M.W.; Silver, R.M.; Hogue, C.J.R.; Willinger, M.; Parker, C.B.; Thorsten, V.R.; Goldenberg, R.L.; Saade, G.R.; Dudley, D.J.; Coustan, D.; et al. Association Between Stillbirth and Illicit Drug Use and Smoking During Pregnancy. *Obstet. Gynecol.* **2014**, *123*, 113–125. [CrossRef] [PubMed]

9. Cornman-homonoff, J.; Kuehn, D.; Aros, S.; Carter, T.C.; Conley, M.R.; Troendle, J.; Cassorla, F.; Mills, J.L. Heavy prenatal alcohol exposure and risk of stillbirth and preterm delivery. *J. Mater.-Fetal Neonatal Med.* **2012**, *25*, 860–863. [CrossRef]

10. Mazor-Dray, E.; Levy, A.; Schlaeffer, F.; Sheiner, E. Maternal urinary tract infection: Is it independently associated with adverse pregnancy outcome? *J. Mater.-Fetal Neonatal Med.* **2009**, *22*, 124–128. [CrossRef]

11. Schieve, L.A.; Handler, A.; Hershow, R.; Persky, V.; Davis, F. Urinary tract infection during pregnancy: Its association with maternal morbidity and perinatal outcome. *Am. J. Public Health* **1994**, *84*, 405–410. [CrossRef] [PubMed]

12. Hosny, A.E.-D.M.S.; El-khayat, W.; Kashef, M.T.; Fakhry, M.N. Association between preterm labor and genitourinary tract infections caused by Trichomonas vaginalis, Mycoplasma hominis, Gram-negative bacilli, and coryneforms. *J. Chin. Med. Assoc.* **2017**, *80*, 575–581. [CrossRef] [PubMed]

13. Mizumoto, B.R.; Moreira, B.M.; Santoro-Lopes, G.; Cunha, A.J.; dos Santos, R.M.R.; Pessoa-Silva, C.L.; Pinheiro, A.A.N.; Ferreira, M.; Leobons, M.B.; Hofer, C.B. Quality of antenatal care as a risk factor for early onset neonatal infections in Rio de Janeiro, Brazil. *Braz. J. Infect. Dis.* **2015**, *19*, 272–277. [CrossRef] [PubMed]

14. Chan, G.J.; Lee, A.C.C.; Baqui, A.H.; Tan, J.; Black, R.E. Risk of Early-Onset Neonatal Infection with Maternal Infection or Colonization: A Global Systematic Review and Meta-Analysis. *PLoS Med.* **2013**, *10*, e1001502. [CrossRef] [PubMed]

15. Salihu, H.M.; Duan, J.; Nabukera, S.K.; Mbah, A.K.; Alio, A.P. Younger maternal age (at initiation of childbearing) and recurrent perinatal mortality. *Eur. J. Obstet. Gynecol. Reprod. Biol.* **2011**, *154*, 31–36. [CrossRef] [PubMed]

16. Lewis, L.N.; Hickey, M.; Doherty, D.A.; Skinner, S.R. How do pregnancy outcomes differ in teenage mothers? A Western Australian study. *Med. J. Aust.* **2009**, *190*, 537–541. [PubMed]

17. Chen, X.K.; Wen, S.W.; Fleming, N.; Demissie, K.; Rhoads, G.G.; Walker, M. Teenage pregnancy and adverse birth outcomes: A large population based retrospective cohort study. *Int. J. Epidemiol.* **2007**, *36*, 368–373. [CrossRef] [PubMed]

18. Fraser, A.M.; Brockert, J.E.; Ward, R.H. Association of young maternal age with adverse reproductive outcomes. *N. Engl. J. Med.* **1995**, *332*, 1113–1117. [CrossRef] [PubMed]

19. Kawakita, T.; Wilson, K.; Grantz, K.L.; Landy, H.J.; Huang, C.C.; Gomez-Lobo, V. Adverse Maternal and Neonatal Outcomes in Adolescent Pregnancy. *J. Pediatr. Adolesc. Gynecol.* **2016**, *29*, 130–136. [CrossRef] [PubMed]

20. Torvie, A.J.; Callegari, L.S.; Schiff, M.A.; Debiec, K.E. Labor and delivery outcomes among young adolescents. *Am. J. Obstet. Gynecol.* **2015**, *213*. [CrossRef]

21. Malabarey, O.T.; Balayla, J.; Klam, S.L.; Shrim, A.; Abenhaim, H.A. Pregnancies in young adolescent mothers: A population-based study on 37 million births. *J. Pediatr. Adolesc. Gynecol.* **2012**, *25*, 98–102. [CrossRef] [PubMed]

22. Kirbas, A.; Gulerman, H.C.; Daglar, K. Pregnancy in Adolescence: Is It an Obstetrical Risk? *J. Pediatr. Adolesc. Gynecol.* **2016**, *29*, 367–371. [CrossRef] [PubMed]

23. Vettore, M.V.; Dias, M.; Vettore, M.V.; Leal, M.D.C. Avaliação do manejo da infecção urinária no pré-natal em gestantes do Sistema Único de Saúde no município do Rio de Janeiro. *Rev. Bras. Epidemiol.* **2013**, *16*, 338–351. [CrossRef] [PubMed]

24. Branum, A.M.; Bailey, R.; Singer, B.J. Dietary Supplement Use and Folate Status during Pregnancy in the United States. *J. Nutr.* **2013**, *143*, 486–492. [CrossRef] [PubMed]

25. DuPlessis, H.M.; Bell, R.; Richards, T. Adolescent pregnancy: Understanding the impact of age and race on outcomes. *J. Adolesc. Health* **1997**, *20*, 187–197. [CrossRef]

26. Tyrberg, R.B.; Blomberg, M.; Kjølhede, P. Deliveries among teenage women—With emphasis on incidence and mode of delivery: A Swedish national survey from 1973 to 2010. *BMC Preg. Child.* **2013**, *13*, 204. [CrossRef] [PubMed]

27. Shrim, A.; Ates, S.; Mallozzi, A.; Brown, R.; Ponette, V.; Levin, I.; Shehata, F.; Almog, B. Is young maternal age really a risk factor for adverse pregnancy outcome in a canadian tertiary referral hospital? *J. Pediatr. Adolesc. Gynecol.* **2011**, *24*, 218–222. [CrossRef] [PubMed]

28. Blomberg, M.; Tyrberg, R.B.; Kjølhede, P. Impact of maternal age on obstetric and neonatal outcome with emphasis on primiparous adolescents and older women: A Swedish Medical Birth Register Study. *BMJ Open* **2014**, *4*, e005840. [CrossRef] [PubMed]

29. Filippov, O.S.; Tokova, Z.Z.; Gata, A.S.; Kuzemin, A.A.; Gudimova, V.V. Abortion: Special statistics in the federal districts of Russian Federation. *Gynecology* **2016**, *18*, 92–96. (In Russian)

30. Bugakova, N.S.; Gelvanovsky, M.I.; Glisin, F.F.; Goryacheva, I.P.; Gokhberg, L.M.; Zghitkov, V.B.; Klimanova, V.V.; Kuznetsova, O.V.; Skatershikova, E.E.; Strukova, V.E.; et al. *Russian Regions. Socioecomomic Indicators*; Rosstat: Moscow, Russia, 2016; p. 1326. (In Russian)

31. UNICEF. *Rosstat Youth in Russia*; UNICEF: Moscow, Russia, 2010; p. 166. (In Russian)

32. Grjibovski, A.M.; Bygren, L.O.; Svartbo, B.; Magnus, P. Social variations in fetal growth in a Russian setting: An analysis of medical records. *Ann. Epidemiol.* **2003**, *13*, 599–605. [CrossRef]

33. Ministry of Health of Arkhangelsk County. Available online: https://www.minzdrav29.ru/ministry/Open_data/ (accessed on 28 November 2017).

34. Rosstart. Available online: http://www.gks.ru/free_doc/new_site/KOUZ16/index.html (accessed on 28 November 2017).

35. Kharkova, O.A.; Krettek, A.; Grjibovski, A.M.; Nieboer, E.; Odland, J.Ø. Prevalence of smoking before and during pregnancy and changes in this habit during pregnancy in Northwest Russia: A Murmansk county birth registry study. *Reprod. Health* **2016**, *13*, 18. [CrossRef] [PubMed]

36. Usynina, A.A.; Odland, I.O.; Pylaeva, Z.A.; Pastbina, I.M.; Grjibovski, A.M. Arkhangelsk County Birth Registry as an important source of information for research and healthcare. *Ekol. Cheloveka [Hum. Ecol.]* **2017**, *2*, 58–64. (In Russian)

37. WHO. *International Statistical Classification of Diseases and Related Health Problems (ICD-10) 10th Revision*, 4th ed.; WHO: Geneva, Switzerland, 2011; Volume 2.

38. WHO. *Adolescent Pregnancy. Issues in Adolescent Health and Development*; WHO: Geneva, Switzerland, 2004.

39. WHO. *Expert Committee on Physical Status: The Use and Interpretation of Anthropometry: Report of a WHO Expert Committee*; WHO: Geneva, Switzerland, 1995.

40. Larivaara, M.M. Pregnancy prevention, reproductive health risk and morality: A perspective from public-sector women's clinics in St. Petersburg, Russia. *Crit. Public Health* **2010**, *20*, 357–371.

41. Mills, M.; Rindfuss, R.R.; McDonald, P.; te Velde, E. Why do people postpone parenthood? Reasons and social policy incentives. *Hum. Reprod. Update* **2011**, *17*, 848–860. [CrossRef] [PubMed]

42. Minjares-Granillo, R.O.; Reza-Lopez, S.A.; Caballero-Valdez, S.; Levario-Carrillo, M.; Chavez-Corral, D.V. Maternal and Perinatal Outcomes among Adolescents and Mature Women: A Hospital-Based Study in the North of Mexico. *J. Pediatr. Adolesc. Gynecol.* **2016**, *29*, 304–311. [CrossRef] [PubMed]

43. Vieira, C.L.; Coeli, C.M.; Pinheiro, R.S.; Brandao, E.R.; Camargo, K.R., Jr.; Aguiar, F.P. Modifying effect of prenatal care on the association between young maternal age and adverse birth outcomes. *J. Pediatr. Adolesc. Gynecol.* **2012**, *25*, 185–189. [CrossRef]

44. Fayed, A.A.; Wahabi, H.; Mamdouh, H.; Kotb, R.; Esmaeil, S. Demographic profile and pregnancy outcomes of adolescents and older mothers in Saudi Arabia: Analysis from Riyadh Mother (RAHMA) and Baby cohort study. *BMJ Open* **2017**, *7*, e016501. [CrossRef] [PubMed]

45. De Vienne, C.M.; Creveuil, C.; Dreyfus, M. Does young maternal age increase the risk of adverse obstetric, fetal and neonatal outcomes: A cohort study. *Eur. J. Obstet. Gynecol. Reprod. Biol.* **2009**, *147*, 151–156. [CrossRef] [PubMed]

46. Salas-Wright, C.P.; Vaughn, M.G.; Ugalde, J.; Todic, J. Substance use and teen pregnancy in the United States: Evidence from the NSDUH 2002–2012. *Addict. Behav.* **2015**, *45*, 218–225. [CrossRef] [PubMed]

47. Linhares, A.O.; Juraci, A.C. Folic acid supplementation among pregnant women in southern brazil: Prevalence and factors associated. *Ciência Saúde Coletiva* **2017**, *22*, 535–542. [CrossRef]

48. Carter, T.C.; Olney, R.S.; Mitchell, A.A.; Romitti, P.A.; Bell, E.M.; Druschel, C.M. Maternal self-reported genital tract infections during pregnancy and the risk of selected birth defects. *Birth Defects Res. Part A Clin. Mol. Teratol.* **2011**, *91*, 108–116. [CrossRef] [PubMed]

Int. J. Environ. Res. Public Health **2018**, *15*, 261

49. Chokephaibulkit, K.; Patamasucon, P.; List, M.; Moore, B.; Rodriguez, H. Genital *Chlamydia trachomatis* Infection in Pregnant Adolescents in East Tennessee: A 7-Year Case-Control Study. *J. Pediatr. Adolesc. Gynecol.* **1997**, *10*, 95–100. [CrossRef]

50. Katz Eriksen, J.L.; Melamed, A.; Clapp, M.A.; Little, S.E.; Zera, C. Cesarean Delivery in Adolescents. *J. Pediatr. Adolesc. Gynecol.* **2016**, *29*, 443–447. [CrossRef] [PubMed]

51. Reichman, N.E.; Pagnini, D.L. Maternal age and birth outcomes: Data from New Jersey. *Fam. Plann. Perspect.* **1997**, *29*, 268–272, 295. [CrossRef]

52. Ganchimeg, T.; Ota, E.; Morisaki, N.; Laopaiboon, M.; Lumbiganon, P.; Zhang, J.; Yamdamsuren, B.; Temmerman, M.; Say, L.; Tuncalp, O.; et al. Pregnancy and childbirth outcomes among adolescent mothers: A World Health Organization multicountry study. *BJOG* **2014**, *121* (Suppl. 1), 40–48. [CrossRef]

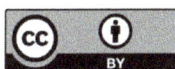

© 2018 by the authors. Licensee MDPI, Basel, Switzerland. This article is an open access article distributed under the terms and conditions of the Creative Commons Attribution (CC BY) license (http://creativecommons.org/licenses/by/4.0/).

International Journal of
*Environmental Research
and Public Health*

MDPI

Article

Factors Associated with Pregnancy among Married Adolescents in Nepal: Secondary Analysis of the National Demographic and Health Surveys from 2001 to 2011

Rina Pradhan *, Karen Wynter and Jane Fisher

Jean Hailes Research Unit, School of Public Health and Preventive Medicine, Monash University,
Melbourne 3800, Australia; Karen.Wynter@monash.edu (K.W.); Jane.Fisher@monash.edu (J.F.)
* Correspondence: Rina.Pradhan@monash.edu

Received: 12 December 2017; Accepted: 23 January 2018; Published: 30 January 2018

Abstract: Pregnancy-related morbidity and mortality are much more prevalent among adolescents than adults, particularly in low-income settings. Little is known about risk factors for pregnancy among adolescents in Nepal, but setting-specific evidence is needed to inform interventions. This study aimed to describe the prevalence, and identify factors associated with pregnancy among adolescents in Nepal between 2001 and 2011. Secondary analyses of Nepal Demographic Health Surveys (NDHS) data from 2001, 2006, and 2011 were completed. The outcome was any pregnancy or birth among married adolescents; prevalence was calculated for each survey year. Although the rate of marriage among adolescent women in Nepal decreased significantly from 2001 to 2011, prevalence of pregnancy and birth among married adolescent women in Nepal remains high (average 56%) in Nepal, and increased significantly between 2001 and 2011. Regression analyses of this outcome indicate higher risk was associated with living in the least resourced region, early sexual debut, and older husband. Despite national efforts to reduce pregnancies among married adolescent women in Nepal, prevalence remains high. Integrated, cross-sectoral prevention efforts are required. Poverty reduction and infrastructure improvements may lead to lower rates of adolescent pregnancy.

Keywords: adolescent pregnancy; risk factors; protective factors; low- and lower-middle income countries

1. Introduction

Pregnancy among adolescent women is associated with high risks to both the mother and her child. Pregnancy-related deaths are twice as common among women aged 15–19 years, than women aged in their twenties [1,2]. Pregnancies during adolescence are also associated with adverse maternal outcomes, including obstructed labour, nutritional anaemia, preterm birth, postpartum infections, unsafe abortion [3], and adverse child outcomes, including infant mortality, foetal growth retardation, and low birth weight [2–5]. Although births to adolescents occur globally, approximately 95% of these births occur in low-income countries. Due to this burden of morbidity and mortality, adolescent pregnancy is recognized as a public health priority.

Global initiatives, in particular the Declaration of the Millennium Development Goals (MDG) in 2000, have focused on decreasing maternal mortality through improving access to antenatal care and health facilities for women to give birth with support from skilled birth attendants [6]. One of the essential MDG indicators for improving maternal health was a reduction in births to adolescents by 2015. Despite this effort, there is still a high prevalence of adolescent births in low-income countries. About one in five adolescent women have a live birth before the age of 18; these young women are mainly from South Asia and sub-Saharan Africa. This suggests that these initiatives might not be recognizing or addressing the determinants of adolescent pregnancy in these settings.

To date, initiatives in low-income countries have generally been based in the health sector, and focused on improved care for adolescents who are pregnant. Kotelchuck [7] proposes that interventions are more likely to be effective if they take a comprehensive life course approach, in which preventive efforts begin from puberty, continue during secondary schooling, and include improved health care during and after pregnancy, in particular, in the most disadvantaged communities, in order to reduce morbidity and prevent mortality [6].

In Nepal, adolescents comprise 23% of the population, and early pregnancy remains very common [8]. Recognizing the gravity of the problem, the Nepal Government developed Adolescent Sexual Reproductive Health (ASRH) Policy in 2000. Programs initiated under this policy have focused on increasing the availability of and access to "adolescent friendly" sexual and reproductive health services, and health information to reduce the incidence of early marriage and childbearing. Currently, the government has extended "adolescent friendly" health services to 732 health facilities in 49 of 75 districts [9]. The government is implementing, monitoring, and scaling up the "adolescent friendly" reproductive health services and health information program at the national level, in partnership with national and international non-governmental organizations [9].

Adolescent pregnancy is not, however, associated only with lack of access to health services. A systematic review of studies from low and lower-middle income countries [10] found that the risk of adolescent pregnancy was also increased by wider socio-demographic and cultural factors, including limited education, low socioeconomic position, insufficient access to and non-use of contraception, early sexual initiation, and belonging to an ethnic and religious minority group. In order to assess the patterns and prevalence of adolescent pregnancy and to target interventions effectively, each country requires comprehensive, specific data about local risk and protective factors. On this basis, evidence-informed programs can be designed to prevent or reduce pregnancy and motherhood among adolescent women, and to manage consequences when pregnancy occurs.

The aim of this study was to identify factors assessed in Nepal Demographic Health Surveys that are associated with pregnancies or births among married adolescents in Nepal.

2. Methods

Secondary analysis of data from the Nepal Demographic Health Surveys (NDHS) in 2001, 2006, and 2011. In this study, the descriptor "adolescent women" is used to refer to married women aged 15–19 years, and "adolescent pregnancy" to pregnancies and births among women aged 15–19 years.

2.1. Ethics

For the NDHS surveys, ethics approval was obtained from the Nepal Health Research Council, Kathmandu, Nepal, and ICF Macro Institutional Review Board, Maryland, USA. Informed consent was obtained prior to the structured face-to-face interview [8,11,12]. For this secondary analysis, ethics approval was obtained from the Monash University Human Research Ethics Committee (reference number CF13/910-2013000428).

2.2. Data Source

The NDHS data are collected every five years by the Nepal Government Ministry of Health and Population [8]. The standard Demographic Health Survey (DHS) questionnaire, modified for country-specific needs, was used [8,11,12]. One of the purposes of the NDHS is to provide current and reliable information on reproductive health both for the country as a whole, and for urban and rural areas separately.

2.3. Procedure

In these surveys, data are collected in a two-stage stratified process: by selecting households first from the ecological divisions of the country, and then, within these, by rural and urban areas [8,11,12].

As most of the population live in rural areas, oversampling of households in urban areas is undertaken to provide estimates with acceptable levels of statistical precision [8,11,12].

Data are collected by trained staff in household-based structured individual interviews with women and men aged 15 to 49 years. All female participants are asked to provide information about their socio-demographic characteristics, marriage, pregnancy history, use of family planning, fertility preferences, antenatal, birth, and postnatal care, child immunization, nutrition, and knowledge on human immunodeficiency virus (HIV) status. For those who are married, data on their husband's socio-demographic characteristics are also collected.

Data for this study were extracted from the NDHS 2001, 2006, and 2011 surveys (http://www.measuredhs.com). The recruitment rate for each of these surveys was at least 98%. Permission was obtained to use these data for further analysis from MEASURE DHS, which is the monitoring and evaluation body of the DHSs globally.

2.4. Study Variables

The outcome variable for the analysis was any pregnancy or birth among married adolescent women. Women were asked their "age at first birth" (in years) and whether they were "currently pregnant", with response options "no or unsure" or "yes". A woman was considered to have had an adolescent pregnancy if her first pregnancy or birth was at any age up to 19 years, or if she was pregnant at the time of the survey, and aged up to 19 years. The analysis was limited to data from married women aged 15–19, because only married women were included in the 2001 survey, even though both married and unmarried women participated in the 2006 and 2011 surveys. The data were weighted to adjust for the stratified cluster sampling design.

Factors which were identified in prior studies as being associated with adolescent pregnancy in lower income settings were selected for this study, providing that the corresponding variables had been collected in all the three waves of the NDHS. Socio-demographic characteristics included women's highest level of education attained, religion, ethnicity, place of residence (urban/rural), ecological region (mountains, hills or Terai (plain land)), developmental region (Eastern, Central, Western, Mid-Western, Far-Western), and occupation. Household wealth quintile was used as an indicator of a woman's socioeconomic position. The DHS wealth quintile is a composite indicator which is derived using principal component analysis based on information about housing characteristics and ownership of household durable goods. Households are classified in five categories based on the wealth quintile: poorest, poorer, middle, richer, and richest. Other variables included the woman's age at first sexual intercourse, and her husband's age, education, and occupation.

Although lack of access to and non-use of modern contraceptives are established risk factors for adolescent pregnancy [13–17], contraceptive use and intention could not be assessed for this study, because the NDHS only assessed current use of contraceptives. It was not possible to determine whether contraception had been used by the young women before pregnancy, or only after having a child. Exposure and access to various forms of media has also been found to be a risk factor for adolescent pregnancy [18], but could not be assessed in this study, as significant amounts of data were missing in the 2001 dataset.

To ensure groups of sufficient sizes, for meaningful analyses, some variables were recoded. There is considerable diversity in the population in Nepal, with over 125 different castes/ethnic groups and 92 languages [19,20]. Ethnicity was recoded to 5 categories from 60 different response options (2001), 90 different response options (2006), and 10 different response options (2011). These categories were used as they are consistent with the Main Nepal Caste and Ethnic Groups with Regional Divisions and Social Groups used in the 2001 Census in Nepal [21]: Brahaman/Chhetri, Terai/Madhesi, Janajati, Dalits and Other.

About 81% of the Nepali population is Hindu, 9% Buddhist, 4% Muslim, 3% Kirat, 1% Christian, and 0.76% other religions [22]. Based on these data, the five response options offered for religion were recoded into four: Hindu, Buddhist, Muslim, and Other.

Respondent's and husband's highest level of education attained were recoded from four to three categories: "no education", "primary", and "secondary or higher education". Respondent's occupation at the time of the survey or in the previous 12 months was recoded from seven to four categories: "agricultural work", "professional work", "not working", and "manual work". In the Nepali context, the term "working" usually refers to income-generating work, and unpaid household or caregiving work is not conceptualised or named as "work". Therefore, "not working" in this context is assumed to mean not having a paid job. Husband's occupation was recoded similarly, except "don't know" was retained as a category; it is not clear whether married adolescent women selected "don't know" as a response to this question, because they did not know whether their husband was working or because their husband was unemployed.

2.5. Statistical Anaysis

The prevalence of adolescent pregnancy was calculated for each survey. Univariate comparisons were conducted to identify possible associations between the relevant socio-demographic and reproductive health factors, and the outcome variable: any adolescent pregnancy. For continuous variables, *t*-tests were conducted, if the variable was normally distributed; if not, non-parametric Mann–Whitney tests were used to test for differences between the two groups (no adolescent pregnancy versus any adolescent pregnancy). Pearson's Chi-squared analysis was used to test for associations between categorical variables and the outcome variable.

To identify a broad range of explanatory variables that might be associated with pregnancy among married adolescent variables, a less restrictive *p*-value of 0.1 was used as cut-off in univariate analysis [23]. Therefore, all variables with *p* values less than 0.1 in univariate analysis were included in a logistic regression model. In addition, some variables which did not meet these statistical significance criteria, but were expected to be associated with married adolescent pregnancy based on existing studies in similar settings, were also included in the logistic regression model. Odds ratios and 95% confidence intervals were calculated. Statistical significance was set at $p < 0.05$ when considering the multivariate model. IBM SPSS Statistics version 20 (Armonk, NY, USA) was used for the data analysis.

3. Results

Data from a total of 2524 married women aged 15–19 from the three NDHS datasets were included in analyses (Table 1).

Table 1. Number of married adolescent women from National Demographic and Household Survey; data from 2001, 2006 and 2011.

Participant Numbers	Year of the Survey			Total
	2001	2006	2011	
Total women participants	8726	10,793	12,674	32,193
Total adolescent women participants	2335	2437	2790	7562
Total married women adolescent women participants	940 (40%)	787 (32%)	797 (29%)	2524

3.1. Characteristics of Married Adolescent Women

The socio-demographic characteristics of the participants are shown in Table 2. In all three surveys, most of the married adolescent women were living in rural areas, and more than half in the Terai ecological zone. A higher proportion lived in the Central region compared with all other regions in all three surveys. In 2006 and 2011, more than half of married adolescent women were educated at least to primary school level. In all three surveys, most of them followed the Hindu religion, and a higher proportion belonged to the Janajati ethnic group compared with other ethnic groups. A smaller proportion of married adolescents were classified as belonging to households in the "richest" wealth quintile, compared to all other wealth quintiles.

In all three surveys, more married adolescent women worked in the agricultural sector or were "not working" than were engaged in non-agricultural income-generating work. The mean age at first sexual intercourse among married adolescent women was almost 16 years. The mean age of the husbands of these married adolescents was 22 years. Amongst the husbands, a higher proportion had secondary or higher education than primary, or no formal education in all three surveys, and in 2001 and 2006, a higher proportion of husbands were involved in agricultural work than in other occupations.

Table 2. Socio-demographic characteristics of married adolescent women and their husbands for each study year.

Socio-Demographic Characteristics of Married Adolescent Women	Year of the Survey					
	2001		2006		2011	
	%	N	%	N	%	N
Residential location						
Urban	5.5 [a]	52	10.9 [b]	86	7.5 [a]	60
Rural	94.5 [a]	889	89.1 [b]	701	92.5 [a]	738
Ecological zone						
Mountain	6.7 [a]	63	9.1 [a]	72	7.4 [a]	59
Hill	38.5 [a]	362	35.8 [a]	282	35.4 [a]	282
Terai (plain land)	54.8 [a]	516	55 [a]	433	57.2 [a]	456
Developmental region						
Central	34.2 [a]	322	29.4 [b]	231	34.1 [a]	272
Eastern	21 [a]	198	20.9 [a]	164	21.9 [a]	175
Western	18.8 [a]	177	20.1 [a]	158	19.4 [a]	155
Mid-Western	15.6 [a]	147	15 [a]	118	14.9 [a]	119
Far-Western	10.3 [a]	97	14.5 [b]	114	9.6 [a]	77
Education						
No education	52.2 [a]	491	37 [b]	291	23.1 [c]	184
Primary	26 [a]	245	30.2 [a]	238	26.2 [a]	209
Secondary or Higher	21.7 [a]	204	32.8 [b]	258	50.7 [c]	404
Religion						
Hindu	86.8 [a]	817	86.4 [a]	680	84.7 [a]	676
Buddhist	6 [a]	56	6.4 [a]	50	7.3 [a]	58
Muslim	5.4 [a]	51	6.4 [a]	50	5.9 [a]	47
Other	1.8 [a,b]	17	0.9 [b]	7	2.1 [a]	17
Ethnicity						
Brahaman/Chhetri	25.9 [a]	244	25.6 [a]	202	23.5 [a]	187
* Terai/Madhesi Castes	19.7 [a]	185	14.1 [b]	111	12.7 [b]	101
Dalit	20.5 [a]	193	18.4 [a]	145	25.3 [b]	202
Janajati	28.2 [a]	265	32.2 [a]	254	32.1 [a]	256
Other	5.7 [a]	54	9.6 [b]	76	6.4 [a]	51
Occupation						
Professional work	2.3 [a]	22	1.9 [a]	15	1.3 [b]	42
Not working	28.2 [a]	265	27.7 [a]	218	36.7 [b]	293
Agricultural work	67.7 [a]	636	67.2 [a]	529	54.2 [b]	433
Manual work	1.8 [a]	17	3.2 [a,b]	25	3.8 [b]	30
Wealth Quintile						
Poorest	23.6 [a]	222	19.3 [b]	152	20.2 [a,b]	161
Poor	21.3 [a]	200	23 [a]	181	23.9 [a]	191
Middle	22.5 [a]	212	26.6 [a,b]	209	29.3 [b]	234
Richer	21.5 [a]	202	19.4 [a]	153	18.4 [a]	147
Richest	11.2 [a]	105	11.7 [a]	92	8.1 [b]	65
Respondent's age at first intercourse (mean (SD))	15.67 [a]	1.44	15.80 [b]	1.6	15.82 [b]	2.27

Table 2. Cont.

Socio-Demographic Characteristics of Married Adolescent Women	Year of the Survey					
	2001		2006		2011	
	%	N	%	N	%	N
Married adolescent women's husbands						
Husband's age (mean (SD))	22.00 [a]	4.05	21.91 [a]	3.44	22.71 [b]	4.07
Husbands Education						
No education	24.3 [a]	228	14.7 [b]	116	15.4 [b]	123
Primary	28.0 [a]	263	30.1 [a]	237	23.8 [b]	190
Secondary or Higher	47.8 [a]	449	55.1 [b]	434	60.8 [c]	485
Husband's Occupation						
Don't know	3.3 [a]	29	3.1 [b]	24	3.2 [a]	25
Professional work	24.7 [a]	220	31.4 [b]	246	38.0 [c]	294
Agricultural work	43.4 [a]	386	35.8 [b]	281	24.8 [c]	192
Manual work	28.7 [a]	255	29.7 [a,b]	233	33.9 [b]	262

* The term "Terai" is used to describe both an ecological region and an ethnic group. An ethnic group originally from the Terai region is also classified as the Terai/Madhesi group. "[a]","[b]","[c]" Within each response category, superscript letters denote significant differences between data collection years.

3.2. Changes in the Socio-Demographic Characteristics of Married Adolescent Women and Their Husbands across Time

There was a significant decrease in the proportion of married adolescent women living in rural areas from 2001 to 2006, and then a significant increase to 2011 (Table 2). A significantly higher proportion of women lived in the Far-Western developmental region, and a significantly lower proportion in the Central developmental region in 2006, compared to 2001 and 2011. There was a significant decrease in the proportion of married adolescent women who had no formal education over the years from 2001 to 2006, and from 2006 to 2011. More than half of married adolescent women were educated to secondary or higher levels in 2011, which reflected a significant increase from 2001. There was also a significant increase in the proportion of husbands with secondary or higher education from 2001 to 2006, and again from 2006 to 2011.

There was a significant decrease in the proportion of married adolescents in the poorest wealth quintile from 2001 to 2006, and a significant increase in the proportion of married adolescents in the middle wealth quintile from 2001 to 2006. There was also a significant decrease in the proportion of married adolescent women reporting their occupation as agricultural work from 2006 to 2011, and an increase in the proportion reporting their occupation as manual work and "not working" from 2001 to 2011. There was a significant decrease in the proportion of married adolescents' husbands working in agricultural jobs from 2001 to 2006, and from 2006 to 2011; a significant increase in proportion of husbands in manual work from 2001 to 2011; and a significant increase in proportion of husbands reported as being in professional work from 2001 to 2006, and again from 2006 to 2011. These findings reflect changes which occurred in standards of living in married adolescent women and their husbands over the decade 2001–2011.

Married adolescent women's mean age at first intercourse, and husbands' age, appeared to be stable over the decade. There was no change in the proportion of married adolescent women within ecological zones and religious groups across the three surveys.

3.3. Prevalence of Pregnancy or Birth among Married Adolescent Women

The prevalence of pregnancy among married adolescent women was calculated for each survey year, and found to be 53% in 2001, 57% in 2006, and 58% in 2011. Although the proportion of adolescent women who were married decreased significantly from 2001 to 2011 (Table 1), in all three surveys, more than half of the married adolescent women in the sample had a child or were pregnant.

The prevalence of adolescent pregnancy or birth among married adolescents increased significantly from 2001 to 2006, but from 2006 to 2011, there was little change.

The following variables were found to be significantly associated with adolescent pregnancy in at least one of the three survey years: place of residence (urban or rural), ecological zone, developmental region, ethnicity, religion, occupation, wealth quintile, participant's age at first intercourse, and husband's age. Respondent's and husband's highest level of education and husband's occupation were not significantly associated with adolescent pregnancy in any of the survey years. However, respondent's and husband's highest level of education were included in the multivariate model, based on evidence from other studies in similar settings.

Place of residence (urban or rural), ecological zone, and developmental region were highly associated with each other. Developmental region was chosen for inclusion in the multivariate model as an indicator of place of residence, as it was most consistently associated with the outcome variable in all three surveys. There was also a strong association between ethnicity and religion, which occurred because "Muslim" describes an ethnic group (included in the "Other" ethnicity category), but also describes a specific religion. Almost all respondents indicated that they were Hindu; the other three response categories for religion included only a few respondents. The respondents were more broadly distributed in terms of ethnicity; thus, this variable was selected for inclusion in the multivariate model.

The final logistic regression model is shown in Table 4. Year of survey was included, because of the significant changes in distribution of demographic characteristics, as shown in Table 2.

Table 3. Logistic regression of factors associated with pregnancy among married adolescent women.

Variables	Proportion of Married Adolescents Who Reported Pregnancy or Birth (%)	Adjusted OR	95% Confidence Interval		*p*-Value
			Lower	Upper	
Developmental Region					
Central (ref)	53.9				
Eastern	64.7	1.59	1.25	2.02	<0.001
Western	53.6	1.04	0.81	1.33	0.78
Mid-Western	55.6	1.28	0.96	1.71	0.09
Far-Western	49.3	1.04	0.76	1.42	0.82
Education					
Secondary or Higher (ref)	54.8				
Primary	57.7	1.09	0.86	1.38	0.49
No education	55.5	1.05	0.81	1.35	0.71
Ethnicity					
Brahaman/Chhetri (ref)	53.6				
Terai/Madhesi Castes	50.5	1.00	0.73	1.37	0.99
Dalit	57.9	1.24	0.94	1.62	0.12
Janajati	59.0	1.49	1.16	1.90	0.001
Other (minority)	60.3	1.29	0.85	1.95	0.24
Occupation					
Professional work (ref)	61.5				
Not working	57.8	0.87	0.51	1.48	0.61
Agriculture work	53.8	0.78	0.47	1.31	0.35
Manual work	72.2	1.69	0.79	3.62	0.17
Wealth Quintile					
Richest (ref)	61.1	0.98	0.55	1.71	0.95
Richer	59.1	0.94	0.68	1.32	0.74
Middle	54.6	0.79	0.56	1.10	0.16
Poor	53	0.80	0.57	1.14	0.22
Poorest	54.7	0.84	0.58	1.21	0.35

Table 4. Logistic regression of factors associated with pregnancy among married adolescent women.

Variables	Proportion of Married Adolescents Who Reported Pregnancy or Birth (%)	Adjusted OR	95% Confidence Interval		*p*-Value
			Lower	Upper	
Respondent's age of first intercourse (mean, SD)					
Adolescent pregnancy	15.52 (1.41)	0.68	0.64	0.73	<0.001
No pregnancy	16.06 (2.15)				
Husband's age (mean, SD)					
Adolescent pregnancy	22.66 (3.76)	1.10	1.08	1.13	<0.001
No pregnancy	21.39 (3.73)				
Husband's Education					
Secondary or Higher (ref)	55.2				
Primary	57	1.01	0.81	1.25	0.95
No education	55.9	0.87	0.67	1.13	0.29
Year of survey					
Year 2001 (ref)	53.2				
Year 2006	57.3	1.24	1.01	1.53	0.041
Year 2011	57.6	1.28	1.028	1.60	0.028

Ref: Reference category.

Only four variables were significantly and independently associated with adolescent pregnancy when other factors were controlled. Higher risk of adolescent pregnancy was associated with living in the Eastern developmental region compared to the Central region. Those living in the Eastern region were 1.6 times more likely to experience adolescent pregnancy or birth as those living in the Central region. Women who experienced sexual intercourse at an older age were significantly less likely to have experienced an adolescent pregnancy. Women who had an older husband were at increased odds of adolescent pregnancy. Pregnancy rates among married adolescents were significantly higher in 2006 and 2011, than in 2001.

4. Discussion

The most striking finding in this study is that the prevalence of pregnancy and childbirth among married adolescent women was significantly higher in the two most recent surveys, than the earliest survey years. Nepal experienced economic deterioration with political instability during the "Maoist insurgency", which lasted from 1996 to 2006. Much of the country's infrastructure was destroyed, and the country's reconstruction and recovery efforts are ongoing, however, these are not distributed evenly, and are incomplete. Vulnerable groups, including adolescents, experience the impacts of resource constraints, but have little power or autonomy to influence or improve their socioeconomic situations. Nevertheless, the Nepali government has implemented policies and programs, which have been supplemented by initiatives from the non-government sector and international donors, to improve access to adolescent friendly health services [9], to increase girls' access to education, and to improve compliance with laws about the minimum legal age for marriage of 18 years. The impact of these efforts could be seen in the steady decline in adolescent marriage rates from 2001 onwards (Table 1). However, the mean prevalence of 56% indicates that pregnancy among married adolescents in Nepal remains common, with its associated risks to the life and health of the mother and her child [24–26].

The strengths of this study include that it used data from nationally representative samples of households included in the Nepal Demographic Health Surveys, which provide specific information for defined health indicators. Sampling, recruitment, and data collection procedures were similar for all three surveys. Selection bias was minimised by a rigorous sampling strategy. Data from all three surveys were collected in structured individual interviews administered in local languages, which enable people with low literacy, or who are unfamiliar with self-report questionnaires, to participate. The only variation among the surveys was that in 2001, data were collected only from married women, whereas both married and unmarried women were included in the 2006 and 2011 surveys. Overall, however, the data are regarded as high-quality indicators of the socio-demographic characteristics and self-reported health status of the population of Nepal.

A limitation of using NDHS data was that inclusion in analyses of two potentially important explanatory factors (use of contraception and exposure to the media) was not possible, because of the way in which the questions had been asked. Despite these, the data provide valuable evidence about the prevalence and factors associated with pregnancy and birth among married adolescent women in Nepal.

A ten-year time frame is considered quite short to identify substantial changes in national health indicators, so testing for significant interactions between the year of survey and socio-demographic characteristics might not be an accurate indicator of change. However, year of survey was included as a predictor in the logistic regression model, and made a significant, independent contribution when controlling for other variables.

The World Health Organization's Social Determinants of Health Framework (SDH) Viner, et al. [27] emphasizes the need to understand personal, family, community, and structural or national factors, in order to address health inequalities. The risk factors for adolescent pregnancy identified in this study fit the multilevel, SDH Framework [27]. Living in the least developed region where there is generally low access to basic needs, including education, transport, health facilities, and income-generating work, and where women experience restrictive gender-based roles and responsibilities, and minority ethnic groups can be marginalized, was associated with the highest rates of adolescent pregnancy, and indicates that the major risk is structural. This is consistent with Choe, et al. [28] finding a decade ago that adolescent pregnancy and birth were most common in the least developed rural areas than in the urban areas of Nepal. Similarly, adolescent women living in rural areas were at higher risk of having a baby than those in urban areas in Ethiopia and Nicaragua [18,29].

Even though univariate analyses revealed individual risk factors associated with pregnancy among adolescents; when other factors were adjusted for in multivariable analyses, these were no longer statistically significant. Factors such as the socioeconomic status and education level of individuals were outweighed by the overall development status of the region. Nevertheless, the associations found here and the evidence from other resource-constrained countries, that lack of or low education and low socioeconomic position increase risk for adolescent pregnancy [10,13,14,18,29], suggest that these remain relevant.

The risk associated with younger age at first sexual intercourse identified in this study can be interpreted as operating at both individual and family/community levels of the SDH Framework [27]. Generally, in Nepal, it is socially unacceptable to be sexually active before marriage. Despite laws which specify the minimum legal age for marriage as 18 with parental consent, and 20 without parental consent, early marriage is widely accepted in Nepali society [30]. It leads to early sexual debut, and, because of lack of knowledge about and access to contraception, increases the likelihood of early pregnancy. This finding is consistent with evidence from Kenya, which documented the association between early sexual debut and adolescent childbearing [16]. Choe, et al. [28] also concluded from a survey in 2000 that early marriage and sexual debut were associated with higher risk of adolescent pregnancy in Nepal. Adhikari, et al. [31] concluded that young age of marriage is one of the important risk factors for unintended pregnancy in Nepal.

Age disparities, in which the husband is older than the young woman (in these data, around seven years), also increased risk of pregnancy. Greater age differences between husbands are commonly associated with greater inequalities in power, and this may mean women lack autonomy to implement their own preferences regarding number and timing of children. Oshiro, et al. [32] reported an association between early marriage and intimate partner violence in Nepal, but data about gender-based violence were only collected in the NDHS 2011. It is likely, however, that when young women are married (probably by family arrangement) to older men, they are less able to make decisions about their reproductive lives.

5. Conclusions

The findings confirm that the prevalence of pregnancy and birth among married adolescent women remains high in Nepal. When other factors were controlled for, the rate of pregnancy among married adolescents increased from 2001 to 2011. The high prevalence of adolescent pregnancy suggests that while increasing access to adolescent friendly reproductive health services might have had benefits for the health of women once pregnant, it has done little to reduce adolescent pregnancy. The major original finding of this study is that it is structural, rather than individual or community level factors, that are most strongly associated with the outcome. This suggests that integrated, cross-sectoral prevention efforts are required. The problem remains most prevalent in the least resourced region, which indicates that poverty reduction, increased access to education and income-generating work, and improved infrastructure, might lead to lower rates of adolescent pregnancy. However, as specified in the Sustainable Development Goals, gender equality and gender empowerment are essential to ensuring that these strategies are designed and implemented in ways that benefit girls and women. These data indicate that in addition to overall structural changes, it will be essential to continue to address the rights of girls to equality of participation in secondary and post-secondary education, with pathways to income-generating work. Education is required for families about the benefits to health, life-expectancy, and economic productivity of enabling young women to delay marriage and child-bearing beyond adolescence. Access to education about fertility and reproductive health for young people and their families, and to contraception for young women and men, remain essential. In addition to the evidence generated by the NDHS surveys, there is a need for evidence from young women's and other stakeholders' perspectives on the cultural and social factors that maintain early marriage and adolescent pregnancy, to inform and increase the effectiveness of national and local strategies.

Acknowledgments: The authors are very grateful to Rosa Gualano for her meticulous review of early drafts of the manuscript.

Author Contributions: Rina Pradhan conceptualized the study and wrote the first draft of the manuscript. Rina Pradhan, Karen Wynter and Jane Fisher contributed to analysis and interpretation. All authors contributed to revisions and read and approved the final manuscript.

Conflicts of Interest: The authors declare no conflict of interest.

Funding: Rina Pradhan was funded by an Australian Award Research Higher Degree Scholarship and Jane Fisher by a Monash University Professorial Fellowship and the Jean Hailes Professorial Fellowship.

Abbreviations

MDG	Millennium Development Goals
ASRH	Adolescent Sexual Reproductive Health
NDHS	Nepal Demographic Health Surveys
DHS	Demographic Health Survey
HIV	Human Immunodeficiency Virus
SDH	Social Determinants of Health Framework

References

1. Paton, D. Exploring the evidence on strategies to reduce teenage pregnancy rates. *Nurs. Times* **2009**, *105*, 22–25. [PubMed]
2. World Health Organization (WHO). *Adolescent Pregnancy: Unmet Needs and Undone Deeds. A Review of the Literature and Programmes*; World Health Organization: Geneva, Switzerland, 2007.
3. World Health Organization (WHO). *Safe and Unsafe Induced Abortion: Global and Regional Levels in 2008, and Trends during 1995–2008*; World Health Organization: Geneva, Switzerland, 2012.
4. Raj, A. When the mother is a child: The impact of child marriage on the health and human rights of girls. *Arch. Dis. Child.* **2010**, *95*, 931–935. [CrossRef] [PubMed]

5.	The United Nations Children's Fund (UNICEF). Progress for Children. Protecting against Abuse, Exploitation and Violence. Child Marriage. Available online: http://www.unicef.org/progressforchildren/2007n6/index_41848.htm (accessed on 13 February 2013).
6.	United Nations. *The Millennium Development Goals Report 2014*; United Nations: New York, NY, USA, 2014.
7.	Kotelchuck, M. Editorial: Building on a life-course perspective in maternal and child health. *Matern. Child Health J.* **2003**, *7*, 5–11. [CrossRef] [PubMed]
8.	Ministry of Health; New ERA; ICF International. *Nepal Demographic and Health Survey (NDHS)*; Ministry of Health; New ERA: Kathmandu, Nepal; ICF International: Calverton, MA, USA, 2011.
9.	Department of Health Services. *Annual Report: Department of Health Services, 2011/2012*; Ministry of Health and Population, Government of Nepal: Kathmandu, Nepal, 2013.
10.	Pradhan, R.; Wynter, K.; Fisher, J. Factors associated with pregnancy among adolescents in low-income and lower middle-income countries: A systematic review. *J. Epidemiol. Community Health* **2015**, *69*, 918–924. [CrossRef] [PubMed]
11.	Ministry of Health; New ERA; ORC Macro. *Nepal Demographic and Health Survey 2001*; Ministry of Health; New ERA: Kathmandu, Nepal; ORC Macro: Calverton, MA, USA, 2001.
12.	Ministry of Health; New ERA; ORC Macro. *Nepal Demographic and Health Survey Report, (NDHS Report)*; Ministry of Health; New ERA: Kathmandu, Nepal; ORC Macro: Calverton, MA, USA, 2006.
13.	Okonofua, F.E. Factors associated with adolescent pregnancy in rural Nigeria. *J. Youth Adolesc.* **1995**, *24*, 419–438. [CrossRef] [PubMed]
14.	Goonewardene, I.M.; Waduge, R.P.D. Adverse effects of teenage pregnancy. *Ceylon Med. J.* **2005**, *50*, 116–120. [CrossRef] [PubMed]
15.	Amoran, O.E. A comparative analysis of predictors of teenage pregnancy and its prevention in a rural town in Western Nigeria. *Int. J. Equity Health* **2012**, *11*, 1–7. [CrossRef] [PubMed]
16.	Were, M. Determinants of teenage pregnancies: The case of Busia district in Kenya. *Econ. Hum. Biol.* **2007**, *5*, 322–339. [CrossRef] [PubMed]
17.	Shrestha, S. Socio-cultural factors influencing adolescent pregnancy in rural Nepal. *Int. J. Adolesc. Med. Health* **2002**, *14*, 101–109. [CrossRef] [PubMed]
18.	Alemayehu, T.; Haider, J.; Habte, D. Determinants of adolescent fertility in Ethiopia. *Ethiop. J. Health Dev.* **2010**, *24*, 30–38. [CrossRef]
19.	National Planning Comission (NPC). *Nepal Millennium Development Goal Progress Report 2010*; National Planing Commission Secretariat: Kathmandu, Nepal, 2010.
20.	Bennett, L.; Dahal, D.R.; Govindasamy, P. *Caste, Ethnic and Regional Identity in Nepal: Further Analysis of the 2006 Nepal Demographic and Health Survey*; Macro International Inc.: Calverton, MA, USA, 2008.
21.	CBS Nepal. *National Population Census 2001*; Central Bureau of Statistics: Kathmandu, Nepal, 2001.
22.	CBS Nepal. *Nepal in Figures*; Central Bureau of Statistics: Kathmandu, Nepal, 2012.
23.	Lang, T.; Secic, M. *How to Report Statistics in Medicine*, 2nd ed.; American College of Physicians: Philadelphia, PA, USA, 2006.
24.	World Health Organization (WHO). *Safe Abortion: Technical and Policy Guidance for Health Systems*; World Health Organization: Geneva, Switzerland, 2012.
25.	United Nations Population Fund (UNFPA). *Motherhood in Childhood: Facing the Challenge of Adolescent Pregnancy*; UNFPA: New York, NY, USA, 2013.
26.	World Health Organization (WHO). *Global Programme on Evidence*; World Health Organization: Geneva, Switzerland, 2000.
27.	Viner, R.M.; Ozer, E.M.; Denny, S.; Marmot, M.; Resnick, M.; Fatusi, A.; Currie, C. Adolescence and the social determinants of health. *Lancet* **2012**, *379*, 1641–1652. [CrossRef]
28.	Choe, M.K.; Thapa, S.; Mishra, V. Early marriage and early motherhood in Nepal. *J. Biosoc. Sci.* **2005**, *37*, 143–162. [CrossRef] [PubMed]
29.	Lion, K.C.; Prata, N.; Stewart, C. Adolescent childbearing in Nicaragua: A quantitative assessment of associated factors. *Int. Perspect. Sex. Reproduct. Health* **2009**, *35*, 91–96. [CrossRef]
30.	Pradhan, A.; Strachan, M. *Adolescent and Youth Reproductive Health in Nepal: Status, Issues, Policies and Programs*; Policy Project; USAID: Kathmandu, Nepal, 2003.

31. Adhikari, R.; Soonthorndhada, K.; Prasartkul, P. Correlates of unintended pregnancy among currently pregnant married women in Nepal. *BMC Int. Health Hum. Rights* **2009**, *9*, 17. [CrossRef] [PubMed]
32. Oshiro, A.; Poudyal, A.K.; Poudel, K.C.; Jimba, M.; Hokama, T. Intimate partner violence among general and urban poor populations in Kathmandu, Nepal. *J. Interpers. Violence* **2011**, *26*, 2073–2092. [CrossRef] [PubMed]

© 2018 by the authors. Licensee MDPI, Basel, Switzerland. This article is an open access article distributed under the terms and conditions of the Creative Commons Attribution (CC BY) license (http://creativecommons.org/licenses/by/4.0/).

International Journal of
*Environmental Research
and Public Health*

MDPI

Article

"Girls Have More Challenges; They Need to Be Locked Up": A Qualitative Study of Gender Norms and the Sexuality of Young Adolescents in Uganda

Anna B. Ninsiima [1,2,*], Els Leye [3], Kristien Michielsen [3], Elizabeth Kemigisha [3,4], Viola N. Nyakato [4] and Gily Coene [1]

[1]   RHEA Centre for Gender, Diversity and Intersectionality, Vrije Universiteit Brussel (VUB), 1050 Brussels, Belgium; gily.coene@vub.ac.be
[2]   School of Women and Gender Studies, Makerere University, 7062 Kampala, Uganda
[3]   International Centre for Reproductive Health, Ghent University, 10 UZ-P114, 9000 Ghent, Belgium; els.leye@ugent.be (E.L.); Kristien.michielsen@ugent.be (K.M.); ekemigisha@must.ac.ug (E.K.)
[4]   Faculty of Interdisciplinary Studies, Mbarara University of Science and Technology, P.O. Box 1410 Mbarara, Uganda; vnyakato@must.ac.ug
*   Correspondence: aninsiim@vub.ac.be

Received: 15 December 2017; Accepted: 19 January 2018; Published: 24 January 2018

Abstract: Unequal power and gender norms expose adolescent girls to higher risks of HIV, early marriages, pregnancies and coerced sex. In Uganda, almost half of the girls below the age of 18 are already married or pregnant, which poses a danger to the lives of young girls. This study explores the social construction of gender norms from early childhood, and how it influences adolescents' agency. Contrary to the mainstream theory of agency, which focuses on the ability to make informed choices, adolescents' agency appears constrained by context-specific obstacles. This study adopted qualitative research approaches involving 132 participants. Of these, 44 were in-depth interviews and 11 were focus group discussions, parcelled out into separate groups of adolescents (12–14 years), teachers, and parents ($n = 88$), in Western Uganda. Data were analysed manually using open and axial codes, and conclusions were inductive. Results show that gender norms are established early in life, and have a very substantial impact on the agency of young adolescents. There were stereotypical gender norms depicting boys as sexually active and girls as restrained; girls' movements were restricted; their sexual agency constrained; and prevention of pregnancy was perceived as a girl's responsibility. Programs targeting behavioural change need to begin early in the lives of young children. They should target teachers and parents about the values of gender equality and strengthen the legal system to create an enabling environment to address the health and wellbeing of adolescents.

Keywords: gender norms; early adolescence; sexual health; agency; Uganda

1. Introduction

Gender and unequal power relations within which sexual identities, beliefs and values are built [1] play a key role in the sexual wellbeing of adolescents [2,3]. Numerous studies indicate that unequal power and gender norms expose girls and women to the risk of HIV, early marriages, pregnancies and sexual violence [2–5]. It should be noted that decisions taken by girls and boys may not only depend on the knowledge they have, but may be influenced by contextual factors like societal values, and financial deprivation [5,6]. Social contexts and interpersonal relationships considerably contribute to the processes that shape adolescents' sexuality [5]. The socialisation in childhood shapes how girls and boys live out their lives as women and men—not only in the reproductive arena, but in the social and economic realm as well [6]. According to Bandura [7], sex role behaviour is promoted by active parental training in sex appropriate interests and expectations. This process is referred to as role modelling, imitation, or observational learning [5]. This takes place 'before young children get an opportunity to observe and discriminate the sexual appropriateness response patterns displayed by adult males and females' [7]. Humans learn prevalent, accepted, or desired behaviours referred to as social norms [5] by observing the behaviours of valued social referents, such as parents, teachers, peers, neighbours and the media [7]. According to Bandura, identifying the sources of emulated behaviour can quite often be problematic given that children are exposed to multiple models [7]. Adolescents might be motivated to conform to behavioural norms because it attracts certain rewards (like acceptance) and contrary to that may attract punishments, such as social rejection, or decrease in social status [5].

The modelling is a continuous process. However, explicitly during adolescence, the world expands for boys by allowing them to enjoy privileges reserved for men; while girls endure new restrictions earmarked for women [6]. The norms that dictate girls to behave like girls [8], and conceptions of female sexuality as passive, devoid of desire, and subordinate to male needs or desires [9] make it difficult for women to negotiate safe sex [10].

Commitment to deal with gender inequalities by embedding gender equality in comprehensive sexuality programmes is a core criterion [11]. The Convention on the Elimination of all Forms of Discrimination Against Women (CEDAW, 1979), is an international human rights convention for the advancement of women and gender equality [12]. The 1994 International Conference on Population and Development (ICPD) Programme of Action focused on promoting human rights, advancing gender equality and improving sexual and reproductive health [13]. Integrating gender is not only a matter of human rights [13] but according to Tolman [9], any intervention that ignores this may be counterproductive or even dangerous.

Some programmes to adolescent health take the individualistic approach where knowledge, and attitudes have become important units of analysis in sexuality programmes [14]. While such approaches may exclusively focus on reducing adolescent risky sexual behaviours, they may fail to explain the multifaceted and multi-determined social processes [2] that facilitate or block such risks. As some studies have indicated [15], there is need to move beyond individualistic approaches towards approaches that address the socio-economic structural dynamics which affect individual risks [14]. Burns [16] indicates that even if girls had the information and skills necessary to have healthy sexual relationships, power imbalances in gender relationships render them powerless in the face of masculine sexual freedom. The dependency syndrome, in particular, the flow of money and gifts being predominantly from males to females renders girls more powerless in African countries [4].

In this paper we examine the degree to which sexual gender norms in Western Uganda are established early in the lives of adolescents; how the norms are perceived; and the effect this has on adolescents' sexual agency, defined as the ability of Uganda's 12–14-year-old adolescents to make purposeful choices and negotiate safe sexual relations in the context of unequal power relations. Authors such as Amartya Sen conceptualize agency as the ability to make purposeful and informed choices [17]. However, this notion has been challenged on the premise that this is rather a Western conceptualization of agency, that relies on individualistic notions of choice and autonomy [18]. For example, Dutta [19] and Kabeer [18] argue that individuals exercise their agency within existing social conventions, values, sanctions and relationships. Social and cultural environments can be constraining or enabling of individual agency [20]. Especially where community structures and cultural traditions are still strong and valued, individualistic and autonomous agency may be constrained by social norms [5].

Few studies have been conducted in Uganda and Sub-Saharan Africa on adolescent sexual agency. For example, Bell argues that young women in Uganda are agentic, using sexual relationships to improve their own situation by extracting money or gifts for sex from men [21]. Michielsen finds older adolescent girls in Rwanda being active agents in transactional sex [22]. Michielsen's finding is similar to Nyanzi's [23] whose participants gave various reasons for transactional sex by arguing that 'nothing is for free'. While Nyanzi interprets this to be agency, she acknowledges the fact that relative poverty has a role to play given that parents are often unable to provide adequately for adolescent girls. It is therefore important to understand that the agency which is considered by Bell, Michielsen and Nyanzi could be very constrained by socio-economic conditions; and thus can only be understood in relative terms and within its relationship with the structures that girls operate in [19]. It should also be noted that the studies above have studied older adolescents, majorly between 15–20 years of age. Other studies, like Muhanguzi [3] and Iyer et al. [24], discuss the norms among older adolescents in central Uganda. It was important to understand the level at which adolescents internalize gender norms to inform programming.

Accordingly, this study brings to light new knowledge on the gendered sexual norms among young adolescents in South Western Uganda—even though some of the findings merely corroborate the general theoretical claims and empirical observations made elsewhere in the developing world on gendered power relations among older adolescents.

Young Adolescents and Sexuality in the Ugandan Context

Uganda has about 46 percent of girls below 18 years already married, and 20–24 percent married or pregnant before they are 15 years [25]. Early marriages and pregnancies account for 20 percent of maternal deaths and those who survive suffer lasting complications like fistula and disability [26]. While sexuality education has been identified as one of the remedies to such risky behaviours [27], in Uganda and many African countries, sex and sexuality are a private matter and openly discussing sexuality is regarded as a taboo [23–26]. Sex is legitimatised in marriage [24] and virginity of girls before marriage is a highly expected cultural norm. Highly gendered sexuality education (SE) was carried out through indigenous institutions of the extended family and the community [16–29] where paternal aunties (known as *Senga* in Central Uganda and *Shwenkazi* in Western Uganda) had an important role in preparing girls for womanhood and marriage. Emphasis was, and still is, on the control of girls' sexuality. Ironically, virginity was, and continues to be, highly valued for girls, but not for boys—even though the emphasis placed on the girl's virginity at the time of marriage appears to be changing [30].

The patriarchal tendencies in Uganda are undeniable and polygamy remains a strong cultural norm in some communities [31]. While polygamy is not acceptable according to the dominant Christian values in Uganda, it is still culturally accepted and has been revitalised as "informal polygamy", in which men have relationships with multiple women under the term "modern polygamy" [32]. Men's control of resources within households persists, with men considered as the heads of the household, main decision-makers and in control of women's sexuality and movements. However, according to Bantebya et al. [32] ideals of marriage are growing more fragile with women taking on new roles, for example, the participation of women in public affairs may leave many men feeling disempowered [32]. Challenging traditional masculinities can contribute to more domestic violence as a response to the cultural shock and unwillingness by some males to adapt to changing roles [32].

Uganda has numerous laws that have been enacted to protect the rights of children and fight gender inequality. These include but are not limited to the Constitution of Uganda 1995. For example, Article 32 (2) provides that the "Laws, cultures, customs and traditions which are against the dignity, welfare or interest of women or any other marginalized group ... or which undermines their status, are prohibited by this Constitution"; The Children's Act (amended in 2016)—under Chapter 59 puts into effect the Constitutional provisions on children and emphasises the protection of the child by upholding their rights; The Domestic Violence Act, 2010, is another gender-friendly piece of legislation in Uganda. The Ugandan defilement law within the Penal Code Act (originally from 1950 which Uganda inherited from British colonial rule), has gone through some changes, whereby the age of sexual consent was increased in 1990 from fourteen to eighteen years. The 1990 edition of the law is very clear in the sense that it is not only illegal for a man to have sexual intercourse with a girl regardless of consent under the age of eighteen years, but also punishable by death [33,34]. As discussed by

Parikh [35], the defilement law was defended by women's rights activists and intended to address the social and health inequalities affecting young women and girls. However, the law was controversial and perceived as undermining men's traditional authority and access to younger women for marriage or sexual relations. It was also criticized on the grounds that it was an encroachment by the state on culturally private matters that should be handled by the community [35]. Although the law intended to prosecute "sugar daddies", Parikh found in her ethnographic study that it rather enforced patriarchal control and class hierarchies.

In 2007, the law was again amended and now includes women offenders and male victims. A person who performs a sexual act with another person who is below the age of 18 years commits an offence punished by a maximum period of life imprisonment. Under aggravating circumstances, the death penalty is sentenced. The law states that where the offender in the case of defilement is below 12 years of age the Children's Act is applied. The Children's Act states that a child above the age of 12 can be arrested and charged if he or she is suspected to have committed an offence, but a child below the age of 12 years cannot be charged with a criminal offence [36].

2. Methods

2.1. Study Design

The study aimed at exploring the gender-related sexuality norms among young adolescents in Uganda. The study used qualitative methods, in particular in-depth interviews (IDIs) and focus group discussions (FGDs). This research is part of a bigger project implementing sexuality education among young adolescents in primary schools in Mbarara district in Western Uganda. The total population of Mbarara district is roughly 472,629 with a total area of 1846 km^2 [37]. The district is occupied largely by the Banyankole ethnic group. The literacy rate for persons above 18 years is about 82%, 87% for persons between 10–17 years and 42% for persons aged 60 and above. Data show that 46.7% of persons above age 10 and 62% above 18 years of age are married in Mbarara District. Agriculture (livestock or crop growing) is the major economic activity engaging 70% of the households [37].

Field work was done between July and August 2016 in Mbarara district with a total of 132 participants. Of these, 44 were in-depth interviews and 11 were focus group discussions, 44 in-depth interviews (IDIs) were done with school adolescent girls ($n = 12$) and, boys ($n = 12$) aged 12–14, teachers ($n = 10$) and parents ($n = 10$). 88 individuals took part in 11 focus group discussions (FGDs) performed in three rural, one semi-urban, and two urban schools. Four FGDs involved school adolescents ($n = 32$), and four FGDs with teachers ($n = 32$) and three FGDs with parents ($n = 24$) were conducted. Purposeful samplings were applied to select the six schools and all the participants. Teachers were selected based on their expertise or involvement in sexuality education. They mainly included senior women, senior men, science teachers, religious education teachers or deputy head teachers. Parents were chairpersons of boards in the school or parent-teacher associations and parents of the children that we interviewed.

The rural–urban divide was purposively designed to account for any differences in sexual behaviours of the pupils, the level of knowledge, the involvement of parents, and the gender norms prevailing among adolescents in rural and urban settings. The parents in the rural setting were mainly small-scale farmers while parents in the urban setting were mainly involved in businesses or formal sector jobs.

For the data collection we used interview guides. The guide for pupils mainly focused on their gender roles, gender and the source of their knowledge and prevailing gender norms regarding sexuality. The guide for teachers mainly focused on their knowledge and attitude towards gender, the prevailing gender norms in the schools and the role of parents. The guide for parents focused on the level of communication with their children, the knowledge they impart in their children (how gendered) and whether they approved sexuality education in schools.

2.2. Data Analysis

Interviews and FGDs were recorded, transcribed, (some) translated from local language (Runyankole) to English. Data was read and re-read and then open coded. In open coding, data were examined on differences and similarities [38] from which concepts were derived. Concepts were based on words or phrases that were used in open coding. Phrases included "like myself", "do not like myself", "menstruation", "aspirations", "domestic chores", "girls leave school when they get pregnant", and "money for sex". Concepts like self-esteem, assertiveness, strong and weaker sex, gender roles, initiation of romantic relationships, among others were identified. We then preceded with axial codes where similar codes from different participants were grouped together, themes created and categories formed from which sections in this paper were derived. Data were identified to find the role played by the context in influencing participants perceptions [38], for example to identify the differences between rural/urban context and male/female perceptions.

2.3. Ethical Clearance

The study obtained approval from the Institutional Research Ethics Committee of Mbarara University (reference MUIRC 1/7) and the Uganda National Council of Science and Technology (reference SS 4045). At the beginning of each interview and focus group, written and verbal informed consent of teachers and parents was sought. Informed written assent of adolescents was obtained plus written informed consent from either the parents or the head teachers of the schools that adolescents attended. We sought consent on whether we could tape record their voices. We also obtained approval from school head teachers of the participating schools and the district administration.

3. Results

3.1. Sexually Active Boys and Restrained Girls

Field findings from Mbarara reveal that masculine behaviour is encouraged among boys and passivity and meekness promoted among girls with particular regard to their sexuality. In the interviews, boys easily talked about their sexual relations. Boys that had girlfriends and those that had engaged in sexual activity were more open about it, compared to the girls. Boys also expressed that they enjoyed larger freedom to explore sexual relations and seemed to be proud with their sexual activity. In one of the rural FGD with eight boys, all boys said they were sexually active except one;

When did you start to sleep with your girlfriend?

Boy 1: *I was 11 years.*

Boy 2: *I was in primary 4 (12 years).*

Boy 3: *As for me, I'm 14 years and still don't have a girlfriend. I need to first grow up and be responsible for my actions.*

Boy 1 (interrogating and ridiculing Boy 3): *What are you waiting for? Are you a tree? Do you think you will be source of timber? Laughter from all ...*

Interviewer: *Does anyone of you have more than one girlfriend?*

Boy 1: *Yes, I have two. One in this school and another in a different school. Just in case one decides to leave me or if she behaves badly, then I have an alternative. Besides, I need to taste different girls.*

Interviewer: *But supposing she finds out that you have another?*

Boy 4: *Ohhh if she sees you that's the end. You can touch them when she is not around.*

Interviewer: *Are these the girlfriends you intend to marry?*

Boy 4: Haaaa, normally you stay with her like for two or three terms and if by that time you have slept with her like three times, you will have gotten tired of her and you leave her. Or she would have developed bad manners of going after other boys.

The quote illustrates how the masculine power of *'tasting girls'* and control of female sexuality has already been formed by the age of 14 years. Boys state that they can have two or three girlfriends but that it is abnormal for a girl to do the same. However, it should not go without mention that girls are not merely passive. Their contestations regarding multiple partners by their boyfriends are an indication that girls are active participants.

However, the social norm that girls need to behave like girls was manifested in their refusal to open up about their own sexual relations during the IDIs or FGDs and to talk solely about other girls in their age group or in the same classes. Societal expectations by elders that girls should stay virgins until marriage, make it difficult for the girls to share such experiences. Even when she is not a virgin, she is supposed to pretend that she is, even among fellow girls:

Interviewer: *Do some of your friends have boy friends?*

Girl: *Yes, some have, but they cannot tell you even if they had (IDI Girl Rural).*

One of the informants revealed that she has a boyfriend who gives her gifts but indicated that she does not have sexual intercourse with him:

Girl: *I cannot let my friend know my secret? Noooooo!! There is no one you can trust under the sun now. So I keep it to myself. I tell my blanket (IDI Girl rural).*

Other informants indicated that when a girl is engaged in sexual relations, even if she is forced, it is still her fault. Furthermore, girls have been taught to be responsible and getting pregnant is solely seen as their responsibility:

I don't know whether there are unwanted pregnancies because one goes there willingly. But I hear people calling it unwanted pregnancies.

(Head teacher semi urban)

Sometimes girls dress inappropriately and cause men to rape them. Others cause it to happen because they eat men's money and accept to meet somewhere not knowing that they may be raped.

(FGD, Girl Rural)

When you get used, spoilt and get pregnant, you stop going to school and start suffering. Your friends start talking about you, you lose respect and you are labelled with ugly names. And if your parents chase you away you become homeless and may become a housemaid ... Nothing happens to the boy. They continue studying, unless they refuse to continue on their own. But getting a girl pregnant does not make them drop out of school.

(IDI Girl rural)

Of course men do not face as many challenges as women. When a girl gets pregnant, that's her end. For me I was told by my mother that girls who get pregnant before marriage are thrown into river Kisiizi. I never wanted a man to touch me because I thought if a man touches me I get pregnant.

(Female Parent, urban)

While there is a law against defilement in Uganda, its enforcement has been ineffective or selective. The men or boys that impregnate girls may either deny paternity, escape, or get into police cells for a few days, only to be released.

A boy who participated in an FGD reported as follows:

> *It is better to impregnate someone's daughter than to steal. Moreover, our parents find a boy who impregnates girl more socially acceptable than a girl who gets pregnant.*
>
> (Boy FGD rural)

A teacher who participated in our focus group discussion rhetorically asked the question:

> *Have you ever heard a defilement case taken serious? She hastened to answer as follows: "No! The laws in Uganda do not work".*

A male parent from rural Uganda—reported:

> *"I took a boy who impregnated my 16 years old daughter to police; he was released in a few days. We get discouraged by the police."*

A female parent from Mbarara municipality faulted government for its incompetence. She argued:

> *"The government is negligent. A young man I know raped an adolescent girl of my daughter's age. Police imprisoned him, but he was released after five days once the parents pleaded with the police. By failing to be tough on offenders, the government itself encourages criminal behaviours. The government should do more. Arrest the criminals and imprison them for a long time."*

Girls are socially expected to take care of their own sexuality but also take responsibility for their male sexual oppressors. It is perceived to be a girl's duty to safeguard herself from the uncontrolled feelings of boys and men. Some girls indicated that when boys write love letters to them or harass them, they dread telling their parents because some parents blame girls for the behaviour of the boys:

> Interviewer: *Do you readily share information with your parents if a boy writes you a love letter or makes advances for a sexual relationship?*
>
> Girl: *No! I received a love letter from a boy. I feared to tell my mother about the letter but I told a teacher. I discerned that my mother might think that I brought the problem upon myself yet that was not the case. There is also a boy in our neighbourhood who touches me inappropriately when my parents are away. I wanted to talk to my mother but I still fear her because she might think I am drawing the advances myself* (IDI Girl semi-urban).
>
> *Some parents can respond harshly by telling you that perhaps you want to sleep with a man if you start sharing information about sexual advances or ask questions about sexuality* (IDI Girl Rural).
>
> *My mother is tough. She is likely to say that the boy would not have approached me if I had not shown interest by familiarizing with boys for example, by smiling in a seductive way* (IDI Girl semi-urban).

Parents and teachers believe that girls' freedoms need to be restricted because girls have more to lose in a relationship than boys. A senior woman (urban) succinctly stated:

> *"Girls have more challenges in this modern world. With this exposure, girls need to be locked up."*

A male rural-based parent seemed to agree. For him:

> *"Girls are like ground nuts, which are a delicacy in Uganda. Everyone wants to pick and eat them. Parents to girl children must take extra effort to control and discipline them."*

Another rural-based parent from a cattle-rearing community, likened girls to milk—another precious but fragile product. For him:

> *"Girls are like milk-it keeps on attracting house flies. As a parent, you have to safeguard your daughters more than you do to your sons. For the boy-child you can send him to school by himself, but the girl child needs to be escorted ... "*

A rural-based girl reported as follows:

"Parents restrict us from visiting our friends. They seem to think that a girl might have a 'deal' to meet a boy and engage in premarital sex. But boys do not get spoilt like girls so they allow them to go. Even if a boy delays to come, he still comes back home without much trouble. Besides girls have many responsibilities, there is always something that you are expected to do at home."

(IDI Girl Rural)

Teachers and parents believed that only girls need sexuality education because they have higher risks than boys. While schools have senior women and senior men who are both responsible for counselling adolescents about maturation, it was only the senior women who were actively involved in sexuality education in all the schools that we visited. The senior women met girls at least 2–3 times a term (three months) while boys could spend a term without meeting the senior man:

As for these old boys, I meet them whenever there is a trigger or a signal that something is wrong. We don't normally give them too much attention as girls because in primary five to primary seven, girls are more sexually advanced than boys, and have more needs for sexuality education.

(senior man-rural)

I meet girls 2–3 times in a term. I teach them to be clean especially during menstruation. Some girls are careless. A man is not supposed to see menstrual blood. I also teach them to respect elders but also to avoid men. I tell them the dangers of AIDS and accepting money from men.

(senior woman rural)

3.2. Gender and Initiation of Sexual Relationships

The sexual relationships that prevail in Mbarara and Uganda depict boys as sexually active and the only beings sanctioned to initiate such relationships. The findings show an overwhelming opposition to girls initiating a love relationship. These are some of the responses from a focus group discussion with girls:

Interviewer: *Who asks for love, a boy or girl?*

Girl: *Boy.*

Interviewer: *What happens when a girl asks a boy?*

Girl: *Can a girl ask a boy for love? I have never heard of that; that would be a prostitute. She will have ashamed us as girls because a girl never advances for sex, even our teacher told us about it in class (FGD Girls semi urban).*

Interviewer: *What would you think of your friend if she asks a boy for love?*

Girl: *I would think she is not normal (Girl, IDI rural).*

Girl: *I would break off that friendship. Her conduct would be regarded as strange (IDI, Girl urban).*

Girl: *If I am a boy I know you want to kill me (IDI, Girl rural).*

It should however be noted that the norm appears to be changing with some girls arguably manifesting some level of agency. It was reported that some girls initiate sexual relationships—only that they typically use subtle but clear ways to convey their message. If a girl admired a boy, she could touch him or struggle to sit with him in class. Sometimes she can send a message by going through her friends or the friends of the boy. According to the boys, it is only brave girls that can advance, and such, are not common. The boys believe that the normal and right procedure is for a boy to ask a girl:

God designed it that a boy should ask a girl and not vice-versa.

(Boy FGD urban)

Some girls can show you signs that they are interested, but it is not normal. You have to be wary of such girls who initiate sexual relationships. They could be having HIV.

(Boy FGD urban)

The only means identified to commence a sexual relationship by boys was giving money or gifts to the girls. For some girls with no economic opportunities for themselves, entering into such relationships is the only way to obtain money to buy food, pads or books. By giving such gift, a boy or man can show his interest in a sexual relationship with a girl. If she does not want the relationship, the girl has to decline those gifts or else she has to account for them by giving in her body:

If you want a girl, however rigid she might be, you give her money or a gift. Once she accepts it, you know you will win her over. You keep giving her in bits and not too much because if she knows you have a lot of money she will always come back for more.

(IDI Boy Rural)

The poverty and economic dependency on the side of girls has led to such constructions that girls can be won over by money, and that boys have the capacity to measure what is just enough for the girls. However, it was also reported that some girls may get the money but still reject sexual activity with those that give them the money. In some instances, such can result into rape or defilement.

3.3. Division of Labour, Strength and Future Aspirations

Findings from this study uphold the widely documented view that girls and boys in Uganda still have different gender roles. The division of roles was stronger in rural areas than urban areas, contrary to the claim by government elites that affirmative action has evened up the gender question. In rural areas, girls reported doing typical traditional work for women like cooking, cleaning, collecting firewood, nursing and babysitting whereas boys go out to graze animals, milk cows, taking products to the market and sometimes fetching water. Findings indicate that whenever boys did not have sisters/girls at home, they performed girls' duties of cooking and washing dishes. However, in the urban areas, while the divide still exists, it was not that substantial mainly because children (boys and girls) in towns have more to do with housework than outdoor activities. According to the boys and girls in the interviews, there are certain activities that need a lot of energy (strength) and therefore have to be done by boys. Thus, adolescents believe in the dominant stereotype that boys are stronger than girls and that outdoor activities are dangerous for girls.

Boys are more energetic. I can carry only a 10 L jerican but for him he can ride with a full milk can of 20–25 L on the bicycle.

(IDI girl urban)

For us girls we do not go out to graze because it is dangerous for us.

(IDI Girl Rural)

Boys are lucky, sometimes you are in the house cooking. You serve them milk and food and for them they are just in the house seated. After the meal, you even clean up the dishes, and often get too exhausted to do your school assignments. You sometimes wish you were a boy who would sit, wait to be served, and have enough time for your school assignments.

(IDI Girl semi-urban)

The gender role divide is reflected in future career aspirations of adolescents. Unlike pupils from the urban areas who have seen women doctors, almost all the girls in the rural areas desire to become nurses and primary school teachers. Some girls expressed with doubt if girls can become doctors:

Interviewer: *What do you want to become in future?*

Girl: *A nurse.*

Interviewer: *Why? Can't you become a doctor?*

Girl: *Most doctors are men (IDI Girl semi-urban).*

Boy: *I want to work in a garage, be a mechanic and get my own garage (boy semi-urban).*

On the other hand, none of the boys mentioned nursing as their preferred profession, but only a handful in the rural area mentioned that they would like to become teachers. The majority of the boys aspire to become doctors, engineers, pilots and police men or soldiers. Because of their socially constructed gender roles (like baby-sitting, cooking), most girls mentioned marriage as an important achievement they want to accomplish. They had a desire to get more information concerning handling men and how to conduct themselves in marriage. While they dream to take on professional courses like teaching, they mainly want to be awarded respect by society if they have a successful marriage:

Interviewer: *What kind of information would you like to hear that is never taught to you?*

They don't tell us how to do things when we get married because we hear that before you get married, you should first visit your aunt to teach you some of these things.

(FGD Girls Rural)

How to conduct yourself when you are going to get married and when you are married

(IDI Girl Rural)

I would like to know how to handle marriage and pregnancy.

(IDI Girl semi-urban)

3.4. Gender and Value Attached to Different Sexes

Our findings indicate that most girls loved being girls but hated the aspect of menstruation:

"For me I hate being in my monthly periods, and I regret being a girl".

(Girl FGD semi-urban)

Given that menstruation of Ugandan girls typically arrives without prior preparation of the adolescents, it is difficult for the girls to psychologically accept it. Others however indicated that they were comfortable with menstruation because it is a sign of fertility. The ability to give birth was one of the most important things that girls loved and valued about themselves:

For me I like experiencing periods. Much as it is painful, I have to endure because you cannot produce if you don't get them and we would like to produce children.

(FGD girls rural)

While some girls endure menstruation, it makes girls hate school because in the context of a poor country like Uganda, girls normally lack sanitary pads and soap to use.

It's not good being a girl because there are problems like menstruation. You feel a lot of pain and boys disturb us asking us very many questions in case they know you have started menstruating.

(Girl semi-urban)

I haven't got my periods but I fear them, they can embarrass you at school.

(IDI Girl 13 rural)

Boys pointed out that it is an honour to be a boy/man:

"No one can ever wish to be a girl in life".

(Boy FGD rural)

While boys are aware that they have to work and become breadwinners for their families, they never wished to be girls because of the hardships associated with painful processes like menstruation and child birth:

"At least wet dreams come and go. But menstrual periods keep coming".

(Boy FGD urban)

Moreover, they indicated that girls perform hard house chores and are never allowed to get out from home.

One of the challenged social norms in the study area however was the reduced segregation between boys and girls in terms of education, care and provisions. Boys complained that girls are favoured when it comes to shopping for clothes, edibles or other items for school. Girls seem to be getting more of what they ask for from parents than the boys. This is different from certain parts of Uganda where girl-child education is not given significance (girls may not continue with school or may be placed in poor schools as compared to boys when parents are faced with financial constraints). In this study, findings from boys, girls, teachers and parents, indicated that there was a more egalitarian tendency in regard to education access.

A parent will send you to a bad school depending on your academic performance; if you have performed badly you go to a bad school. Not because you are a boy or girl .

(IDI Girl urban)

We don't segregate our children (boys and girls) like our parents and grandparents did. We know that when a girl gets education she becomes an important person.

(Male parent FGD Rural)

However, differences in values attached to a boy and girl child were persistent. Boys expressed that it was powerful to be a boy because they learnt from their parents that boys take over from their fathers when their fathers are away. And in case the father died, boys inherit property and look after the home rather than the girls:

A woman's role is to remain at home only.

(Boy FGD Urban)

A girl also expressed the value attached to the boy child:

Girl: *I want to have 2 children, a boy and a girl.*

Interviewer: *Supposing you get only girls?*

Girl: *Ai bambe!!! (Meaning Uhhhhh); In our society when you produce girls only it's like you have no children. You know that* (IDI Girl rural).

A parent stated:

I have five girls. People say I have produced nothing but prostitutes. That I have no child because I have no boys. I feel bad that I have not yet given my husband a boy. When girls grow, they get married to other families. But a boy stays home and makes the family grow and continue. With girls, the family is no more. My husband is now sleeping with other women looking for a boy. He has already brought me one boy from another woman. I am looking after him. I am also still producing may be God will bless me with a boy. While I would be happy getting a boy, I still love my girls. And I want them to study. When they study, they can become important persons and help me.

(Female parent semi-urban)

4. Discussion

The study aimed at understanding sexuality gender norms among young adolescents, parents and teachers and how they influence adolescents' sexual dynamics. While Muhanguzi [3] and Iyer et al. [24] discuss the norms among older adolescents in central Uganda, this study explored whether these norms already manifest among the age of 12–14 years in western Uganda. Findings indicate that the agency of an individual actor is challenged by gender norms and stereotypes governing the attitudes and behaviour of adolescents. These gender norms are an important mediating factor in their sexual and reproductive experience [39]. Gendered norms are taught at home by parents. But as Bandura argues, learning and modelling takes place in different ways by different social referents which include extended family, teachers, peers and the media [7]. Various aunties play a complementary role by ensuring that girls become well-versed in the socially "appropriate" feminine behaviours and roles. These include the "proper" ways of how a good girl should sit, prepare food, conduct herself, respect elders and so on [40]. On the other hand, boys typically perform duties largely outside the home and are not very restricted in their movements. This finding is similar to that of Ngabaza [40] who found that boys and girls are socialised to perform different roles, have different expectations from parents, aunties and the wider communities. The differences exhibited in their aspirations like the values girls attach to motherhood, marriage, care giving and admiration for formal-sector jobs like nursing and teaching are a significant part of long-term gender ideals [14]. Such aspirations are both drivers to, and results of, unequal power relations [14], which are key aspects of sexuality.

The masculine behaviour was already present among boys aged 12–14. Boys engage with multiple partners, enjoy free movement, engage in economic activities and have the capacity to use the money to win over girls into sexual activity. By contrast, neither the boys nor the wider society expect the same behaviour from the girl-child. Girls are socially expected to be nice, submissive, and have restricted movements. The control of resources by men leads to un-equal power relations whereby girls/women cannot negotiate safer sex [4]. Unequal economic power restricts a girl's sexual agency and could result in coercive sexual practices [3]. However, the norm or practice of multiple partners and polygamy for boys/men is contested by girls and women. Thus this is a practice that is done without girl's knowledge, which can be considered as a sign of girl's agency. While polygamy or multiple partners is legitimised by cultural norms, and thus providing the conduit through which agency is realised [19], girls/women continuously interact and live within these structures and participate in avenues to challenge them [19]. Other studies like Haberland [41] and De Meyer [39] reveal that more egalitarian gender attitudes are related to higher use of protection/contraceptives and easier communication about sex within the couple than those that had negative gender norms.

Results from this study indicate that female sexual activity is restricted and girls who express sexual agency are considered to be prostitutes or abnormal. Both boys and girls agreed that it was quite abnormal and strange if a girl proposed a sexual relationship to a boy. This is similar to what Muhanguzi [3] found in her study among older adolescents in Uganda. It should however be noted that girls have continuously expressed their sexual feelings though using subtle ways to convey their message. This has also been reported by Nyanzi [23] in her study among older adolescents in Uganda where girls are no longer expected to be amateurs but at the same time not lose their virginity. The stereotypical gender norm depicting boys as sexually active and girls as dormant with less (sexual) agency was also reflected in De Meyer et al. [39]. Our findings show that girl's movement was more restricted compared to that of boys. Manifested in quotes like *"girls need to be locked up"* and gender stereotypes that girls naturally attract men, the dominant social norms give parents and teachers a mandate to control the girl-child more seriously than their male counterparts. Girls are socially expected to control their own sexuality but also take responsibility for boys' sexualities because pregnancy is deemed to be girl's responsibility. Moreover, as [37] reports, girls who get pregnant may get disowned by their families and have no guarantee that they will be accepted by the boy's/man's family. The notion of girls being punished for becoming pregnant was also found in Rwanda [22].

This is also reflected in Varga's study where it was found that nothing ever happens to a boy if he does not accept paternity [42].

Moreover, while sexuality education should involve teaching of gender equality, to assist in changing patriarchal attitudes towards women/girls, our study suggests that sexuality education by teachers and parents gave preferentially higher attention to the girls compared to the boys. From this perspective, sexuality education mainly focused on biological aspects like hygiene, and control of girls' sexuality. Girls were taught how to control themselves from male advances, respecting elders and helping with household chores. Tamale [31] shows that sexuality education taught in Uganda basically reinforces patriarchal control of female sexuality where girls are taught to be submissive to men. Teachers' perceptions are shaped by gendered values which shape girls and boys differently [9]. A study done by Iyer and Aggleton, [43] (p. 6) in central Uganda found that teachers believed that boys need to behave like men and be in control while girls' first responsibility is " … " having respect, and value for, their bodies … they are the "Mothers of Tomorrow". Moreover, findings of this study also indicated that parents did not give girls an environment to express their worries regarding their sexuality. According to Svanemyr, et al. [15], gender norms that emphasize silence mostly for girls in obtaining information do not create a safe environment for their agency and wellbeing.

The legal system which would be supportive of addressing child protection and gender inequalities from local councils (courts), the police, and probation officers to Courts of Judicature is still weak (thanks to the high level of corruption in the Ugandan police force) and patriarchal. It is undermined by cultural values where sexuality is treated as a private matter [35]. This, coupled with poverty among the parents who may forego legal procedures when the culprits offer money [35] or choose to get their daughter married and save them the shame of keeping a pregnant daughter [33], has reinforced, not transformed, socially embedded patriarchal norms.

5. Conclusions

Our findings point to several potential target areas for programming to improve sexual and reproductive health among adolescents. One is that gender norms form early in life and create unequal power relations that constrain adolescents from exercising agency with regard to their sexuality and health. Thus, any program targeting behavioural change needs to begin early in the lives of young children. Second, the sexuality education that should address the unequal gender relations seems to be propagated by teachers and parents in Uganda. Thus, any program that aims at behavioural change without addressing the socio-cultural norms that perceive men as strong and all-knowing, and girls as passive and only designed for reproduction and men's consumption will be counterproductive. A comprehensive gender-sensitive sexuality education focusing on values like equality, reciprocity, self-esteem and respect would be important. Such programs we argue will only be effective if they do not only target the teachers, but also parents and the community. This is because the primary agents of socialisation are families first, and then schools. Decisions taken by an individual are influenced by the socio-structure in which they live. Targeting schools with gender sensitive sexuality education, for example, without targeting the family would have diminutive impact. Third, in addition to educating children, teachers and parents about the values of gender equality, there is need for Uganda to strengthen the legal framework. An enabling legislative and policy framework is critically important in supporting adolescents, teachers and parents to address the health and wellbeing of adolescents.

Limitations of the Study

The study focused on how social/gender norms constrain young adolescents' agency regarding sexuality. While we may not authoritatively claim that the sample selected for this study is representative of the whole country, we can claim that results can be moveable to most parts of Uganda and other parts of Africa and Asia that have similar levels of economic development and similar patriarchal norms.

Future research needs to explain the difference between the norms that adolescents practice (actual or perceived) and the norms expected of them by others/referents (injunctive). It would also be helpful to explain the extent to which parents and teachers influence and the extent to which peer pressure influences adolescents. More studies are needed to explain dynamics like the level of household income, the dynamics of accessing the legal system and the policy environment surrounding sexuality in Uganda.

Acknowledgments: This work is part of a project—"Who am I" aiming at Mitigating Adverse Sexual and Reproductive Health Outcomes through a Comprehensive Primary School Sexuality Education Program in South-Western Uganda. It was funded by VRIL-UOS team under Project Grant Number ZEIN2015PR411. Special thanks go to VLIR-UOS for the financial support without which this work would not have been done. Sincere gratitude is extended to our research assistants—Isaac Ahimbisiibwe and Clara Atuhaire, who did tremendous work. We sincerely thank the research participants for their time and eagerness to take part in the study; the inputs of the adolescents that we interacted with, their parents and the teachers are gratefully acknowledged.

Author Contributions: Anna B. Ninsiima wrote the proposal, collected data, analyzed and wrote the first draft of this manuscript. Gily Coene, Kristien Michielsen, and Els Leye participated in proposal writing, and substantially contributed to the intellectual development of the manuscript. Elizabeth Kemigisha, and Viola N. Nyakato participated in editing of the manuscript.

Conflicts of Interest: The authors declare no conflict of interest.

References

1. Tolman, D.L.; Striepe, M.I.; Harmon, T. Gender matters: Constructing a model of adolescent sexual health. *J. Sex Res.* **2003**, *40*, 4–12. [CrossRef] [PubMed]
2. De Meyer, S.; Jaruseviciene, L.; Zaborskis, A.; Decat, P.; Vega, B.; Cordova, K.; Temmerman, M.; Degomme, O.; Michielsen, K. A cross-sectional study on attitudes toward gender equality, sexual behavior, positive sexual experiences, and communication about sex among sexually active and non-sexually active adolescents in Bolivia and Ecuador. *Glob. Health Action* **2014**, *1*, 1–10. [CrossRef] [PubMed]
3. Muhanguzi, F.K. Gender and sexual vulnerability of young women in Africa: Experiences of young girls in secondary schools in Uganda. *Cult. Health Sex* **2011**, *13*, 713–725. [CrossRef] [PubMed]
4. Madise, N.; Zulu, E.; Ciera, J. Is poverty a driver for risky sexual behaviour? Evidence from national surveys of adolescents in four African countries. *Afr. J. Reprod. Health* **2007**, *11*, 83–98. [CrossRef] [PubMed]
5. Van de Bongardt, D.; Reitz, E.; Sandfort, T.; Deković, M. A meta-analysis of the relations between three types of peer norms and adolescent sexual behavior. *Personal. Soc. Psychol. Rev.* **2015**, *19*, 203–234. [CrossRef] [PubMed]
6. Mensch, B.S.; Bruce, J.; Greene, M.E. *The Uncharted Passage Girls' Adolescence in the Developing World*; The Population Council: New York, NY, USA, 1998.
7. Bandura, A. Social-Learning theory of identificatory processes. In *Handbook of Socialization Theory and Research*; Rand McNally: Chicago, IL, USA, 1969; pp. 213–262.
8. Ngabaza, S.; Shefer, T.; Catriona, I.M.; Ngabaza, S.; Shefer, T.; Macleod, I. "Girls need to behave like girls you know": The complexities of applying a gender justice goal within sexuality education in South African schools applying a gender justice goal within sexuality education in South African schools. *RHM* **2016**, *24*, 71–78.
9. Tolman, D.L. Female adolescents, sexual empowerment and desire: A missing discourse of gender inequity. *Sex Roles* **2012**, *66*, 746–757. [CrossRef]
10. Holland, J.; Ramazanoglu, C.; Scott, S.; Sharpe, S.; Thomson, R. Risk, power and the possibility of pleasure: Young women and safer sex. *AIDS Care* **1992**, *4*, 273–283. [CrossRef] [PubMed]
11. Ketting, E.; Friele, M.; Michielsen, K. Evaluation of holistic sexuality education: A European expert group consensus agreement. *Eur. J. Contracept. Reprod. Health Care* **2016**, *21*, 68–80. [CrossRef] [PubMed]
12. McCracken, T.K.K.; Márquez, S.; Priest, S.; Ana, F. *Sexual and Reproductive Health and Rights*; European Union: Brussels, Belgium, 2016.
13. UNFPA. *Operational Guidance for Comprehensive Sexuality Education: A Focus on Human Rights and Gender*; UNFPA: New York, NY, USA, 2014; pp. 1–76.

14. Wamoyi, J.; Mshana, G.; Mongi, A.; Neke, N.; Kapiga, S.; Changalucha, J. A review of interventions addressing structural drivers of adolescents' sexual and reproductive health vulnerability in Sub-Saharan Africa: Implications for sexual health programming. *Reprod. Health* **2014**, *11*, 88. [CrossRef] [PubMed]
15. Svanemyr, J.; Amin, A.; Robles, O.J.; Greene, M.E. Creating an enabling environment for adolescent sexual and reproductive health: A framework and promising approaches. *J. Adolesc. Health* **2015**, *56*, S7–S14. [CrossRef] [PubMed]
16. Burns, K. Sexuality education in a girls' school in Eastern Uganda. *Agenda Empower Women Gend. Equity* **2002**, *53*, 81–88.
17. Sen, A. Introduction "Development as freedom". In *Development as Freedom*; Oxford University Press: Oxford, UK, 2001; pp. 3–11.
18. Kabeer, N. "Chapters 1–5". In *Reversed Realities: Gender Hierarchies in Development Thought*; Verso: London, UK; New York, NY, USA, 1994.
19. Dutta, M.J.; Basu, A. Meanings of health: Interrogating structure and culture. *Health Commun.* **2008**, *23*, 560–572. [CrossRef] [PubMed]
20. Giddens, A. Agency, institution and time-space analysis. In *Advances in Social Theory and Methodology toward an Integration of Macro and MicroSociologies*; Routledge & Kegan Paul: Abingdon, UK, 1981; pp. 161–174.
21. Bell, S.A. Young people and sexual agency in Rural Uganda. *Cult. Health Sex* **2012**, *14*, 283–296. [CrossRef] [PubMed]
22. Michielsen, K.; Remes, P.; Rugabo, J.; van Rossem, R.; Temmerman, M. Rwandan young people's perceptions on sexuality and relationships: Results from a qualitative study using the "mailbox technique". *Sahara J.* **2014**, *11*, 51–60. [CrossRef] [PubMed]
23. Nyanzi, S.; Pool, R.; Kinsman, J. The negotiation of sexual relationships among school pupils in South-Western Uganda. *AIDS Care Psychol. Socio-Med. Asp. AIDS/HIV* **2001**, *13*, 83–98. [CrossRef] [PubMed]
24. Iyer, P.; Clarke, D.; Aggleton, P. Barriers to HIV and sexuality education in Asia. *Health Educ.* **2014**, *114*, 118–132. [CrossRef]
25. Ahikire, J.; Madanda, A. *A Survey on Re-Entry of Pregnant Girls in Primary and Secondary Schools in Uganda*; FAWE: Kampala, Uganda, 2011.
26. Schlecht, J.; Rowley, E.; Babirye, J. Early relationships and marriage in conflict and post-conflict settings: Vulnerability of youth in Uganda. *Reprod. Health Matters* **2013**, *21*, 234–242. [CrossRef]
27. Kirby, D.; Laris, B.A.; Rolleri, L. *Sex and HIV Education Programs for Youth: Their Impact and Important Characteristics*; Family Health International (FHI): Durham, NC, USA, 2006; pp. 1–166.
28. Neema, S.; Musisi, N.; Kibombo, R. *Adolescent Sexual and Reproductive Health in Uganda: A Synthesis of Research Evidence*; Alan Guttmacher Institute: Washington, DC, USA, 2004.
29. Muyinda, H.; Nakuya, J.; Whitworth, J.A.G.; Pool, R. Community sex education among adolescents in rural Uganda: Utilizing indigenous institutions. *AIDS Care Psychol. Socio-Med. Asp. AIDS/HIV* **2004**, *16*, 69–79. [CrossRef] [PubMed]
30. Tamale, S. Eroticism, sensuality and "women's secrets" among the Baganda. *IDS Bull.* **2006**, *37*, 89–97. [CrossRef]
31. Tamale, S. *African Sexualities: A Reader*; Pambazuka Press: Cape Town, South Africa, 2011.
32. Bantebya, G.; Muhanguzi, F.; Watson, C. *Adolescent Girls in the Balance: Changes and Continuity in Social Norms and Practices around Marriage and Education in Uganda*; Overseas Development Institute: London, UK, 2014.
33. Ghimire, A.; Samuels, F. *Changes and Continuity in Social Norms and Practices around Marriage and Education in Uganda*; Overseas Development Institute: London, UK, 2014.
34. Wilhelmsson, T. *What about the Law? A Case Study of the Protective Structures Concerning Young Girls Sexual and Reproductive Health and Rights in Mbarara, Uganda*; Lunds University: Lund, Sweden, 2004.
35. Parikh, S.A. "They arrested me for loving a schoolgirl": Ethnography, HIV, and a feminist assessment of the age of consent law as a gender-based structural intervention in Uganda. *Soc. Sci. Med.* **2012**, *74*, 1774–1782. [CrossRef] [PubMed]
36. Government of Uganda (GoU). *Children (Amendment) Act, 2016*; GoU: Kampala, Uganda, 2016.
37. UBOS. *Uganda National Population and Housing Census Report: Population Growth Rates Non-Household Population and Sex Composition of the Population*; UBOS: Kampala, Uganda, 2014.
38. Strauss, A.; Corbin, J. Basics of qualitative research. In *Basics of Qualitatice Research*, 2nd ed.; SAGE Publishing: Thousand Oaks, CA, USA, 1990; pp. 3–14.

39. De Meyer, S.; Kågesten, A.; Mmari, K.; McEachran, J.; Chilet-Rosell, E.; Kabiru, C.W.; Maina, B.; Jerves, E.M.; Currie, C.; Michielsen, K. Temporary removal: "Boys should have the courage to ask a girl out": Gender norms in early adolescent romantic relationships. *J. Adolesc. Health* **2017**, *61*, S42–S47. [CrossRef] [PubMed]
40. Ngabaza, S.; Shefer, T.; Macleod, C.I. "Girls need to behave like girls you know": The complexities of applying a gender justice goal within sexuality education in South African schools. *Reprod. Health Matters* **2016**, *24*, 71–78. [CrossRef] [PubMed]
41. Timreck, E.; Rogow, D.; Haberland, N. *Addressing Gender and Rights in Your Sex/HIV Education Curriculum: A Starter Checklist*; Population Council: New York, NY, USA, 2007.
42. Varga, C.A. How gender roles influence sexual and reproductive health among South African adolescents. *Stud. Fam. Plan.* **2003**, *34*, 160–172. [CrossRef]
43. Iyer, P.; Aggleton, P. "Sex education should be taught, fine ... but we make sure they control themselves": Teachers' beliefs and attitudes towards young people's sexual and reproductive health in a Ugandan secondary school. *Sex Educ.* **2013**, *13*, 40–53. [CrossRef]

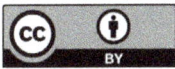

© 2018 by the authors. Licensee MDPI, Basel, Switzerland. This article is an open access article distributed under the terms and conditions of the Creative Commons Attribution (CC BY) license (http://creativecommons.org/licenses/by/4.0/).

International Journal of
Environmental Research and Public Health

MDPI

Article

STI Knowledge in Berlin Adolescents

Frederik Tilmann von Rosen [1,2,*,†], **Antonella Juline von Rosen** [1,2,†],
Falk Müller-Riemenschneider [1,3], **Inken Damberg** [2] **and Peter Tinnemann** [1,4]

[1] Charité—Universitätsmedizin Berlin, Institute for Social Medicine, Epidemiology and Health Economics, 10117 Berlin, Germany; an_pa@uni-bremen.de (A.J.v.R.); falk.mueller-riemenschneider@nuhs.edu.sg (F.M.-R.); peter.tinnemann@charite.de (P.T.)
[2] Institute for Public Health and Nursing Research, University of Bremen, 28359 Bremen, Germany; idamberg@uni-bremen.de
[3] Saw Swee Hock School of Public Health, National University of Singapore, Singapore 117549, Singapore
[4] Akademie für Öffentliches Gesundheitswesen, 40472 Düsseldorf, Germany
* Correspondence: rosen@uni-bremen.de; Tel.: +49-421-89771192
† These authors contributed equally to this work.

Received: 26 November 2017; Accepted: 19 December 2017; Published: 10 January 2018

Abstract: Sexually transmitted infections (STIs) pose a significant threat to individual and public health. They disproportionately affect adolescents and young adults. In a cross-sectional study, we assessed self-rated and factual STI knowledge in a sample of 9th graders in 13 secondary schools in Berlin, Germany. Differences by age, gender, migrant background, and school type were quantified using bivariate and multivariable analyses. A total of 1177 students in 61 classes participated. The mean age was 14.6 (SD = 0.7), 47.5% were female, and 52.9% had at least one immigrant parent. Knowledge of human immunodeficiency virus (HIV) was widespread, but other STIs were less known. For example, 46.2% had never heard of chlamydia, 10.8% knew of the HPV vaccination, and only 2.2% were aware that no cure exists for HPV infection. While boys were more likely to describe their knowledge as good, there was no general gender superiority in factual knowledge. Children of immigrants and students in the least academic schools had lower knowledge overall. Our results show that despite their particular risk to contract an STI, adolescents suffer from suboptimal levels of knowledge on STIs beyond HIV. Urgent efforts needed to improve adolescent STI knowledge in order to improve the uptake of primary and secondary prevention.

Keywords: sexual health; sexually transmitted diseases; sexually transmitted infections; adolescent health; Berlin; Germany

1. Introduction

Sexually transmitted infections (STIs) are a serious public health problem worldwide, with an estimated one million new infections each day [1]. They have a wide range of negative consequences on individual health, ranging from physical discomfort to infertility, malignancy, severe maternal and foetal pregnancy complications, and loss of life [2]. Beyond the detrimental effect on individual health, STIs also represent a significant economic burden. It is estimated that more than ten billion dollars per year are spent on STIs other than human immunodeficiency virus (HIV) in the United States alone [3]. The most frequent viral STI pathogens are human papillomavirus (HPV), herpes simplex virus 2 (HSV-2), HIV, and Hepatitis B. The most widespread bacterial STIs are chlamydia trachomatis, gonorrhoea, and syphilis [4,5].

Although HIV prevalence in Germany is still low compared to most other European countries [6], there has been a marked rise in the number of newly diagnosed cases of HIV resulting from both homosexual and heterosexual intercourse, as well as intravenous drug use over the last five years [7]. An even higher increase in incidence has been observed in other STIs: chlamydia, commonly regarded as the most frequent cause of female infertility in developed countries [8,9], is becoming widespread in Germany [10,11]. The number of newly diagnosed syphilis cases in Germany has risen more than fourfold since 2000 [12,13], and gonorrhoea cases are becoming more widespread, with increasing antibiotic resistance being an additional problem [14,15]. Furthermore, HPV-related neoplasia is a growing problem. For example, vulvar cancer, often linked to an infection with HPV, has greatly increased in Germany over the last decade [16]. HPV is also frequently transmitted in oral and anal sexual practice, causing high rates of local infection of the oropharyngeal and anal regions [17,18]. This is likely to be the cause of the increasing rates of HPV-related neoplasia of the head and neck [19], and of the anus [20].

Despite increasing numbers of new infections with STIs, the limited existing research indicates a considerable ignorance regarding the existence and dangers of STIs other than HIV in Germany. One study found that in a representative sample of adults across Germany, a majority had never heard of syphilis, gonorrhoea, hepatitis, genital herpes, chlamydia, and HPV. Only 6% were aware of HPV and 14% of chlamydia as the two most frequent viral and bacterial STIs [21]. Another study amongst adolescents in two cities in Northern Germany discovered that participants perceive the likelihood of infection with HIV much higher than that of the much more prevalent infection with HPV [22]. Furthermore, adolescents were found to be largely ignorant of the existence of chlamydia, even in an urban setting of particularly high prevalence [23].

One reason for this large-scale ignorance might be that STIs other than HIV escaped the attention of German public health authorities and sexual health educators for a long time. For example, over the last two decades, the Federal Centre for Health Education (Bundeszentrale für gesundheitliche Aufklärung, BZgA) as the national authority for health education and health promotion has launched a multitude of campaigns warning of the risk of HIV, but an awareness campaign for other STIs, such as hepatitis B or chlamydia, was only launched in 2016 [24].

Due to more frequently changing sexual partners and lower rates of correct and consistent contraceptive use, adolescents and young adults are particularly at risk of contracting and transmitting STIs [25–27]. For women it has been argued that, the risk of infection in adolescence or early adulthood is elevated further due to a greater anatomical susceptibility to certain STIs at young age [28,29]. Indeed, studies show a higher incidence of STIs in this age bracket [30–32]. One review estimated that adolescents and young adults account for 50% of new infections with STIs, while representing only 25% of the sexually active population [33]. Young people are also likely to suffer most from long-term sequelae, for example if an infection with an oncogenic type of HPV leads to neoplasia years or decades later [34], or if they experience hypofertility at a later stage caused by untreated infection with chlamydia [35]. Therefore, adolescents can be regarded as a particularly suitable audience for primary and secondary STI prevention.

Condom use is an effective method to prevent infection with an STI [36,37]. Moreover, several STIs can be readily prevented through vaccination (Hepatitis B, HPV) [38,39]. Others, such as chlamydia, gonorrhoea, or syphilis, are curable with appropriate antibiotic regimens, thus enabling the prevention of long-term sequelae [40–42]. However, awareness of the existence and risk of different STIs are prerequisites to actual utilization of preventive and curative options.

Currently, readily available prevention methods are not widely utilized in Germany. One study found that only 39% of boys and 31% of girls used a condom in their last sexual contact [43]. Only 11.3% of women under 25 participated in the recommended chlamydia screening in 2015 [24], and less than a third of girls are vaccinated against HPV at the average age of sexual debut [44]. This is despite the fact that both adolescent HPV vaccination and chlamydia screening are strongly endorsed by German medical bodies and are fully covered by statutory health insurance [45,46].

Considering the limited existing research on adolescent STI knowledge in Germany, we assessed self-reported and factual knowledge on different STIs amongst 9th-graders in Berlin, Germany. Specifically, we assessed the extent to which participants were aware of different STIs and how they self-rated their knowledge. Factual knowledge on STI curability and on the existence of vaccines for STIs was tested. Results could help schools, parents, and other sexual health educators to address particular "areas of need", in order to raise awareness and knowledge amongst a population disproportionately at risk of acquiring STIs.

2. Methods

2.1. Study Design

Data on STI awareness was collected within the framework of a larger survey on the knowledge of sexual health issues amongst Berlin adolescents. Details of the study and its population and methodology have been partially described elsewhere. It was demonstrated that adolescents were ill-informed on the important issue of emergency contraception [47]. Furthermore, adolescents' preferences regarding online sexual health resources were assessed [48]. The survey was conducted throughout the year 2012 in grade nine of secondary schools in Berlin.

The study was conducted with the approval of the Ethics Committee of the Charité-Universitätsmedizin Berlin and the Berlin Senate's Department for Education, Youth and Science. In accordance with Berlin state law, written parental consent was mandatory for all students who had not yet reached 14 years of age, and a favourable vote of the parent-teacher-conference was a prerequisite for a school's participation.

2.2. Sampling and Data Collection

All public secondary schools in Berlin were contacted by telephone and email with in-depth information on the study and a request to include the school in the sample. Schools allocated regular lessons in which the study was conducted using paper questionnaires. Students were informed of the aim of the study and the range of topics addressed. It was pointed out that participation was voluntary and anonymous, and that the survey did not represent a formal school assignment or otherwise affected school grades. Following the collection of questionnaires, students were provided with the correct answers to all knowledge questions.

2.3. Questionnaire

The questionnaire was designed by the authors to assess self-evaluated and actual knowledge on different STIs, amongst other sexual health questions. A pre-test in one school class was conducted and the comments led to minor modifications in the wording of questions.

In the general part of the questionnaire, students were requested to state their age and gender. Furthermore, students were asked to provide their parents' place of birth to assess migratory background. To safeguard parental informational self-determination in accordance with Berlin Senate policy, options were limited to "Germany" and "abroad", and no information on the time of migration was collected.

Furthermore, the variable of school type was coded for each participant to assess the differences between the three types of Berlin secondary schools: the most academically selective type of University-Preparatory Schools (Gymnasium), Comprehensive Secondary Schools (Integrierte Gesamtschule) with the option to qualify for university access, and the least academic school type—Comprehensive Secondary Schools without this option. For clarity, these three school types were reported below as "highest academic tier", "intermediate academic tier", and "lowest academic tier".

In the part on STIs, students were first asked to self-evaluate their knowledge of the seven most frequent bacterial and viral STIs: HIV/AIDS, syphilis, genital herpes, hepatitis B, gonorrhoea, chlamydia, and HPV. A Likert-Scale was employed, with the options to rate knowledge as "good", "rather good", "mediocre", "rather bad", and "bad", and a further option to select "I have never heard of this STI". Furthermore, factual knowledge was tested by asking students to state whether a reliable cure and/or a vaccination exists for the following STIs (correct responses in brackets, according to the current Centers for Disease Control and Prevention (CDC) Guidelines [49]): HIV (no cure, no vaccination), hepatitis B (no cure, vaccination exists), chlamydia (curable, no vaccination), HPV (no cure, vaccination exists), and genital herpes (no cure, no vaccination).

2.4. Statistical Analysis

IBM SPSS Statistics Version 25 (SPSS Inc., Chicago, IL, USA) was employed for data analysis. Frequencies were computed for all items. We used chi-square statistics to test for bivariate relationships between the independent variables gender, migratory background, and school type, and the outcomes of self-reported awareness and knowledge in the factual questions on STIs.

Using multiple regression models, we quantified the effect of demographic variables on outcomes. Since age, gender, migratory background, and academic standing had all been shown to be predictors of sexual health knowledge in different previous studies [50–52], they were maintained as factors in all of the analyses. To account for the possible effect of clustering by school or class, a mixed multilevel regression model (SPSS GENLINMIXED) was employed and school and class included as random effects. Odds ratios and confidence intervals were calculated from regression. For clarity of results, outcome categories were dichotomized for regression. The regression outcome variables were thus "high knowledge" (response either "good" or "rather good" knowledge) on individual STIs, "never heard" for individual STIs, and "correct response" for each of the knowledge questions. Robust estimation was used to take into account possible violations of model assumptions. Missing cases were excluded from statistical analyses.

The Strengthening the Reporting of Observational Studies in Epidemiology (STROBE) statement [53] was followed in the presentation of the methods and results of this study. The statistical methodology used was approved by the Competence Center for Clinical Trials of the University of Bremen.

The original dataset of the study cannot be made available to the general public due to the constraints placed on data availability by the Berlin Senate's Department for Education, Youth and Science. The dataset can be obtained upon reasonable request from the corresponding author.

3. Results

3.1. Study Participants

We successfully contacted the heads of the biology departments in 142 out of 287 schools. Subsequently, 13 schools with a total of 61 ninth grade classes agreed to participate. The limited time to teach the demanding state curriculum was most frequently given as the reason for non-participation.

Participating schools hailed from seven of the twelve Berlin City Districts (Mitte, Pankow, Charlottenburg-Wilmersdorf, Spandau, Steglitz-Zehlendorf, Treptow-Köpenick, and Marzahn-Hellersdorf) and included very diverse settings. Schools in former East and West Berlin were included, as were schools from inner-city to suburban, and from the most wealthy to relatively impoverished city areas [54].

During the lessons that were allocated by participating schools, 1190 students were in attendance. Ten students aged 13 failed to provide parental consent and could thus not participate. Two students elected not to take part, and one very recently arrived immigrant was unable to read German. Thus, a total of 1177 students participated.

Of participants providing gender information, 547 were female (46.5%) and 605 (51.4%) were male. Age ranged from 13 to 16 years, with a mean age of participants of 14.6 (SD 0.8). For migratory background, 544 (46.2%) had two German-born parents, 260 (22.5%) participants reported one, and 352 (30.4%) two parents of foreign birth. Participants were virtually equally spread across the three school types, with 390 (33.1%) participants attending a school of the lowest, 395 (33.6%) of the intermediate, and 392 (33.3%) of the highest academic tier.

3.2. Self-Reported STI Knowledge

Self-evaluated knowledge regarding the most widespread bacterial and viral STIs, sorted in order of decreasing awareness is shown in Table 1. This order will be followed in subsequent tables. HIV was known to virtually all participants, with many stating good or rather good knowledge. Knowledge and awareness were visibly lower for other STIs, of which the most frequently known infection was hepatitis B. Despite being the bacterial STI with the highest prevalence, chlamydia was the infection with the lowest proportion of participants claiming good knowledge and the lowest rate of awareness.

Table 1. Self-rated knowledge of sexually transmitted infections (STIs) in order of decreasing awareness.

STI	Self-Rated Knowledge					
	Good n (%)	Rather Good n (%)	Mediocre n (%)	Rather Bad n (%)	Bad n (%)	Never Heard n (%)
HIV n = 1148 *	438 (38.2%)	379 (33.0%)	217 (18.9%)	58 (5.1%)	39 (3.4%)	17 (1.5%)
Hepatitis B n = 1136 *	142 (12.5%)	170 (15.0%)	292 (25.7%)	231 (20.3%)	150 (13.2%)	151 (13.3%)
Genital herpes n = 1130 *	109 (9.7%)	129 (11.4%)	264 (23.4%)	219 (19.4%)	143 (12.7%)	266 (23.5%)
Syphilis n = 1131 *	80 (7.1%)	129 (11.4%)	238 (21.0%)	188 (16.6%)	116 (10.3%)	380 (33.6%)
HPV n = 1129 *	66 (5.9%)	82 (7.3%)	163 (14.4%)	218 (19.3%)	178 (15.8%)	422 (37.4%)
Gonorrhoea n = 1125 *	84 (7.5%)	76 (6.8%)	170 (15.1%)	173 (15.4%)	141 (12.5%)	481 (42.8%)
Chlamydia n = 1134 *	63 (5.6%)	71 (6.3%)	154 (13.6%)	174 (15.3%)	148 (13.1%)	6.2%)

* number of responses included.

Distribution of self-evaluated knowledge by gender is shown in Table 2. Association between gender and reported knowledge was statistically significant for all STIs, except for hepatitis B and chlamydia. Female respondents reported lower knowledge and were more likely to state complete lack of awareness for each of the STIs apart from chlamydia. While chlamydia was the STI with the lowest awareness overall and amongst male participants, gonorrhoea was the infection least known to girls in the sample.

Table 2. Self-rated knowledge by gender.

STI	Gender	Self-Rated Knowledge						p (from χ^2)
		Good	Rather Good	Mediocre	Rather Bad	Bad	Never Heard	
HIV	female	32.0%	35.1%	22.6%	5.5%	3.9%	0.9%	0.001
n = 1134 *	male	43.3%	31.0%	15.9%	4.7%	3.0%	2.0%	
Hepatitis B	female	11.3%	15.6%	25.6%	21.2%	13.2%	13.2%	0.96
n = 1122 *	male	12.9%	14.6%	25.9%	20.0%	13.2%	13.4%	
Genital herpes	female	6.8%	9.7%	23.7%	20.6%	13.1%	26.1%	0.03
n = 1116 *	male	11.4%	13.1%	23.1%	18.5%	12.2%	21.6%	
Syphilis	female	5.1%	8.1%	19.4%	16.0%	11.1%	40.3%	<0.001
n = 1117 *	male	8.2%	14.3%	22.7%	17.4%	9.2%	28.2%	
HPV	female	3.8%	5.3%	14.0%	19.8%	15.5%	41.6%	0.01
n = 1116 *	male	7.2%	9.2%	14.8%	19.1%	15.8%	33.9%	
Gonorrhoea	female	4.2%	6.2%	12.5%	15.7%	13.4%	48.0%	<0.001
n = 1112 *	male	9.6%	7.4%	17.5%	15.4%	11.7%	38.4%	
Chlamydia	female	5.8%	6.2%	11.6%	17.1%	13.1%	46.2%	0.45
n = 1121 *	male	4.8%	6.5%	15.1%	14.1%	12.9%	46.6%	

* number of responses included.

A table of differences by gender, migrant status and school type of participants who selected the "never heard of" option for the presented STIs can be found in Supplementary File 1. Students from the intermediate tier of schools were generally least likely to have never heard of the different STIs.

Students of two foreign-born parents were most likely to be fully unaware of the existence of all STIs, bar hepatitis B.

3.3. Factors Associated with Self-Reported STI Knowledge in Multivariable Analysis

Table 3 depicts the results of the regression model for high self-evaluated knowledge. For all STIs bar hepatitis B and chlamydia, female respondents were significantly less likely to evaluate their knowledge as "good" or "rather good".

Table 3. Factors associated with high self-evaluated knowledge in multivariable analysis.

Variable	HIV n = 1127 **	Hepatitis B n = 1115 **	Genital Herpes n = 1109 **	Syphilis n = 1110 **
	OR (95% CI)	OR (95% CI)	OR (95% CI)	OR (95% CI)
Age (per year increase)	1.00 (0.83–1.19)	1.12 (0.89–1.41)	1.23 (0.92–1.66)	1.20 (0.83–1.74)
Female Gender *	0.71 (0.52–0.97) ***	1.03 (0.73–1.45)	0.65 (0.51–0.82) ***	0.55 (0.4–0.75) ***
Migratory Background *	0.58 (0.45–0.74) ***	0.96 (0.75–1.23)	1.04 (0.71–1.51)	0.69 (0.49–0.97) ***
Intermediate School Tier *	1.51 (0.72–3.17)	0.92 (0.76–1.10)	1.62 (0.59–4.43)	1.30 (0.66–2.55)
Highest School Tier *	1.13 (0.51–2.50)	0.66 (0.44–0.98) ***	0.66 (0.25–1.74)	1.19 (0.59–2.40)

Variable	HPV n = 1109 **	Gonorrhoea n = 1106 **	Chlamydia n = 1114 **
	OR (95% CI)	OR (95% CI)	OR (95% CI)
Age (per year increase)	1.20 (0.87–1.65)	1.41 (1.07–1.86) ***	0.97 (0.72–1.32)
Female Gender *	0.56 (0.40–0.78) ***	0.65 (0.43–0.99) ***	1.15 (0.69–1.91)
Migratory Background *	1.05 (0.78–1.43)	0.77 (0.5–1.21)	0.89 (0.57–1.39)
Intermediate School Tier *	1.12 (0.54–2.33)	0.69 (0.33–1.43)	1.09 (0.60–1.99)
Highest School Tier *	0.44 (0.22–0.88) ***	0.58 (0.28–1.21)	0.44 (0.23–0.82) ***

OR: Odds ratio; CI: Confidence interval; * Reference categories are male gender, no migrant background, and lowest school tier. ** number of participants included in the regression model; *** $p < 0.05$.

The results of the regression model for the outcome of "unawareness" of the different STIs are presented in Table 4. While there were no significant differences for HIV, hepatitis B, and chlamydia, female students were significantly more likely to have never heard of HPV, syphilis, and gonorrhoea. Students with an immigrant background were more likely to have never heard of genital herpes and syphilis.

Table 4. Factors associated with unawareness of STIs in multivariable analysis.

Variable	HIV n = 1127 **	Hepatitis B n = 1115 **	Genital Herpes n = 1109 **	Syphilis n = 1110 **
	OR (95% CI)	OR (95% CI)	OR (95% CI)	OR (95% CI)
Age (per year increase)	0.96 (0.70–1.32)	0.92 (0.66–1.28)	0.86 (0.67–1.11)	0.87 (0.68–1.11)
Female Gender *	0.88 (0.65–1.19)	1.00 (0.61–1.65)	1.27 (0.85–1.92)	1.74 (1.37–2.22) ***
Migratory Background *	1.34 (0.96–1.88)	1.48 (0.87–2.51)	1.95 (1.52–2.49) ***	1.70 (1.08–2.67) ***
Intermediate School Tier *	0.61 (0.34–1.08)	0.81 (0.30–2.19)	0.47 (0.19–1.19)	0.63 (0.39–1.01)
Highest School Tier *	0.66 (0.36–1.24)	1.08 (0.48–2.42)	0.97 (0.42–2.24)	0.91 (0.52–1.56)

Variable	HPV n = 1109 **	Gonorrhoea n = 1106 **	Chlamydia n = 1114 **
	OR (95% CI)	OR (95% CI)	OR (95% CI)
Age (per year increase)	0.95 (0.78–1.16)	0.77 (0.60–0.997) ***	0.85 (0.66–1.10)
Female Gender *	1.29 (1.01–1.66) ***	1.39 (1.02–1.91) ***	0.92 (0.66–1.28)
Migratory Background *	1.4 (0.94–2.09)	1.49 (0.98–2.26)	1.44 (0.94–2.20)
Intermediate School Tier *	0.83 (0.38–1.85)	1.11 (0.49–2.47)	0.73 (0.44–1.18)
Highest School Tier *	1.78 (0.78–4.08)	1.33 (0.64–2.78)	1.33 (0.83–2.11)

OR: Odds ratio; CI: Confidence interval; * Reference categories are male gender, no migrant background, and lowest school tier. ** number of participants included in the regression model; *** $p < 0.05$.

3.4. Factual STI-Knowledge

3.4.1. Bivariate Analyses

Correct response rates to the knowledge questions on the curability and existence of vaccines for STIs are presented in Table 5. While it was widely known that no reliable cure has been found for HIV to date, knowledge was much lower regarding the curability of other STIs. For vaccination, again a majority knew that no vaccination protects from HIV, and slightly less than half knew that a vaccination exists for hepatitis B. Knowledge was low for the other STIs, and only 10.8% of participants were aware of the existence of an HPV vaccine.

Table 5. Correct answers on STI cures and vaccinations.

Question	Correct Response	n (%) Correct
HIV cure (n = 1131 *)	no reliable cure	946 (83.6%)
Hepatitis B cure (n = 1122 *)	no reliable cure	245 (21.8%)
Genital herpes cure (n = 1121 *)	no reliable cure	88 (7.9%)
HPV cure (n = 1126 *)	no reliable cure	25 (2.2%)
Chlamydia cure (n = 1125 *)	cure exists	212 (18.8%)
HIV vaccination (n = 1133 *)	no vaccination	716 (63.2%)
Hepatitis B vaccination (n = 1134 *)	vaccination exists	552 (48.7%)
Genital herpes vaccination (n = 1125 *)	no vaccination	200 (17.8%)
HPV vaccination (n = 1133 *)	vaccination exists	122 (10.8%)
Chlamydia vaccination (n = 1130 *)	no vaccination	113 (10.0%)

* number of responses included.

Results by gender varied depending on the STI and there was no trend suggesting general knowledge superiority of either gender. While awareness of the HPV vaccine was low overall, it was significantly higher among boys than girls.

Students with migratory background overall tended to have lower rates of correct responses. For example, of students with two German-born parents, 370 out of 528 (70.1%) were aware that no vaccination was available for HIV and 463 out of 529 (87.5%) knew that HIV could not reliably be cured. Corresponding numbers with both parents born abroad were 177/343 (51.6%) for vaccination and 252/339 (74.3%) for curability (p (from χ^2) <0.001 and <0.001). While association was not significant for most STIs, lower proportions of children of immigrants selected the correct response on all of the questions but on curative options for HPV and genital herpes. A table with STI knowledge by migratory background can be found in Supplementary File 2.

For all questions bar on the curability of infection with HPV, it was students from the intermediate academic tier of schools who had the highest rate of correct responses. There was no clear knowledge difference between students from the lowest or the highest tier of schools. The full results for knowledge differences by school type can be found in Supplementary File 3.

3.4.2. Multivariable Analyses

Multivariate analysis was performed for the questions on curability and vaccination options for HIV, Hepatitis B, HPV, genital herpes, and chlamydia. The dichotomous outcome categories were "correct response" vs. "other response". Results are presented in Table 6.

Table 7 shows the results from the multivariable regression model for the outcome variable of correct responses on cure and vaccination questions. As in bivariate analyses, autochthonous German students were more likely to know the lack of curative and vaccination options for HIV, as were students from the intermediate tier of schools. Male students were again significantly more likely to know that a vaccination exists for HPV.

Table 6. Correct answers on STI cures and vaccinations by gender.

Question	Gender	Percentage Correct	p (from χ^2)
HIV cure	male	82.5%	0.29
n = 1116 *	female	85.0%	
Hepatitis B cure	male	24.4%	0.03
n = 1108 *	female	19.0%	
Genital herpes cure	male	11.0%	<0.001
n = 1107 *	female	4.2%	
HPV cure	male	2.6%	0.41
n = 1113 *	female	1.7%	
Chlamydia cure	male	18.3%	0.76
n = 1112 *	female	19.1%	
HIV vaccination	male	66.8%	0.02
n = 1119 *	female	59.8%	
Hepatitis B vaccination	male	45.5%	0.02
n = 1120 *	female	52.4%	
Genital herpes vaccination	male	17.4%	0.70
n = 1111 *	female	18.3%	
HPV vaccination	male	12.9%	0.01
n = 1119 *	female	7.9%	
Chlamydia vaccination	male	8.8%	0.23
n = 1116 *	female	11.0%	

* number of responses included.

Table 7. Factors associated with correct responses on cure and vaccination questions.

Variable	HIV n = 1109 * OR (95% CI)	Hepatitis B n = 1101 * OR (95% CI)	Genital Herpes n = 1100 * OR (95% CI)	HPV n = 1106 * OR (95% CI)	Chlamydia n = 1105 * OR (95% CI)
Age (per year increase)	1.00 (0.82–1.22)	1.23 (0.94–1.61)	1.14 (0.90–1.45)	1.02 (0.86–1.22)	1.29 (1.08–1.54) **
Female Gender *	1.14 (0.82–1.58)	0.93 (0.71–1.22)	0.37 (0.22–0.61) **	0.91 (0.68–1.21)	1.13 (0.83–1.52)
Migratory Background *	0.73 (0.47–1.12)	0.82 (0.53–1.28)	1.22 (0.82–1.81)	1.50 (1.06–2.12) **	0.86 (0.65–1.14)
Intermediate School Tier *	3.14 (1.56–6.29) **	1.55 (1.02–2.34) **	1.89 (0.79–4.55)	0.98 (0.55–1.77)	1.62 (1.16–2.26) **
Highest School Tier *	2.32 (1.11–4.84) **	1.43 (0.88–2.32)	0.41 (0.13–1.29)	0.83 (0.57–1.22)	1.05 (0.60–1.83)

Variable	HIV n = 1112 * OR (95% CI)	Hepatitis B n = 1113 * OR (95% CI)	Genital Herpes n = 1104 * OR (95% CI)	HPV n = 1109 * OR (95% CI)	Chlamydia n = 1109 * OR (95% CI)
Age (per year increase)	1.10 (0.98–1.25)	1.07 (0.89–1.27)	1.13 (0.86–1.49)	1.29 (0.93–1.79)	1.14 (0.88–1.47)
Female Gender *	0.70 (0.47–1.04)	1.30 (0.99–1.70)	1.09 (0.80–1.47)	0.60 (0.41–0.88) **	1.24 (0.94–1.64)
Migratory Background *	0.61 (0.43–0.88) **	0.82 (0.69–0.98)	0.75 (0.53–1.07)	0.74 (0.45–1.23)	0.71 (0.47–1.07)
Intermediate School Tier *	2.59 (1.71–3.94) **	1.31 (0.83–2.07)	1.61 (0.79–3.29)	1.77 (1.10–2.87) **	1.88 (1.34–2.63) **
Highest School Tier *	1.70 (1.01–2.86) **	1.14 (0.77–1.68)	1.12 (0.43–2.92)	0.65 (0.29–1.46)	1.12 (0.72–1.73)

OR: Odds ratio; CI: Confidence interval; * number of participants included in the regression model; ** $p < 0.05$.

4. Discussion

We measured self-rated and factual knowledge regarding different STIs in the framework of a cross-sectional study assessing the sexual health knowledge of Berlin adolescents. We encountered a high participation rate (1177/1179) despite the explicit emphasis on the voluntary nature of participation. It was assessed whether students had heard of different STIs, how they would describe their own knowledge, and whether they were able to state which STIs were curable and for which a vaccination exists.

With a mean participant age of 14.6 years, population-level data suggests that a majority of adolescents in our study had already experienced some form of sexual contact or intimacy, although most have not engaged in penetrative sexual intercourse [43]. Across Germany, the mean age of sexual debut is 14.9 years for female and 15.1 years for male adolescents [55].

As expected, nearly all of the students had heard of HIV, and a majority rated their knowledge as (rather) good and knew that HIV could neither be cured nor vaccinated against. However, overall knowledge for other STIs was much less satisfactory, with low self-reported knowledge and high levels of ignorance regarding individual STIs. For example, more than 46% of participants had never heard of chlamydia and merely 18% knew that chlamydia can be cured. This widespread lack of knowledge is in line with previous studies in Germany on both adolescents and the population at large [21,22]. Results from adolescents in South-East England point towards a similar level of ignorance [56], whereas Swedish studies show between 86% [57] and 96% [58] of adolescents to be aware of chlamydia. This lack of awareness that is shown by our study is particularly noteworthy given the fact that chlamydia is the most frequent bacterial STI [4], has a particularly high incidence among adolescents and young adults [59,60], and is a frequent reason for infertility later in life [9]. Despite the ready and cost-free availability of chlamydia screening and treatment to German adolescents, our results show the target population is hardly aware of the disease's existence.

Another STI for which there was a widespread lack of knowledge was HPV. Despite being the STI with the highest prevalence [4], more than a third of students responded to have never heard of it, and fewer than 13% described high knowledge. Results for the factual questions were dire, with less than 2.2% of respondents knowing that there is currently no treatment to cure HPV infection, and that the HPV vaccine is only known to 10.8% of respondents. This is visibly lower than the rates that are found amongst adolescents in a previous study in Germany [51] and in other European countries [61–63]. In contrast to these previous studies, the male participants in our sample were significantly more likely to be aware of the HPV vaccine, shown both in bivariate and regression analysis. This is especially surprising given that the HPV vaccine is primarily marketed to a female audience in Germany: in all German states except for Saxony, HPV vaccination is exclusively recommended for female adolescents [64], and only few statutory health insurance providers cover male HPV vaccination [65].

Condoms can prevent infection with STIs. However, their use requires motivation. Research shows that adolescents regard condoms primarily as a method to prevent pregnancy. If STI prevention is considered at all, it is mainly the risk of HIV that is taken into account [56,66]. However, most sexually active adolescents in Germany rely on hormonal methods of contraception to prevent pregnancy, with only a minority employing condoms instead or concurrently [43]. HIV, due to its low prevalence in Germany, is unlikely to be an effective motivator for condom use, at least in heterosexual intercourse. Our results show, that other STIs—most of which are much more prevalent than HIV—are relatively little known to adolescents. This lack of knowledge is likely to diminish motivation to use condoms and/or access other methods of STI prevention, both primary (such as HPV or hepatitis B vaccination) and secondary (such as Pap tests or chlamydia screening). If adolescents and young adults are to make a truly informed choice on the uptake of preventive options, the level of STI awareness and knowledge needs to be improved.

In our results, for most STIs, even groups that are usually shown to have superior sexual health proficiency (such as female adolescents, the academically-advantaged, and non-ethnic minority students [43,51,67,68]) have only non-satisfactory knowledge. We regard this as indicative that schools, parents, primary care physicians, public health authorities, and other providers of sexual health information fail to communicate the most basic facts about STIs beyond HIV, even to the most accessible population groups. The recent launch of the first (non-HIV) STI awareness campaign by the BZgA is a much needed initiative towards improving STI knowledge. However, in a country with compulsory school education, we regard schools as the most promising vector to multiply relevant health information and reach virtually all adolescents. For this, it is imperative that STIs and STI prevention are explicitly included in the school curriculum. The current state curriculum in Berlin, unfortunately, falls short in this respect Condoms are the only prevention method, and "HIV/AIDS" the sole STI specifically included in the curriculum [69]. Comprehensive teacher-delivered school tuition on STIs and preventive instruments could address the widespread information gap that is highlighted by our study, as could the co-optation of external providers of STI prevention education into schools [70].

Beyond schools, STI information can—and should—also be spread through other means, for example through healthcare professionals [71], social media channels [72], mass media campaigns [73], and through peer education programmes [74]. A multidimensional approach combining different channels of access to adolescents bears the promise to improve STI knowledge, and thus potentially curtail the increasing rates of new infections and lower the rate of long-term sequelae of infection.

Strengths and Limitations

The relatively large number of participants from a sample of schools of all three types of Berlin public schools represents a strength of the study, as does the virtually complete rate of participation.

Only 13 out of a total of 287 eligible schools, however, took part in the study. Despite schools hailing from very diverse social and geographical settings, there might be a systemic difference between participating and non-participating schools, for example in terms of the teaching bodies' interest and openness regarding sexual health education.

Furthermore, students were asked to evaluate their knowledge regarding STIs on a multiple choice questionnaire, which might have led to the over-reporting of knowledge as compared to a questionnaire in which participants were to list STIs in an open question.

5. Conclusions

Sexually transmitted infections pose a serious threat to individual as well as public health. Despite different effective instruments of primary and secondary prevention being readily available, their uptake is impeded by widespread lack of knowledge. This is especially true for adolescents and young adults, an age group that is particularly at risk of contracting an STI. Our study shows that across demographic divides, adolescents in Berlin, Germany suffer from a low level of knowledge on all of the most frequent STIs apart from HIV, despite their growing incidence. It is crucial that this lack of knowledge is addressed and that adolescents are educated on the threats that are posed by different infections, and on the existing and readily available methods to prevent, detect, and cure STIs. Knowledge is a necessary prerequisite to making an informed choice regarding STI prevention, screening, and treatment and schools as well as health information providers need to address current knowledge deficits.

Supplementary Materials: The following are available online at www.mdpi.com/1660-4601/15/1/110/s1, Supplementary File 1: lack of awareness of STIs by gender, migrant background, and school type, Supplementary File 2: Correct answers on STI cures and vaccinations by migrant background, Supplementary File 3: Correct answers on STI cures and vaccinations by school type.

Acknowledgments: This study is part of a project to improve adolescent sexual health, partially funded by a grant from the German Federal Ministry of Education and Research. The funding sponsor had no role in the design of the study; in the collection, analyses, or interpretation of data; in the writing of the manuscript, and in the decision to publish the results. We acknowledge support from the German Research Foundation (DFG) and the Open Access Publication Fund of the University of Bremen.

Author Contributions: F.T.v.R. and A.J.v.R. contributed equally to this work.

Conflicts of Interest: The authors declare no conflicts of interest.

References

1. World Health Organization. Sexually Transmitted Infections (STIs). Available online: http://www.who.int/mediacentre/factsheets/fs110/en/ (accessed on 20 September 2017).
2. World Health Organization. Global Health Sector Strategy on Sexually Transmitted Infections, 2016–2021. Available online: http://www.who.int/reproductivehealth/publications/rtis/ghss-stis/en/ (accessed on 20 September 2017).
3. Institute of Medicine; Committee on Prevention and Control of Sexually Transmitted Diseases. *The Hidden Epidemic: Confronting Sexually Transmitted Diseases*; Butler, W.T., Eng, T.R., Eds.; National Academies Press: Washington, DC, USA, 1997; ISBN 978-0-309-05495-9.

4. National Prevention Information Network. Incidence, Prevalence, and Cost of Sexually Transmitted Infections in the United States. Available online: https://npin.cdc.gov/publication/incidence-prevalence-and-cost-sexually-transmitted-infections-united-states (accessed on 20 September 2017).
5. Schmidt-Petruschkat, S. Allgemeine Gynäkologie. Zunahme von Geschlechtskrankheiten in Deutschland—Ein bislang unbeachtetes Risiko? *Geburtshilfe Frauenheilkd.* **2009**, *69*, 429–432. [CrossRef]
6. Murray, C.J.L.; Ortblad, K.F.; Guinovart, C.; Lim, S.S.; Wolock, T.M.; Roberts, D.A.; Dansereau, E.A.; Graetz, N.; Barber, R.M.; Brown, J.C.; et al. Global, regional, and national incidence and mortality for HIV, tuberculosis, and malaria during 1990–2013: A systematic analysis for the Global Burden of Disease Study 2013. *Lancet* **2014**, *384*, 1005–1070. [CrossRef]
7. Robert Koch-Institut. Archiv 2016—Schätzung der Zahl der HIV-Neuinfektionen und der Gesamtzahl von Menschen mit HIV in Deutschland. Available online: https://www.rki.de/DE/Content/Infekt/EpidBull/Archiv/2016/45/Art_01.html (accessed on 17 July 2017).
8. Mårdh, P.-A. Tubal factor infertility, with special regard to chlamydial salpingitis. *Curr. Opin. Infect. Dis.* **2004**, *17*, 49–52. [CrossRef] [PubMed]
9. Westrom, L.V. Chlamydia and its effect on reproduction. *J. Br. Fertil. Soc.* **1996**, *1*, 23–30.
10. Griesinger, G.; Gille, G.; Klapp, C.; von Otte, S.; Diedrich, K. Sexual behaviour and Chlamydia trachomatis infections in German female urban adolescents, 2004. *Clin. Microbiol. Infect.* **2007**, *13*, 436–439. [CrossRef] [PubMed]
11. Stock, C.; Guillén-Grima, F.; Prüfer-Krämer, L.; Serrano-Monzo, I.; Marin-Fernandez, B.; Aguinaga-Ontoso, I.; Krämer, A. Sexual behavior and the prevalence of Chlamydia trachomatis infection in asymptomatic students in Germany and Spain. *Eur. J. Epidemiol.* **2001**, *17*, 385–390. [CrossRef] [PubMed]
12. Robert Koch-Institut. Epidemisches Bulletin 44/2013. Available online: https://www.rki.de/DE/Content/Infekt/EpidBull/Archiv/2013/Ausgaben/44_13.pdf (accessed on 17 September 2017).
13. Jansen, K.; Schmidt, A.J.; Drewes, J.; Bremer, V.; Marcus, U. Increased incidence of syphilis in men who have sex with men and risk management strategies, Germany, 2015. *Eurosurveillance* **2016**, *21*. [CrossRef] [PubMed]
14. Abraham, S.; Poehlmann, C.; Spornraft-Ragaller, P. Gonorrhea: Data on antibiotic resistance and accompanying infections at the University Hospital Dresden over a 10-year time period. *J. Dtsch. Dermatol. Ges. J. Ger.* **2013**, *11*, 241–249. [CrossRef] [PubMed]
15. Regnath, T.; Mertes, T.; Ignatius, R. Antimicrobial resistance of Neisseria gonorrhoeae isolates in south-west Germany, 2004 to 2015: Increasing minimal inhibitory concentrations of tetracycline but no resistance to third-generation cephalosporins. *Eurosurveillance* **2016**, *21*. [CrossRef] [PubMed]
16. Holleczek, B.; Sehouli, J.; Barinoff, J. Vulvar cancer in Germany: Increase in incidence and change in tumour biological characteristics from 1974 to 2013. *Acta Oncol.* **2017**, 1–7. [CrossRef] [PubMed]
17. Ciccarese, G.; Herzum, A.; Rebora, A.; Drago, F. Prevalence of genital, oral, and anal HPV infection among STI patients in Italy. *J. Med. Virol.* **2017**, *89*, 1121–1124. [CrossRef] [PubMed]
18. Drago, F.; Herzum, A.; Ciccarese, G.; Bandelloni, R. Prevalence of oral human papillomavirus in men attending an Italian sexual health clinic. *Sex. Health* **2016**, *13*, 597–598. [CrossRef] [PubMed]
19. Tanaka, T.I.; Alawi, F. Human Papillomavirus and Oropharyngeal Cancer. *Dent. Clin. N. Am.* **2018**, *62*, 111–120. [CrossRef] [PubMed]
20. Lin, C.; Franceschi, S.; Clifford, G.M. Human papillomavirus types from infection to cancer in the anus, according to sex and HIV status: A systematic review and meta-analysis. *Lancet Infect. Dis.* **2017**. [CrossRef]
21. Bundeszentrale für Gesundheitliche Aufklärung. AIDS im Öffentlichen Bewusstsein der Bundesrepublik Deutschland 2016. Available online: https://www.infodienst.bzga.de/?id=teaserext2.13&idx=7018 (accessed on 27 September 2017).
22. Samkange-Zeeb, F.; Pöttgen, S.; Zeeb, H. Higher risk perception of HIV than of chlamydia and HPV among secondary school students in two German cities. *PLoS ONE* **2013**, *8*, e61636. [CrossRef] [PubMed]
23. Gille, G.; Klapp, C.; Diedrich, K. Chlamydien—Eine Heimliche Epidemie unter Jugendlichen Prävalenzbeobachtung bei Jungen Mädchen in Berlin (18 July 2005). Available online: http://www.aerzteblatt.de/archiv/47702 (accessed on 30 December 2012).
24. Bremer, V.; Dudareva-Vizule, S.; Buder, S.; an der Heiden, M.; Jansen, K. Sexuell übertragbare Infektionen in Deutschland. *Bundesgesundheitsblatt Gesundheitsforschung Gesundheitsschutz* **2017**, *60*, 948–957. [CrossRef] [PubMed]

25. Kan, M.L.; Cheng, Y.A.; Landale, N.S.; McHale, S.M. Longitudinal Predictors of Change in Number of Sexual Partners across Adolescence and Early Adulthood. *J. Adolesc. Health* **2010**, *46*, 25–31. [CrossRef] [PubMed]

26. Santelli, J.S.; Brener, N.D.; Lowry, R.; Bhatt, A.; Zabin, L.S. Multiple Sexual Partners among U.S. Adolescents and Young Adults. *Fam. Plan. Perspect.* **1998**, *30*, 271–275. [CrossRef]

27. Panatto, D.; Amicizia, D.; Lugarini, J.; Sasso, T.; Sormani, M.P.; Badolati, G.; Gasparini, R. Sexual behaviour in Ligurian (Northern Italy) adolescents and young people: Suggestions for HPV vaccination policies. *Vaccine* **2009**, *27*, A6–A10. [CrossRef] [PubMed]

28. Hwang, L.Y.; Ma, Y.; Benningfield, S.M.; Clayton, L.; Hanson, E.N.; Jay, J.; Jonte, J.; Godwin de Medina, C.; Moscicki, A.-B. Factors that influence the rate of epithelial maturation in the cervix in healthy young women. *J. Adolesc. Health* **2009**, *44*, 103–110. [CrossRef] [PubMed]

29. Lee, V.; Foley, E.; Tobin, J.M. Relationship of cervical ectopy to chlamydia infection in young women. *J. Fam. Plan. Reprod. Health Care* **2006**, *32*, 104–106. [CrossRef] [PubMed]

30. Bremer, D.V.; Hofmann, A.; Hamouda, O. Epidemiologie der Chlamydia-trachomatis-Infektionen. *Hautarzt* **2007**, *58*, 18–23. [CrossRef] [PubMed]

31. Fortenberry, J.D. Unveiling the Hidden Epidemic of Sexually Transmitted Diseases. *JAMA J. Am. Med. Assoc.* **2002**, *287*, 768–769. [CrossRef]

32. Kraut, A.A.; Schink, T.; Schulze-Rath, R.; Mikolajczyk, R.T.; Garbe, E. Incidence of anogenital warts in Germany: A population-based cohort study. *BMC Infect. Dis.* **2010**, *10*, 360. [CrossRef] [PubMed]

33. Siracusano, S.; Silvestri, T.; Casotto, D. Sexually transmitted diseases: Epidemiological and clinical aspects in adults. *Urologia* **2014**, *81*, 200–208. [CrossRef] [PubMed]

34. McCredie, M.R.E.; Sharples, K.J.; Paul, C.; Baranyai, J.; Medley, G.; Jones, R.W.; Skegg, D.C.G. Natural history of cervical neoplasia and risk of invasive cancer in women with cervical intraepithelial neoplasia 3: A retrospective cohort study. *Lancet Oncol.* **2008**, *9*, 425–434. [CrossRef]

35. Land, J.A.; Van Bergen, J.E.A.M.; Morré, S.A.; Postma, M.J. Epidemiology of Chlamydia trachomatis infection in women and the cost-effectiveness of screening. *Hum. Reprod. Update* **2010**, *16*, 189–204. [CrossRef] [PubMed]

36. Centers for Disease Control and Prevention (CDC). Update: Barrier protection against HIV infection and other sexually transmitted diseases. *MMWR Morb. Mortal. Wkly. Rep.* **1993**, *42*, 589–591, 597.

37. Pierce Campbell, C.M.; Lin, H.-Y.; Fulp, W.; Papenfuss, M.R.; Salmerón, J.J.; Quiterio, M.M.; Lazcano-Ponce, E.; Villa, L.L.; Giuliano, A.R. Consistent condom use reduces the genital human papillomavirus burden among high-risk men: The HPV infection in men study. *J. Infect. Dis.* **2013**, *208*, 373–384. [CrossRef] [PubMed]

38. Peto, T.J.; Mendy, M.E.; Lowe, Y.; Webb, E.L.; Whittle, H.C.; Hall, A.J. Efficacy and effectiveness of infant vaccination against chronic hepatitis B in the Gambia Hepatitis Intervention Study (1986–1990) and in the nationwide immunisation program. *BMC Infect. Dis.* **2014**, *14*, 7. [CrossRef] [PubMed]

39. Herweijer, E.; Sundström, K.; Ploner, A.; Uhnoo, I.; Sparén, P.; Arnheim-Dahlström, L. Quadrivalent HPV vaccine effectiveness against high-grade cervical lesions by age at vaccination: A population-based study. *Int. J. Cancer* **2016**, *138*, 2867–2874. [CrossRef] [PubMed]

40. Geisler, W.M.; Uniyal, A.; Lee, J.Y.; Lensing, S.Y.; Johnson, S.; Perry, R.C.W.; Kadrnka, C.M.; Kerndt, P.R. Azithromycin versus Doxycycline for Urogenital Chlamydia trachomatis Infection. *N. Engl. J. Med.* **2015**, *373*, 2512–2521. [CrossRef] [PubMed]

41. Kerani, R.P.; Stenger, M.R.; Weinstock, H.; Bernstein, K.T.; Reed, M.; Schumacher, C.; Samuel, M.C.; Eaglin, M.; Golden, M. Gonorrhea treatment practices in the STD Surveillance Network, 2010–2012. *Sex. Transm. Dis.* **2015**, *42*, 6–12. [CrossRef] [PubMed]

42. Clement, M.E.; Okeke, N.L.; Hicks, C.B. Treatment of Syphilis: A Systematic Review. *JAMA* **2014**, *312*, 1905–1917. [CrossRef] [PubMed]

43. Heßling, A. *Youth Sexuality 2010: Repeat Survey of 14 to 17-Year-Olds and Their Parents*; Bundeszentrale für Gesundheitliche Aufklärung (BZgA): Cologne, Germany, 2010; ISBN 978-3-937707-80-8.

44. Robert Koch-Institut. Archiv 2017—Aktuelles aus der KV-Impfsurveillance: Impfquoten der Rotavirus-, Masern-, HPV- und Influenza-Impfung in Deutschland. Available online: https://www.rki.de/DE/Content/Infekt/EpidBull/Archiv/2017/01/Art_01.html (accessed on 6 September 2017).

45. Mund, M.; Sander, G.; Potthoff, P.; Schicht, H.; Matthias, K. Introduction of Chlamydia trachomatis screening for young women in Germany. *JDDG J. Dtsch. Dermatol. Ges.* **2008**, *6*, 1032–1037. [CrossRef] [PubMed]

46. Pathirana, D.; Hillemanns, P.; Petry, K.-U.; Becker, N.; Brockmeyer, N.H.; Erdmann, R.; Gissmann, L.; Grundhewer, H.; Ikenberg, H.; Kaufmann, A.M.; et al. Short version of the German evidence-based Guidelines for prophylactic vaccination against HPV-associated neoplasia. *Vaccine* **2009**, *27*, 4551–4559. [CrossRef] [PubMed]

47. Von Rosen, F.T.; von Rosen, A.J.; Müller-Riemenschneider, F.; Tinnemann, P. Awareness and knowledge regarding emergency contraception in Berlin adolescents. *Eur. J. Contracept. Reprod. Health Care* **2017**, *22*, 45–52. [CrossRef] [PubMed]

48. Von Rosen, A.J.; von Rosen, F.T.; Tinnemann, P.; Müller-Riemenschneider, F. Sexual Health and the Internet: Cross-Sectional Study of Online Preferences among Adolescents. *J. Med. Internet Res.* **2017**, *19*, e379. [CrossRef] [PubMed]

49. Center for Disease Control and Prevention. Sexually Transmitted Diseases Treatment Guidelines, 2015. *MMWR Recomm. Rep.* **2015**, *64*, 1–137.

50. Hoff, T.; Greene, L.; Davis, J. National Survey of Adolescents and Young Adults: Sexual Health Knowledge Attitudes and Experiences. Available online: https://kaiserfamilyfoundation.files.wordpress.com/2013/01/national-survey-of-adolescents-and-young-adults.pdf (accessed on 14 September 2017).

51. Samkange-Zeeb, F.; Mikolajczyk, R.T.; Zeeb, H. Awareness and knowledge of sexually transmitted diseases among secondary school students in two German cities. *J. Community Health* **2013**, *38*, 293–300. [CrossRef] [PubMed]

52. Sheeran, P.; Taylor, S. Predicting intentions to use condoms: A meta-analysis and comparison of the theories of reasoned action and planned behavior. *J. Appl. Soc. Psychol.* **1999**, *29*, 1624–1675. [CrossRef]

53. Von Elm, E.; Altman, D.G.; Egger, M.; Pocock, S.J.; Gøtzsche, P.C.; Vandenbroucke, J.P. Strengthening the reporting of observational studies in epidemiology (STROBE) statement: Guidelines for reporting observational studies. *BMJ* **2007**, *335*, 806–808. [CrossRef] [PubMed]

54. Amt für Statistik Berlin-Brandenburg. *Regionaler Sozialbericht Berlin und Brandenburg 2015*; Amt für Statistik Berlin-Brandenburg: Berlin, Germany, 2016.

55. Bundeszentrale für Gesundheitliche Aufklärung. Jugendsexualität. Wiederholungsbefragung von 14-bis 17-Jährigen und Ihren Eltern. Available online: https://publikationen.sexualaufklaerung.de/index.php?docid=227 (accessed on 17 September 2017).

56. Garside, R.; Ayres, R.; Owen, M.; Pearson, V.A.H.; Roizen, J. "They never tell you about the consequences": Young people's awareness of sexually transmitted infections. *Int. J. STD AIDS* **2001**, *12*, 582–588. [CrossRef] [PubMed]

57. Höglund, A.T.; Tydén, T.; Hannerfors, A.K.; Larsson, M. Knowledge of human papillomavirus and attitudes to vaccination among Swedish high school students. *Int. J. STD AIDS* **2009**, *20*, 102–107. [CrossRef] [PubMed]

58. Andersson-Ellstrom, A.; Forssman, L. Sexually transmitted diseases—Knowledge and attitudes among young people. *J. Adolesc. Health* **1991**, *12*, 72–76. [CrossRef]

59. Gale, M.; Hayen, A.; Truman, G.; Varma, R.; Forssman, B.L.; MacIntyre, C.R. Demographic and geographical risk factors for gonorrhoea and chlamydia in greater Western Sydney, 2003–2013. *Commun. Dis. Intell. Q. Rep.* **2017**, *41*, E134–E141. [PubMed]

60. Torrone, E.; Papp, J.; Weinstock, H.; Centers for Disease Control and Prevention (CDC). Prevalence of Chlamydia trachomatis genital infection among persons aged 14–39 years—United States, 2007–2012. *MMWR Morb. Mortal. Wkly. Rep.* **2014**, *63*, 834–838. [PubMed]

61. Balla, B.C.; Terebessy, A.; Tóth, E.; Balázs, P. Young Hungarian Students' Knowledge about HPV and Their Attitude toward HPV Vaccination. *Vaccines* **2016**, *5*, 1. [CrossRef] [PubMed]

62. Sopracordevole, F.; Cigolot, F.; Gardonio, V.; Di Giuseppe, J.; Boselli, F.; Ciavattini, A. Teenagers' knowledge about HPV infection and HPV vaccination in the first year of the public vaccination programme. *Eur. J. Clin. Microbiol. Infect. Dis.* **2012**, *31*, 2319–2325. [CrossRef] [PubMed]

63. Drago, F.; Ciccarese, G.; Zangrillo, F.; Gasparini, G.; Cogorno, L.; Riva, S.; Javor, S.; Cozzani, E.; Broccolo, F.; Esposito, S.; et al. A Survey of Current Knowledge on Sexually Transmitted Diseases and Sexual Behaviour in Italian Adolescents. *Int. J. Environ. Res. Public Health* **2016**, *13*, 422. [CrossRef] [PubMed]

64. Robert Koch-Institut. Mitteilung der Ständigen Impfkommission am RKI: Anwendung des Neunvalenten Impfstoffs Gegen Humane Papillomviren (HPV). Available online: https://search.datacite.org/works/10.17886/EPIBULL-2016-027 (accessed on 29 October 2017).

65. Deutsches Ärzteblatt. Urologen Empfehlen HPV-Impfung für Jungen. Available online: https://www.aerzteblatt. de/nachrichten/69265/Urologen-empfehlen-HPV-Impfung-fuer-Jungen (accessed on 29 October 2017).

66. De Visser, R. One size fits all? Promoting condom use for sexually transmitted infection prevention among heterosexual young adults. *Health Educ. Res.* **2005**, *20*, 557–566. [CrossRef] [PubMed]

67. De Graaf, H.; Vanwesenbeeck, I.; Meijer, S. Educational Differences in Adolescents' Sexual Health: A Pervasive Phenomenon in a National Dutch Sample. *J. Sex Res.* **2015**, *52*, 747–757. [CrossRef] [PubMed]

68. Santelli, J.S.; Lowry, R.; Brener, N.D.; Robin, L. The association of sexual behaviors with socioeconomic status, family structure, and race/ethnicity among US adolescents. *Am. J. Public Health* **2000**, *90*, 1582–1588. [PubMed]

69. Berliner Senatsverwaltung für Bildung, Jugend und Familie. Allgemeine Hinweise zu den Rahmenplänen für Unterricht und Erziehung in der Berliner Schule a V 27: Sexualerziehung. Available online: https://www.berlin.de/sen/bildung/unterricht/faecher-rahmenlehrplaene/rahmenlehrplaene/ mdb-sen-bildung-schulorganisation-lehrplaene-av27_2001.pdf (accessed on 17 September 2017).

70. Phillipson, L.; Gordon, R.; Telenta, J.; Magee, C.; Janssen, M. A review of current practices to increase Chlamydia screening in the community—A consumer-centred social marketing perspective. *Health Expect.* **2016**, *19*, 5–25. [CrossRef] [PubMed]

71. Millstein, S.G.; Igra, V.; Gans, J. Delivery of STD/HIV preventive services to adolescents by primary care physicians. *J. Adolesc. Health* **1996**, *19*, 249–257. [CrossRef]

72. Jones, K.; Baldwin, K.A.; Lewis, P.R. The potential influence of a social media intervention on risky sexual behavior and Chlamydia incidence. *J Community Health Nurs.* **2012**, *29*, 106–120. [CrossRef] [PubMed]

73. Oh, M.K.; Grimley, D.M.; Merchant, J.S.; Brown, P.R.; Cecil, H.; Hook, E.W. Mass media as a population-level intervention tool for Chlamydia trachomatis screening: Report of a pilot study. *J. Adolesc. Health* **2002**, *31*, 40–47. [CrossRef]

74. Stephenson, J.; Strange, V.; Forrest, S.; Oakley, A.; Copas, A.; Allen, E.; Babiker, A.; Black, S.; Ali, M.; Monteiro, H.; et al. Pupil-led sex education in England (RIPPLE study): Cluster-randomised intervention trial. *Lancet* **2004**, *364*, 338–346. [CrossRef]

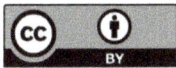

© 2018 by the authors. Licensee MDPI, Basel, Switzerland. This article is an open access article distributed under the terms and conditions of the Creative Commons Attribution (CC BY) license (http://creativecommons.org/licenses/by/4.0/).

International Journal of
Environmental Research and Public Health

MDPI

Article

Parents' Perspectives on Family Sexuality Communication from Middle School to High School

Jennifer M. Grossman *, Lisa J. Jenkins and Amanda M. Richer

Wellesley Centers for Women, Wellesley College, Wellesley, MA 02481, USA; ljenkins@wellesley.edu (L.J.J.); aricher@wellesley.edu (A.M.R.)
* Correspondence: jgrossma@wellesley.edu

Received: 18 December 2017; Accepted: 7 January 2018; Published: 10 January 2018

Abstract: Parents' conversations with teens about sex and relationships can play a critical role in improving teenage reproductive health by reducing teens' risky sexual behavior. However, little is known about how teen-parent communication changes from early to middle adolescence and how parents can tailor their communication to address their teens' changing development and experiences during these periods. In this longitudinal qualitative study, U.S. parents ($N = 23$) participated in interviews when their teens were in early adolescence, then again when the teens were in middle adolescence. Participants were largely mothers and were from diverse racial/ethnic and educational backgrounds. Thematic analysis was used to assess continuity and change in parents' perceptions of teen-parent communication. Findings showed that many parents adapted their conversations with their teens about sex and relationships as teens developed. Once teens had entered high school, more parents described feeling comfortable with their conversations. However, parents also more often reported that their teens responded negatively to the communication in high school than they had in middle school. These findings may help parents to anticipate their own as well as their teens' responses to family conversations about sex at different developmental time points and to strategize how to effectively talk with their teens about sex and relationships to improve their teens' overall reproductive health.

Keywords: teenage reproductive health; teen-parent relationships; family sexuality communication; adolescent development

---

1. Introduction

Teens' risky sexual behaviors, such as early sex, sex without a condom and having multiple partners have negative health outcomes [1]. Despite historically low birth rates for U.S. teens [2], rates continue to be higher than in other developed countries [3], and three out of four teen pregnancies in the U.S. are unintended [4]. Family conversations about sex and relationships provide one way to improve teen reproductive health by reducing teens' sexual risk behavior [5,6]; however, teen-parent conversations about sex are only effective at reducing teens' risk behavior when parents' match their messages about sex with their teen's developmental level and sexual experience [7,8]. Addressing teens' developmental level is particularly important as teens transition from early to middle adolescence, as youth experience rapid developmental change in identity, sexuality and relationships during this time period [9]. Family sexuality communication can be further inhibited by many parents' under-estimation of their teens' sexual behavior [10], which may make it difficult for parents' to effectively address teens' developmental needs and could prevent teens from obtaining knowledge they need to reduce their sexual risk behavior [11]. Despite the need for developmentally appropriate family conversations about sex and the challenges parents face in achieving this goal, with few exceptions [12] little research assesses family sexuality communication over the transition from early (11–14) to middle adolescence (15–17).

Shifts in teens' development from early to middle adolescence may complicate how parents talk with their teens about sex and how teens respond to these conversations. The transition from middle school to high school is a pivotal one for teen sexual activity. While 5–13% of adolescents report having had sex by 8th grade [13], 36% are sexually active by 10th grade [1]. By age 12, approximately 25% of teens report having had a romantic relationship, which doubles by age 15 [14]. To effectively navigate these changing roles and behaviors, many adolescents need information and support to negotiate social situations related to sex and relationships.

To support teens' health, parents may face challenges related to noticing changes in their teens' development and adapting their approaches to talking about sex and relationships to address them. Parents also need to be aware that teens' growth from early to middle adolescence brings shifts in teen-parent relationships [15] such as growing independence and expanding social networks [16,17], which may lead to less openness or engagement with parents on the issues going on in their lives. Teens also show increasing influence of peer versus parent relationships from early to middle adolescence [18]. Therefore, teens' questions and concerns related to sex and relationships, their willingness to talk with parents about sexual issues, and their ways of talking may change during this transition.

Many parents face their own challenges to talking effectively with their teens about sex and relationships. Barriers to parents' talk with their teens about sex include parents' lack of accurate information regarding sexual health, discomfort in talking about sex, and perceptions that their teens are not ready to talk about sex or engage in sexual activity [11,19]. Under-estimation of teens' sexual activity is an area where some parents' discomfort with their teens' sexuality can intersect with teens' development to impede effective teen-parent communication about sex. A large-scale study found that among sexually active teens, 55% of their parents incorrectly reported that their teens had not had sex, which may relate to social norms or parental beliefs against teen sex [10]. This has implications if parents' messages about sexuality do not match teens' needs and development. Inaccurate perceptions of teens' sexual experience may prevent parents from providing key guidance to their teens on sexual issues [11]. For example, parents' focus on delaying sex can be health-promoting for teens who have not had sex, but this message may miss the boat for sexually active teens, who might benefit more from information about protection methods to avoid pregnancy and sexually transmitted infections.

Parents' and teens' backgrounds also shape the content and style of sexuality communication, as well as its impact [20–25]. Much research investigates the role of teen and parent gender in family sexuality communication. The gender of both teens and parents can shape the frequency, content and impact of conversations. For example, parents are more likely to share messages with female than male teens that focus on abstinence and resisting a partner's advances [20]. Other research shows that teen girls are more likely than boys to talk with family members about sex [21]. Findings are mixed as to whether family communication about sex is more likely to affect sexual behavior of male or female teens [5,21]. Few studies have explored change over time in parents' sexuality communication with male and female teens. Family sexuality communication is also shaped by families' racial and ethnic backgrounds [22,23], and research suggests that this communication can protect teens of different racial and ethnic groups from risky sexual behavior [24,25]. The current study explores family communication about sex and relationships within a racially and ethnically diverse sample, but a comparison of racial/ethnic groups is beyond the scope of this paper.

While few studies assess continuity and change in parent-teen talk about sex and relationships, one quantitative study that followed adolescents over a 12-month period found that once teens became sexually active, parents' messages about sex focused more on issues such as how to choose a birth control method and recognize symptoms of sexually transmitted infections [12]. At the same time, cross-sectional research suggests that once teens become sexually active, they may be less likely to talk with parents about their sexual thoughts and experiences due to fear that their parents might judge them or worry about their sexual behavior [26,27] or concern that their parents may try to control their developing sexuality [28]. In contrast, a 4-year longitudinal study of late adolescents found that participants felt that both themselves and their parents became more comfortable and open in talking about sex over the course of college as they developed [29], consistent with growing mutuality in teen-parent relationships during emerging adulthood [30]. These studies suggest the importance of adolescents' development when understanding how parents and teens talk about sexuality. While the periods of early and middle adolescence include significant change in identity, sexuality and relationships, there is a gap in research assessing change in teen-parent talk about sex during this developmental transition.

The lack of studies on change over time in teen-parent sexuality communication and the critical importance of developmentally appropriate parental conversations with teens show the need for longitudinal research in this area. The current study provides a unique longitudinal examination of parents' perceptions of continuity and change in teen-parent communication from middle school to high school. The knowledge gained from this study will guide our understanding of how parents do or do not adapt their approaches to sexuality communication to teens' changing development and sexuality. It also explores the role of teen gender in shaping parents' approaches to talk with teens about sex and relationships and the content of these conversations.

2. Materials and Methods

2.1. Recruitment and Participants

Our interview sample consisted of parents of adolescents from three schools that participated in an evaluation of *Get Real: Comprehensive Sex Education That Works*, a three-year program developed by Planned Parenthood League of Massachusetts. *Get Real* is a comprehensive sexuality communication program which emphasizes delaying sex while providing medically accurate information about protection. It identifies parents as the primary sexuality educators of their children and includes supports for teens and their family members to talk with each other about sexuality and relationships. *Get Real* has been shown to be effective in delaying sex for middle school students [5]. Researchers interviewed participating parents twice: once when teens were in seventh grade and again when teens were in tenth grade. Schools were selected for the interview study because their student populations were demographically representative of the larger evaluation, which included 24 schools (see [5] for a further description of the evaluation study). Active consent was required for interview participation. A letter was distributed to inform parents about the interview study and to invite them to participate. Each school decided how consent forms were distributed (see Grossman and colleagues for details [31]). Approximately 177 parents/guardians were invited to participate in interviews, and 38 consent forms were returned, with four parents not consenting to participate. All parents who provided consent were contacted for an interview; 94% of those (32 parents/guardians) completed interviews (Time 1). Only one parent in each family was interviewed. Given the focus of the current study on teen-parent communication, three participating guardians (great aunt, grandmother, older sister) were excluded from this analysis. Each parent completed a demographic questionnaire.

Participating parents were invited to participate in follow–up interviews three years later, when parents had high school-aged teens (Time 2). Parents were contacted by e-mail and phone and asked to complete active consent forms for the follow-up study. Of the 29 original parent participants, 23 agreed to participate and completed interviews at Time 2, representing 79% of the original parent sample; 6 families were unreachable. For both Time 1 and Time 2, interviews were conducted over the phone primarily in English (2 were conducted in Spanish), took 30–45 min and were later transcribed and translated as needed. Parents were each given $25 in appreciation of their participation. Each participant was asked to create a code name to protect confidentiality; those pseudonyms are used here. All participating parents were provided with a resource list with contact information for organizations supporting youth and family social, emotional, and sexual health. At each time point, human subjects approval was granted from The Institutional Review Board at Wellesley College to conduct this work (January 2011 and December 2013). Only parents who participated in both Time 1 and Time 2 interviews were included in this paper. Within our sample of 23 parents, 20 parents were mothers and three parents were fathers. Fifty percent of participants self-identified as Black/African American, 13% as Hispanic/Latino, and 37% as White. Thirty-eight percent of participants reported completing high school or less education, 25% reported some college education, 29% reported college or additional education, and 8% did not respond to this question. Thirty-seven percent of participants reported single-parent status, 46% reported living in two-parent families, and 17% reported living with a parent as well as another adult family member. Demographics of participants who participated in both Time 1 and Time 2 interviews were similar to the 29 participants who participated in Time 1 interviews [31].

2.2. Interview Protocol

Prior to interviews, participants were reminded of the purpose of the study and reassured that it would be normal to feel a bit embarrassed or uncomfortable, and that they could choose not to answer any questions. Interview questions addressed parents' communication with their adolescent children about sex and relationships at each time point. Specifically, we asked parents about the content of their communication with their teens, their comfort with this communication, and their understanding and experiences of talking with their teens about sexual issues.

2.3. Data Analysis

We used thematic analysis to systematically identify themes in the interview data [32]. The first and second authors closely read the transcribed interviews and separately identified overarching themes in parents' Time 1 and Time 2 data that represented patterns in parents' perceptions and experiences of sexuality communication with their teens. The authors then coded interview data, reviewed and revised themes based on how they fit with coded data, defined and named them and developed sub-themes [33]. The themes were then compared across parents' Time 1 and Time 2 interviews to explore continuity and change in parents' perceptions of sexuality communication when teens were in middle school and high school. The themes were not mutually exclusive, in that one participant's responses could generate more than one code. The 1st and 3rd authors conducted reliability checks [34]. The intercoder reliability of 94% represented a high level agreement between the two coders. NVivo 10.0 (QSR International, Melbourne, Australia) [35] was used to facilitate coding.

3. Results

Six overarching themes emerged from parent interviews. The first three themes reflect parents' experiences of and approaches to communication with their teens about sex and relationships: Reasons for sexuality communication, Comfort (or discomfort) talking about sex, and Perceptions of teens' experiences of sexuality communication. The remaining themes focus on whether and how parents talk with their teens about specific content areas, namely Talk about dating & relationships, Talk about readiness for sex, and Talk about sexual risk and protection. See Table 1 for a comparison of themes for Time 1 and Time 2 interviews.

Table 1. Parents' perceptions of parent-teen sexuality communication at Time 1 and Time 2 (*N* = 23).

Theme	Time 1	Time 2
Reasons for sexuality communication		
Why talk more	18 (78%)	15 (65%)
Why talk less	9 (39%)	10 (43%)
Comfort talking about sex		
Comfort	15 (65%)	22 (96%)
Discomfort	9 (39%)	1 (4%)
Perceptions of teens' experiences of sexuality communication		
Positive Engagement	16 (70%)	15 (65%)
Negative Engagement	9 (39%)	15 (65%)

Table 1. *Cont.*

Theme	Time 1	Time 2
Talk about dating and relationships	21 (91%)	22 (96%)
Talk about readiness for sex		
Concrete reasons to delay sex	14 (61%)	9 (39%)
Emotional & relational reasons to delay sex	11 (48%)	11 (48%)
Talk about sexual risk & protection	22 (96%)	23 (100%)

3.1. Reasons for Sexuality Communication

In the *Reasons for sexuality communication* theme, parents talked about the reasons they talked more or talked less with their teens about sex and relationships with sub-themes of *Why talk more* and *Why talk less*. At Time 1, 78% (18/23) of parents described their reasoning for why they talked with their teens about sex, whereas 65% (15/23) of parents at Time 2 did so. Parents of male and female teens reported similar rates of why they talk at Time 1 and Time 2. Parents at both time points described a focus on protecting teens from future risk. At Time 1, Jada explained why she talked with her teens about sex, "I wanted to empower my kids by giving them the tools, the language, the understanding, because no matter how much you prepare your kids for situations that you would rather they not have an experience with, sometimes it doesn't pan out". Judy shared, "I would much rather [my children] ask me questions than just be blindsided by reality". Parents at Time 2 shared similar responses. Julia explained, "They're going to face all those things in life, so you have to talk about everything. I don't want them to be in pain and I want them to stay to school for their education and find someone to marry, to continue their life and have a family". Derrick explained, "I constantly always bring it [sex] up, you know, just to make sure she don't do nothing that I consider stupid".

Differences in reasons parents gave for talking with their teens about sex at Time 1 compared to Time 2 emerged. At Time 1, parents talked about the importance of teens getting accurate information about sexual issues and described teens initiating conversations about sex, whereas at Time 2, parents described talk about sex because of teens' interest or involvement in romantic and/or sexual relationships. For example, at Time 1 Maria explained, "I want my son to learn from me before he learns from one of his friends in school". Ellen explained why she talks with her daughter about sex, "so she's educated and she has the right information, and not the wrong information". Parents at Time 1 also described their teens' questions as a motivation for talking with them about sex. For example, Kevi said, "He [my son] actually brought it up. He had a few questions about sex and he wasn't sure if what he had heard was true". Another parent (Barbara) shared, "[My son] asked me the names of the parts of the penis and the names of the parts of the vagina, and then it was time to tell him how things really are." At Time 2, parents identified teens' interest or involvement in relationships as a reason for talking with them about sex. Alex explained her increased communication with her son about sex, "because he has a girlfriend, so we talk a lot more now." Susan shared, "I thought it was not necessary too much before because she wasn't really hooking up with people. But now she's more social and she's going to be more adult now. She wants to have a boyfriend, that's when I know it's probably the time".

A similar number of parents at Time 1 (39%, 9/23) and Time 2 (43%, 10/23) described why they rarely or never talked with their teens about sex. Parents at both time points described not talking with their teens because they perceived them as not being ready or mature enough to talk about sexual issues or due to perceptions that the teens were not interested or engaged in dating. At Time 1, parents were more likely to describe reasons why they did not talk with female (55%) than male teens (17%) about sex, but differences were less evident at Time 2 (females = 36%, males = 50%). At Time 1, Carmel explained, "She's too young right now. I don't want to put ideas in her head". Similarly, Rose shared, "We didn't go over details because she's just waiting to get her period, so she's kind of like a little girl still". At Time 2, Jasmine described why she doesn't talk with her daughter about sex, "I don't think she's ready. When she's ready, she'll come to me," Another parent at Time 2 (Marcia) explained why she rarely talks with her son about sex, "[Dating] is not one of his interests right now … so we don't have to talk about it".

3.2. Comfort Talking about Sex

The second theme relates to parents' Comfort (or discomfort) in talking with teens about sex with sub-themes of *Comfort* and *Discomfort*. More parents expressed comfort with sexuality communication at Time 2 (96%, 22/23) than at Time 1 (65%, 15/23). At Time 1, *Comfort talking about sex* was described more frequently by parents of female (82%) than male teens (50%), but differences were not evident at Time 2 (females = 100%, males = 92%). At Time 1, Cordelia shared, "I don't have any trouble talking to my kids about sex", while Julia stated, "I'm pretty comfortable, it's just that sometimes I don't know exactly what to say". At Time 2, many parents discussed ways in which their comfort talking about sex had grown since their children were in middle school, often related to perceived changes in their teens' increased age and maturity. For example, Jenny described talking with her daughter about sex, "I'm really comfortable. I feel she's older so she's able to understand a little bit more than she did in middle school". Barbara described what it's like to talk with her son in high school, "I feel more comfortable because [my son] is more of an adult. And he knows more about sex and about relationships". A third parent, Maria, described her growing ease in talking with her son about sex, "I think the maturity. He's bigger and it's he's somewhat more serious now. So we have good communication".

Several parents described discomfort in talking with their teens about sex at Time 1, (39%, 9/23), whereas only one parent described discomfort at Time 2 (4%, 1/23). At Time 1, parents more often described discomfort in talking with male (50%) than female teens (27%), but these differences were not evident at Time 2 (males = 8%, females = 0%). Some female parents at Time 1 described difficulties in talking with their sons about sexual issues. One mother, Alex, explained, "It's just the comfort of him being the male child. It feels weird for me to sit with my son and have these conversations". Some parents at Time 1 discussed the importance of talking with their children about sex despite their discomfort with these conversations. Jada explained, "I'm still somewhat uncomfortable … to me it's more the awkwardness of finding the right words at the right time. But, you know, the sigh of relief is, no matter how uncomfortable I am, I'm willing to do it". A father (Ryan) explained, "[My daughter] will just randomly ask like how old was I, or what age you think is too young [to have sex] and it kind of throws me off. But I do appreciate that it's open enough for her to ask me something like that".

3.3. Perceptions of Teens' Experiences of Sexuality Communication

The third theme, *Perceptions of teens' experiences of sexuality communication*, focuses on how parents perceive teens' behavioral and emotional responses to talking with a parent about sex with sub-themes of *Positive engagement* and *Negative engagement*. At both time points, parents described variation in teens' responses to talking with parents about sex, ranging from comfort and engagement to discomfort and avoidance. At Time 1 (70%, 16/23) and Time 2 (65%, 15/23) more than half of parents described ways their teens showed positive engagement in talking with them about sex. There were no evident differences in parents' reports of positive engagement of male or female teens at either Time 1 or Time 2. At Time 1, parents often described teens asking them questions, such as Ellen, whose daughter asked, "Mom, what's a dental dam?" Kevi described her son's communication about sex at Time 1, "He is continually asking questions. He's very open." Alex described her son's engagement when they talked about sexually transmitted infections, "I was like, 'That's the way that you can catch something that you can never, ever, ever get rid of because there's no medicine for it.' He was like 'For real?' I was like, 'Yeah, for real.'" At Time 2, parents described their perceptions of teens' engagement primarily through showing they were listening and seeming open and comfortable with conversations. For example, Jada described her son's response to her communication, "He kind of listens and just doesn't say anything. It's like he's putting it in his pocket somewhere, and maybe he'll use it someday." Marie talked about her children's response to her talk about sex, "They're so used to it that I think talking to me is just like, 'Oh, I'm talking to one of my friends'".

More parents described negative teen responses to talk about sex at Time 2 (65%, 15/23) than Time 1 (39%, 9/23), which include avoidance or negative reactions to parent talk about sex, such as appearing embarrassed or uncomfortable and saying they already knew the information parents provided. There were no evident differences in parents' reports of negative engagement of male or female teens at either time point. At Time 1, Jean described her son's response to her and her husband raising the topic of sex "He just kind of looked at us with a blank look like, 'Shut up. I don't want to hear it.'" Parents described similar struggles at Time 2, and some pointed out an increased level of discomfort with talking about sex as teens got older. For example, Kevi shared about her son, "he just seemed more open when he was younger than he is now. I think he gets more embarrassed." Lynn stated, "I talk all the time [about sex] and he rolls his eyes." Jasmine described her daughter's response to her raising sexual topics, "She'll say, 'Ma, I already know. I already know'".

3.4. Talk about Dating and Relationships

The next three themes described the content of parents' conversations with their teens related to sex and relationships. The first content theme addresses how parents and teens *Talk about dating and relationships*. Almost all participating parents at Time 1 (91%, 21/23) and Time 2 (96%, 22/23) reported talking with their teens about this topic. However, the content of these conversations differed for Time 1 and Time 2. At Time 1, the most common focus of conversation described by parents was rules for teen dating and relationships, while at Time 2 conversations focused more on teens' interest or involvement in dating and how to have a healthy relationship. There were no evident differences in parents' frequency of talk with male or female teens about dating and relationships at either Time 1 or Time 2. At Time 1, Jean explained how she talks with her son about dating: "He's girl-crazy right now and my husband and I are very adamant about there's no need for thirteen year olds to have relationships. 'It's normal to have those feelings. It's the self-control and acting on them that you have to really remember what you were taught and realize that that's not okay, because it can go further.'" Cordelia shared a similar message with her daughter about dating at Time 1: "I think it's premature now, they're 13. I tell them I don't know the number because I don't know how mature they're going to be at age X. So I'd rather not put an age out there until I see them at that age." Other parents at Time 1 described giving their children permission to do some level of dating, but set limits on what activities were permitted. For example, Tiffany explained her message to her son, "If you see a girl that you particularly like, okay fine. You can go to McDonalds, you can go to the movies. But you know, that's pretty much it".

In contrast, at Time 2 many parents described conversations about teens' interest or involvement in relationships and how to have a healthy relationship as opposed to rules about dating. Parents also reported that some of these conversations were initiated by teens. For example, Jasmine shared, "I can say she's a teenager right now and she tells me things like people like her or this boy likes her." Cordelia reported, "We're constantly having discussions about their feelings—they find this one attractive, they find that one attractive." Parent-teen conversations about healthy relationships often included feedback to teens on how to be in a healthy relationship. For example, Daisy shared the messages she passes on to her son, "I gave him advice about dating, that he's young and he's going to meet a lot of girls but don't get into a really serious relationship. Just get to know the person." Kevi described a conversation with her son, "I always tell him how to have respect for his girlfriend and it will come back to him as well, and never to be in a bad relationship".

3.5. Talk about Readiness for Sex

The second content theme, *Talk about readiness for sex*, includes sub-themes of *Concrete reasons to delay sex* and *Emotional and relational reasons to delay sex*. Concrete reasons for delay focus on specific time points or life events such as finishing school, getting married, or reaching a certain age (e.g., 18, 21) before having sex. At Time 1, 61% (14/23) of parents described talking with their teens about concrete reasons to delay sex, whereas only 39% (9/23) of parents at Time 2 reported talking about this issue. At both Time 1 (males = 75%, females = 46%) and Time 2 (males = 50%, females = 27%), parents more often described talking with male than female teens about concrete reasons to delay sex. At Time 1, delaying sex until finishing school or getting married were the two primary points of discussion. For example, Daisy shared, "Before you make any decisions about having sex, I really want you to have your education finished, go to college." Jean stated, "For us sex comes after marriage, which is a covenant with God. So there's nothing outside of marriage that makes sex okay." Some parents raised both these issues, such as Barbara, "I told him he has to wait until getting married to start a relationship with a girl. I think education comes first." As with Time 1, at Time 2 some parents described conversations about finishing school and waiting until a teen was older before having sex. For example, Ellen stated, "You're too young; you need to live life. Get an education; go to college. Leave the state; see the world." Jada described a conversation with her children about when they're old enough to have sex, "I tell them 'I hope you're at least twenty-one before you do.'" In contrast, delaying sex until marriage was rarely discussed at Time 2.

The second sub-theme for *Talk about readiness for sex* addressed emotional or relational reasons for delay focused on teens' emotional maturity and being in a close, committed relationship before having sex. Half of parents at both Time 1 (48%, 11/23) and Time 2 (48%, 11/23) described talking with their teens about emotional or relational reasons for delay. At Time 1 parents more often described talking with male (58%) than female teens (36%) about emotional or relational reasons to delay sex, but this was not evident at Time 2 (males = 50%, females = 46%). Parents described similar content of conversations at both time points. For example, at Time 1 Lynn shared, "I have stressed to both of my sons the importance of being really ready and really in love before having sex. That it's not something to be casual about." Similarly, Rose explained how she talks with her daughter about sex, "I want her to be in love, not to feel cheap or any of that type of thing. I want her to be really ready." At Time 2, Marie shared her advice to her daughter, "I feel like if you have self-respect and maturity, that's going to really help you decide when the time's right for you. If you love yourself enough, you're not going to need to have sex with someone to define yourself." Cordelia described her advice to her daughter about sex, "focus on being in a loving relationship with somebody that doesn't hurt you, that you're committed to and he's committed to you".

3.6. Talk about Sexual Risk and Protection

The third content theme addresses how parents and teens *Talk about sexual risk and protection*. Most parents at Time 1 (96%; 22/23) and all parents at Time 2 (100%; 23/23) reported talking with their teens about this topic often emphasizing teen pregnancy and parenting, sexually transmitted infections (STIs), and protection methods. There were no evident differences in parents' frequency of talk with male or female teens about sexual risk and protection at either Time 1 or Time 2.

Parents at both time points described talking with teens about teen pregnancy and parenting, focusing on the hardships of teen parenthood. Some parents talked with their children about the challenges that they or other family members faced as teen parents. At Time 1, Ellen described talking with her daughter about her own mother's struggles as a teen parent, "My mother had me at 15. We talk about that a lot, and I tell her how my mother's life was not easy. She had a really, really hard time for a lot of years." At Time 2, Marcia described how she talks with her son about her own experiences, "I just always tell him, 'Don't be like me, because life is hard.' You know? And probably if I had waited until I was older, then I would have more education and stuff like that and then now it wouldn't be such struggle." At Time 2, many parents elaborated on the importance of taking responsibility for teen parenting roles. For example, Carmel shared, "I say, 'You're going to take care of the child yourself. You and your partner—wherever he is—are going to take care of it [your child] yourself. I have raised mine, so that's your responsibility." Similarly, Julia explained what she said to her son about getting someone pregnant, "If you have a lady who gets pregnant, you know what's going to happen? In tenth grade? You have to leave school. You have to work at McDonalds, because I'm not going to take care of more people than what I'm taking care of now".

Parents at both time points talked about risks of sexually transmitted infections (STIs). At Time 1, Tiffany warned her son about STIs, "I try to let that be known that you hear about the girls going around doing blowjobs and stuff, but you can still pick up STDs through blowjobs. So I know it seems so open, but I really feel like they need to know this." Marie shared, "I tell my children, 'It's so much more than you just laying down and having sex.' there could be unwanted pregnancies, it could be a death sentence, or an STD." Similarly, at Time 2, Rose explained to her daughter, "You just have to be careful of sex with different people and people carry diseases and that type of thing".

Parents at both time points described talk with their teens about the importance of using protection methods, particularly condoms, to avoid pregnancy and STIs. Parents' description of conversations with their teens at both time points included general directives to use protection and specific plans to access condoms. At Time 1, Daisy described her comments to her son, "You've got to be careful. There's a lot of diseases. You've got to wear a condom.' Tiffany explained, "I can tell him 'no' until I'm blue in the face, but you know, he gets that urge and he still wants to try it, he's going to try it regardless. We try to let him know when that time comes, just come to us and his dad will give him the condoms or he gets some sort of access to condoms." Parents at Time 2 passed on similar messages. For example, Carmel recalled a conversation with her daughter, "All I say is: 'If you do get ready [to have sex], make sure your partner has condoms, and if they don't, you're not having any. You might get anything: gonorrhea, syphilis, anything that it has no cure for. Then, what you going to do?'" Judy explained how she talked about protection with her son, "When he's ready to take that step [having sex], he made that vow that he's going to come to me and I told him it may seem weird to some people, but I'll be the first one to go out and buy him condoms." In contrast, a small minority of parents expressed concerns that providing condoms might encourage their teens to have sex. For example, at Time 1, Marcia recalled a conversation with her son, "He tells me that he has it [a condom] in his locker at school. I said, 'Uh-uh. Don't keep it there at school. Bring it home. When you have it in school, you might get ideas'".

4. Discussion

This study is one of the few to longitudinally investigate teen-parent communication about sex and relationships and the only one to our knowledge that explores continuity and change in parents' perspectives of sexuality communication. It provides an opportunity to explore how parents navigate talking with their teens about sex and relationships among a diverse group of parents in the context of change in teens' development as well as teen-parent relationships from early to middle adolescence. This study explores how parents approach conversations with their teens about sex and relationships, what they talk about, how they perceive their teens' reactions to these conversations and finally, the role of teen gender in this communication.

This study's findings show that many parents adapted their conversations with their teens about sex and relationships as teens developed. For example, parents at Time 2 noted that teens' expressed interest in dating motivated parents to talk with their teens about sex and relationships, which was not evident at Time 1. Similarly, parents' approaches to talking with teens about dating shifted from rules and restrictions at Time 1 to discussions of relationship experiences and how to have healthy relationships at Time 2, which suggests an awareness of teens' changing developmental needs from middle school to high school. Further, more parents at Time 1 than Time 2 talked with their teens about concrete landmarks for delaying sex (e.g., finishing school, turning 18, getting married). This may indicate parents' awareness of teens' growing autonomy in making their own decisions about sexual behavior or growing acceptance of sex as a normative part of teens' experience as they get older. With few exceptions, parents in this sample showed shifting approaches to talk with teens from middle school to high school which suggest parents' responsiveness to teens' development. Despite parents' shifts over time toward more positive approaches to teens' relationships, their conversations with teens about sex remained focused on its negative consequences, rather than addressing any potential benefits.

A complexity with parents' responsiveness to perceived changes in teens' development is that parents may not always accurately perceive teens' interest in or readiness for relationships and sex. For example, some parents described delaying talk with their teens about sex due to a belief that their child was not interested in dating. Whereas some parents may accurately perceive their teens' lack of interest in dating or relationships, other parents may under-estimate teens' involvement in relationships and sexual activity [10]. A longitudinal study of the timing of parent-teen conversation about sex found that over 40% of teens have sex before having conversations with parents about protection methods or sexually transmitted infections [12]. Waiting until teens themselves raise questions about sex or until teens are perceived as "ready" may prevent parents from providing key guidance to their teens on sexual issues [11,36].

In contrast to changing parental approaches to conversations with teens about dating and sex, communication about teen pregnancy, STIs, and protection methods showed little change in frequency or content over time. The high level of parent communication about these topics indicates that parents see these issues as educational for their teens. However, the lack of change in content from early to middle adolescence suggests that parents may not yet perceive their teens as immediately at risk for pregnancy or STIs even in the high school sample. Further interviews with parents of teens who are later in high school or post-high school could inform whether parents approach these conversations differently with a late adolescent/emerging adult sample.

The findings from this paper also show a complex interplay between parents' and teens' shifting responses to talk about sex over time. Many parents described their own growing comfort in talking with teens about sex and relationships as teens got older and they described high school-aged teens as more able to understand and discuss sexual issues. However, more parents at Time 2 than Time 1 noticed teens' negative responses to parents' comments about sex or relationships, consistent with prior research identifying teens' reluctance to talk with parents about sex when adolescents become sexually active [26,27]. These findings may help to explain challenges parents and teens face in talking with each other about sex and relationships, particularly later in adolescence. Parents' level of comfort (or discomfort) and teens' engagement (or lack of) with talk about sex may fluctuate over time and could impede effective communication. However, even when parents expressed discomfort with talking with teens about sex and relationships, they often described their commitment to talking despite this discomfort. Similarly, a study of mothers' communication with teens about sex found that "mothers push through their discomfort . . . because they believe the stakes are too high" (p. 317) [36]. Elliot suggests that by anticipating and normalizing teens' resistance to talking with parents about sex, parents can more effectively overcome these barriers.

Teen gender also shaped parent comfort and engagement with sexuality communication as well as its content, particularly at Time 1. Parents were more likely to describe reasons for not talking with their daughters than sons about sex and relationships, often referring to their daughters' lack of readiness to discuss sexual issues and perceptions of them as "little girls". This may reflect parents' reluctance to see their teen daughters as sexual beings, which has been suggested in prior work on parents' attitudes toward teen girls' sexuality [20]. This may also be reflected in parents' lower frequency of reported talk with their daughters than sons at Time 1 about delaying sex. While research suggests that parents are more likely to talk with daughters than sons about abstinence [20], some parents may postpone these conversations with daughters until middle adolescence as they don't yet perceive early adolescent girls as ready to engage with sexual issues. Interestingly, despite parents' lower frequency of talk with their daughters than sons, they describe more comfort in talking about sex with daughters than sons. Some mothers specifically discussed discomfort in talking with sons because of their gender. This complements prior findings that teens can be more comfortable talking with same-sex family members about sex and relationships [37].

Parents' and teens' struggles to talk with one another about sex and relationships and the role of gender in these interactions suggest the importance of exploring other teen resources for conversations about sex, in addition to parents. Research shows that over half of teens talk with extended family, such as stepmothers, grandparents, uncles, cousins, and siblings about sex [38,39]. This is particularly relevant for Black and Latino teens, who more often have non-parental family members involved in their upbringing [40,41]. Teens also talk with peers about sex and relationships, although findings suggest that these conversations are not always health-promoting [42,43]. Further research is needed to understand the role non-parental relationships play in talking with teens about sex and relationships and whether and how this communication can support teens' health.

In the current sample of highly engaged parents, parents were likely to talk with teens despite their own and their teens' discomfort in addressing sexual issues. However, this persistence may not be typical among a more representative parent sample. Families' participation in a school-based sex education program may also have increased their engagement with family sexuality communication. Finding ways to include parents who are less engaged in family sexuality communication in research studies would help to assess to what extent this study's findings are generalizable to a broader population. In addition, the sample size is small and results should therefore be seen as preliminary. Future research would also benefit from a matched, longitudinal design that includes perspectives on family sexuality communication from both parents and teens when teens are in early and middle adolescence, which would provide a comparison to how parents may perceive (or misperceive) their teens' responses to conversations about sex and relationships. While analysis by racial and ethnic group is beyond the scope of this study, their role in shaping family conversations about sex and relationships [22,23] suggests that future studies would benefit from exploring similarities and differences across racial and ethnic groups. Additionally, interactions of family sexuality communication and social class would help to understand variation across family contexts. Finally, it is important to include more fathers in research on family sexuality communication, a group that is under-represented in this area of study [24]. Inclusion of fathers could provide insight into how their perspectives on talking with teens about sex and relationships over time are similar or different than those of mothers, who represented the majority of the current sample.

These findings provide evidence of parents' responsiveness to their teens' age, development and experiences in their conversations with teens about sex and relationships. However, combined with prior research on parents' under-reporting of teens' sexual behavior [11], this study's findings raise questions about whether some parents may wait too long to begin talking with their teens about sex and relationships, which could impact teen's sexual health by resulting in unwanted teen pregnancies or sexually transmitted infections. This study also reiterates the challenges of talking with teens about issues that often make both teens and their parents uncomfortable and highlights developmental shifts that may make parent-teen conversations easier or more difficult at different stages of adolescent development. To counter teen resistance, parents may need to make extra efforts to engage teens in open and non-judgmental ways. These findings may help parents to anticipate their own as well as their teens' responses to family conversations about sex at different developmental time points, normalizing potential negative responses and helping parents to strategize how to overcome both their own and teens' discomfort to achieve effective communication about sex and relationships.

5. Conclusions

Family sexuality communication can provide a protective tool to improve public health outcomes by reducing teen pregnancy and sexually transmitted infections. However, in order to talk effectively with teens about sex and relationships, parents need to talk with teens in ways that developmentally fit their age and experiences. Talking with teens about sex is a challenge for many parents [11,19] and the added complexity of matching it with teens' development is not an easy task. Health education programs that include outreach to parents can help to increase parents' skills and comfort in talking with teens about sex and relationships [44,45]. While some school and community-based programs provide guidance for parents, more resources/supports are needed to provide parents with the tools they need to support teens' reproductive health and reduce these public health concerns. Since parents are one key resource for teens' sexuality communication [46], helping them to talk in open and

Int. J. Environ. Res. Public Health **2018**, *15*, 107

developmentally appropriate ways with their teens and manage potential challenges of their own and their teens' discomfort in talking about sex and relationships can make a difference in supporting teens' reproductive health.

Acknowledgments: This work was supported by the Eunice Kennedy Shriver National Institute of Child Health and Human Development: R03HD073381 and by Wellesley Centers for Women. The authors are grateful for editorial feedback from the Wellesley Centers for Women Writing Group.

Author Contributions: Jennifer M. Grossman conceived of the paper, collected the data and wrote the majority of the paper. Jennifer M. Grossman and Lisa J. Jenkins analyzed the data and wrote up study findings. Amanda M. Richer did a reliability check on study analyses, contributed to writing the discussion section and made major edits to the paper.

Conflicts of Interest: The authors declare no conflict of interest. The founding sponsors had no role in the design of the study; in the collection, analyses, or interpretation of data; in the writing of the manuscript, and in the decision to publish the results. The content is solely the responsibility of the authors and does not necessarily represent the official views of the National Institutes of Health.

References

1. Kann, L.; McManus, T.; Harris, W.A.; Shanklin, S.L.; Flint, K.H.; Hawkins, J.; Queen, B.; Lowry, R.; Olsen, E.O.; Chyen, D.; et al. Youth risk behavior surveillance—United States, 2015. *MMWR Surveill. Summ.* **2016**, *65*, 26–28.

2. Martin, J.A.; Hamilton, B.E.; Osterman, M.J.; Driscoll, A.K.; Mathews, T.J. Births: Final data for 2015. *Nat. Vital Stat. Rep.* **2017**, *66*, 1–70.

3. Sedgh, G.; Finer, L.B.; Bankole, A.; Eilers, M.A.; Singh, S. Adolescent pregnancy, birth, and abortion rates across countries: Levels and recent trends. *J. Adolesc. Health* **2015**, *56*, 223–230. [CrossRef] [PubMed]

4. Finer, L.B.; Zolna, M.R. Declines in unintended pregnancy in the United States, 2008–2011. *N. Engl. J. Med.* **2016**, *374*, 843–852. [CrossRef] [PubMed]

5. Grossman, J.M.; Tracy, A.J.; Charmaraman, L.; Ceder, I.; Erkut, S. Protective effects of middle school comprehensive sex education with family involvement. *J. Sch. Health* **2014**, *84*, 739–747. [CrossRef] [PubMed]

6. Murry, V.M.; McNair, L.D.; Myers, S.S.; Chen, Y.-F.; Brody, G.H. Intervention induced changes in perceptions of parenting and risk opportunities among rural African American youth. *J. Child Fam. Stud.* **2014**, *23*, 422–436. [CrossRef]

7. Clawson, C.L.; Reese-Weber, M. The amount and timing of parent-adolescent sexual communication as predictors of late adolescent sexual risk-taking behaviors. *J. Sex Res.* **2003**, *40*, 256–265. [CrossRef] [PubMed]

8. Miller, K.S.; Levin, M.L.; Whitaker, D.J.; Xu, X. Patterns of condom use among adolescents: The impact of mother-adolescent communication. *Am. J. Public Health* **1998**, *88*, 1542–1544. [CrossRef] [PubMed]

9. Greydanus, D.E.; Pratt, H.D.; Merrick, J. Sexuality in childhood and adolescence. In *Sexuality: Some International Aspects*; Merrick, J., Greydanus, D.E., Eds.; Nova Science: Hauppauge, NY, USA, 2016; pp. 1–31.

10. Mollborn, S.; Everett, B. Correlates and consequences of parent-teen incongruence in reports of teens' sexual experience. *J. Sex Res.* **2010**, *47*, 314–329. [CrossRef] [PubMed]

11. Malacane, M.; Beckmeyer, J.J. A review of parent-based barriers to parent–adolescent communication about sex and sexuality: Implications for sex and family educators. *Am. J. Sex. Educ.* **2016**, *11*, 27–40. [CrossRef]

12. Beckett, M.K.; Elliott, M.N.; Martino, S.; Kanouse, D.E.; Corona, R.; Klein, D.J.; Schuster, M.A. Timing of parent and child communication about sexuality relative to children's sexual behaviors. *Pediatrics* **2010**, *125*, 34–42. [CrossRef] [PubMed]

13. Centers for Disease Control and Prevention (CDC), 1995–2015 Middle School Youth Risk Behavior Survey Data. Available online: http://nccd.cdc.gov/youthonline/ (accessed on 8 December 2017).

14. Carver, K.; Joyner, K.; Udry, J.R. National estimates of adolescent romantic relationships. In *Adolescent Romantic Relations and Sexual Behavior: Theory, Research, and Practical Implications*; Florsheim, P., Florsheim, P., Eds.; Lawrence Erlbaum: Mahwah, NJ, USA, 2003; pp. 23–56, ISBN 978-0805838305.

15. Grotevant, H.D.; Cooper, C.R. Patterns of interaction in family relationships and the development of identity exploration in adolescence. *Child Dev.* **1985**, *56*, 415–428. [CrossRef] [PubMed]

16. Wray-Lake, L.; Crouter, A.C.; McHale, S.M. Developmental patterns in decision-making autonomy across middle childhood and adolescence: European American parents' perspectives. *Child Dev.* **2010**, *81*, 636–651. [CrossRef] [PubMed]

17. Zimmerman, B.; Cleary, T. Adolescents' development of personal agency: The role of self-efficacy beliefs and self-regulatory skill. In *Self-Efficacy Beliefs of Adolescents*; Pajares, F., Urdan, T., Eds.; Information Age: Charlotte, NC, USA, 2006; pp. 45–70.

18. Dishion, T.J.; Piehler, T.F.; Myers, M.W. Dynamics and ecology of adolescent peer contagion. In *Understanding Peer Influence in Children and Adolescents*; Prinstein, M.J., Dodge, K.A., Eds.; Guilford: New York, NY, USA, 2008; pp. 72–93.

19. Pariera, K.L. Barriers and prompts to parent-child sexual communication. *J. Fam. Commun.* **2016**, *16*, 277–283. [CrossRef]

20. Kuhle, B.X.; Melzer, D.K.; Cooper, C.A.; Merkle, A.J.; Pepe, N.A.; Ribanovic, A.; Verdesco, A.L.; Wettstein, T.L. The 'birds and the bees' differ for boys and girls: Sex differences in the nature of sex talks. *Evol. Behav. Sci.* **2015**, *9*, 107–115. [CrossRef]

21. Kapungu, C.T.; Baptiste, D.; Holmbeck, G.; McBride, C.; Robinson-Brown, M.; Sturdivant, A.; Crown, L.; Paikoff, R. Beyond the 'birds and the bees': Gender differences in sex-related communication among urban African-American adolescents. *Fam. Proc.* **2010**, *49*, 251–264. [CrossRef] [PubMed]

22. Hutchinson, M.K.; Montgomery, A.J. Parent communication and sexual risk among African Americans. *West. J. Nurs. Res.* **2007**, *29*, 691–707. [CrossRef] [PubMed]

23. Moncloa, F.; Wilkinson-Lee, A.M.; Russell, S.T. Cuídate sin pena: Mexican mother-adolescent sexuality communication. *J. Ethn. Cult. Divers. Soc. Work* **2010**, *19*, 217–234. [CrossRef]

24. Guilamo-Ramos, V.; Goldberg, V.; Lee, J.J.; McCarthy, K.; Leavitt, S. Latino adolescent reproductive and sexual health behaviors and outcomes: Research informed guidance for agency-based practitioners. *Clin. Soc. Work J.* **2012**, *40*, 144–156. [CrossRef] [PubMed]

25. Fletcher, K.D.; Ward, L.M.; Thomas, K.; Foust, M.; Levin, D.; Trinh, S. Will it help? Identifying socialization discourses that promote sexual risk and sexual health among African American youth. *J. Sex Res.* **2015**, *52*, 199–212. [CrossRef] [PubMed]

26. Golish, T.; Caughlin, J. "I'd rather not talk about it": Adolescents' and young adults' use of topic avoidance in stepfamilies. *J. Appl. Commun. Res.* **2002**, *30*, 78–106. [CrossRef]

27. Crohn, H.M. Communication about sexuality with mothers and stepmothers from the perspective of young adult daughters. *J. Divorce Remarriage* **2010**, *51*, 348–365. [CrossRef]

28. O'Sullivan, L.F.; Meyer-Bahlburg, H.F.L.; Watkins, B.X. Mother-daughter communication about sex among urban African American and Latino families. *J. Adolesc. Res.* **2001**, *16*, 269–292. [CrossRef]

29. Morgan, E.M.; Thorne, A.; Zurbriggen, E.L. A longitudinal study of conversations with parents about sex and dating during college. *Dev. Psychol.* **2010**, *46*, 139–150. [CrossRef] [PubMed]

30. Koepke, S.; Denissen, J.J.A. Dynamics of identity development and separation-individuation in parent-child relationships during adolescence and emerging adulthood—A conceptual integration. *Dev. Rev.* **2012**, *32*, 67–88. [CrossRef]

31. Grossman, J.M.; Charmaraman, L.; Erkut, S. Do as I say, not as I did: How parents talk with early adolescents about sex. *J. Fam. Issues* **2016**, *37*, 177–197. [CrossRef]

32. Braun, V.; Clarke, V. Using thematic analysis in psychology. *Qual. Res. Psychol.* **2006**, *3*, 77–101. [CrossRef]

33. Sandelowski, M. Theoretical saturation. In *The Sage Encyclopedia of Qualitative Research Methods*; Given, L., Ed.; SAGE: Thousand Oaks, CA, USA, 2008; pp. 875–876.

34. Miles, M.B.; Huberman, A.M. *Qualitative Data Analysis: An Expanded Sourcebook*, 2nd ed.; SAGE: Thousand Oaks, CA, USA, 1994.

35. QSR International. *NVivo Qualitative Data Analysis Software*; Version 10; QSR International: Melbourne, Australia, 2012.

36. Elliott, S. Talking to teens about sex: Mothers negotiate resistance, discomfort, and ambivalence. *Sex. Res. Soc. Policy* **2010**, *7*, 310–322. [CrossRef]

37. Caughlin, J.P.; Golish, T.D.; Olson, L.N.; Sargent, J.E.; Cook, J.S.; Petronio, S. Intrafamily secrets in various family configurations: A communication boundary management perspective. *Commun. Stud.* **2000**, *51*, 116–134. [CrossRef]

38. Grossman, J.M.; Tracy, A.J.; Richer, A.M.; Erkut, S. The role of extended family in teen sexual health. *J. Adolesc. Res.* **2015**, *30*, 31–56. [CrossRef] [PubMed]
39. Harper, G.W.; Timmons, A.; Motley, D.N.; Tyler, D.H.; Catania, J.A.; Boyer, C.B.; Dolcini, M.M. 'It takes a village': Familial messages regarding dating among African American adolescents. *Res. Hum. Dev.* **2012**, *9*, 29–53. [CrossRef] [PubMed]
40. Jones, D.J.; Zalot, A.A.; Foster, S.E.; Sterrett, E.; Chester, C. A review of childrearing in African American single mother families: The relevance of a coparenting framework. *J. Child Fam. Stud.* **2007**, *16*, 671–683. [CrossRef]
41. Stanton-Salazar, R.D. *Manufacturing Hope and Despair: The School and Kin Support Networks of U.S.-Mexican Youth*; Teachers College Press: New York, NY, USA, 2001.
42. Epstein, M.; Ward, L.M. 'Always use protection': Communication boys receive about sex from parents, peers, and the media. *J. Youth Adolesc.* **2008**, *37*, 113–126. [CrossRef]
43. Trinh, S.L.; Ward, L.M.; Day, K.; Thomas, K.; Levin, D. Contributions of divergent peer and parent sexual messages to Asian American college students' sexual behaviors. *J. Sex Res.* **2014**, *51*, 208–220. [CrossRef] [PubMed]
44. Kirby, D.; Miller, B.C. Interventions designed to promote parent teen communication about sexuality. In *Talking Sexuality: Parent-Adolescent Communication*; Feldman, S., Rosenthal, D., Eds.; Jossey-Bass: San Francisco, CA, USA, 2002; pp. 93–110.
45. Santa Maria, D.; Markham, C.; Bluethmann, S.; Mullen, P.D. Parent-based adolescent sexual health interventions and effect on communication outcomes: A systematic review and meta-analyses. *Perspect. Sex. Reprod. Health* **2015**, *47*, 37–50. [CrossRef] [PubMed]
46. Albert, B. *With One Voice 2010: America's Adults and Teens Sound Off About Teen Pregnancy*; The National Campaign to Prevent Teen and Unplanned Pregnancy: Washington, DC, USA, 2010.

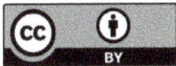

© 2018 by the authors. Licensee MDPI, Basel, Switzerland. This article is an open access article distributed under the terms and conditions of the Creative Commons Attribution (CC BY) license (http://creativecommons.org/licenses/by/4.0/).

International Journal of
Environmental Research and Public Health

MDPI

Article

"I Am Ready and Willing to Provide the Service . . . Though My Religion Frowns on Abortion"— Ghanaian Midwives' Mixed Attitudes to Abortion Services: A Qualitative Study

Prince Oppong-Darko [1,*], Kwame Amponsa-Achiano [2] and Elisabeth Darj [1,3,4]

[1]   Department of Public Health and Nursing, NTNU, Norwegian University of Science and Technology, 7491 Trondheim, Norway; elisabeth.darj@ntnu.no
[2]   Public Health Division, Ghana Health Service, Accra, Ghana; kaash8@yahoo.com
[3]   Department of Obstetrics and Gynecology, St Olav's Hospital, 7030 Trondheim, Norway
[4]   Department of Women's and Children's Health, Uppsala University, 75185 Uppsala, Sweden
*   Correspondence: quaqudarko@yahoo.co.uk; Tel.: +47-9189-7729

Received: 27 October 2017; Accepted: 28 November 2017; Published: 4 December 2017

Abstract: Background: Unsafe abortion is a major preventable public health problem and contributes to high mortality among women. Ghana has ratified international conventions to prevent unwanted pregnancies and provide safe abortion services, legally authorizing midwives to provide induced abortion services in certain circumstances. Objective: The aim of the study was to understand midwives' readiness to be involved in legal induced abortions, should the law become less restricted in Ghana. Methods: A qualitative study design, with a topic guide for individual in-depth interviews of selected midwives, was adopted. The interviews were tape-recorded and analyzed using content analysis. Results: Participants emphasized their willingness to reduce maternal mortalities, their experiences of maternal deaths, and their passion for the health of pregnant women. Knowledge of Ghana's abortion law was generally low. Different views were expressed regarding readiness to engage in abortion services. Some expressed it as being sinful and against their religion to assist in abortion care, whilst others felt it was good to save the lives of women. Conclusion: The midwives made it clear that unsafe abortions are common, stigmatizing and contributing to maternal mortality, issues that must be addressed. They made various suggestions to reduce this preventable tragedy.

Keywords: unsafe abortions; midwives perception; authorization; Ghana

1. Introduction

Despite agreeing to adhere to international conventions, unsafe abortion remains a major public health challenge in Ghana [1]. The World Health Organization (WHO) defines unsafe abortion as a procedure for terminating an unintended pregnancy carried out either by persons lacking the necessary skills or in an environment that does not conform to minimal medical standards, or both. This definition comprises practices that create hazardous circumstances before, during, or after an abortion [2].

It is estimated that around 22 million unsafe abortions occur annually worldwide, and almost all of these are in developing countries [3]. Recent data estimate that 44,000 deaths occur due to unsafe abortion and that a disproportionate two-thirds of all abortion-related deaths occur in Africa [4].

Ghana has ratified numerous international charters and conventions, including the Universal Declaration of Human Rights and the United Nations Sustainable Development Goals (SDG). All countries are responsible for achieving SDGs, including the reduction of the global maternal mortality ratio to 70 per 100,000 live births by 2030, and unsafe abortion is one of the most common causes of maternal morbidity and mortality. However, many countries have laws that are generally against induced abortion, and abortion is only permitted to be performed under certain circumstances [3].

The Provincial National Defence Council Law, section 58 of Act 29 of 1960, amended 1985, regulates abortion in Ghana. The Act states that, "Abortion is unlawful and both the woman and anyone who abets the offence by facilitating the abortion by whatever means, are guilty of an offense of causing abortion" [1]. However, abortion is permitted under some circumstances: when pregnancy is the result of rape, defilement, or incest; if its continuation would involve risk to the life of the pregnant woman; if the pregnancy will injure the woman's physical or mental health; or there is a substantial risk that the child may suffer from a serious physical abnormality or disease. Under any of these circumstances, abortion is permitted [1]. In 2006, the Ministry of Health and Ghana's Health Service developed standards for the provision of comprehensive abortion care. Midwives have since then been authorized to provide early legal abortion in accordance with the law. The main idea behind the authorization was the shortage of physicians in the country. The WHO has established the minimum threshold of doctors, nurses, and midwives deemed necessary to deliver essential maternal and child health services at 23 per 10,000 people. Ghana, with limited numbers of health worker resources, currently has only 11 per 10,000, serving 28 million inhabitants [5]. The aim of shifting the task of performing abortions from physicians to midwives is to reduce the number of illegal and unsafe abortions.

Realizing that authorized and well-trained midwives can provide competent and safe abortion-related services and that providing these safe services may reduce the amount of maternal deaths, governments have modified their laws and policies so as to include and empower midwives in providing abortion services [6] and some are considering the expansion of these services to include non-essential abortions. Unsafe abortions account for 11% of all maternal deaths, which is currently 319 per 100,000 live births in Ghana [5]. Midwives are trained as part of their curriculum to use manual vacuum aspiration (MVA) for post-abortion care in case of complications after miscarriage. However, little is known about midwives' readiness and willingness to offer abortion services in Ghana. A successful expansion of the provision of safe abortion services would largely depend on the midwives and their motivation, knowledge, and readiness to provide abortion services. Studies have been performed in Ghana to explore the potential providers' perceptions of abortion services [7], but none have specifically looked at midwives' readiness to engage in these services, should the law be changed to make abortion less restricted. In order to frame the interpretation of the results from this present study, the socio-ecological model, first introduced by Bronfenbrenner, will be used in the discussion [8,9]. This model will make it easier to understand midwives' views at different levels in society, as well as their own and others' roles in preventing unnecessary and preventable maternal mortalities caused by unsafe and illegal abortions. The aim of this study was to explore midwives' readiness for the provision of safe abortion services in Ghana.

2. Material and Methods

2.1. Study Design

A qualitative study design was used for the study. This design was chosen due to its ability to explore the participants' attitudes and perceptions, through a prepared topic guide, covering areas of interest. Further, for a deeper understanding of issues, which were brought up by the respondents, their narratives were structured in subcategories and categories. A qualitative study aims to explore a phenomenon by answering questions of "how" instead of by counting numbers and answering questions of "what" or "how many" [10]. The midwives perceptions, experiences, and views would not have been able to catch using a quantitative survey. Individual in-depth interviews were preferred and employed, due to the sensitive nature of the topic. We anticipated that discussing potential illegal matters in a group could be a hindrance to obtaining open and in-depth information about their perceptions.

2.2. Study Setting

The study was conducted in a district in Western Ghana, with the majority of the inhabitants living in rural areas. The district has one government health center and nine smaller clinics.

2.3. Study Participants

The single inclusion criterion was that participants were practicing midwives in the district. All midwives were invited to take part voluntarily, with the aim of gaining a broad variation of views. No specific exclusion criteria were set in relation to age, gender, or length of work experience; however, no retired midwives were invited to participate. Mobile phone numbers for the eligible midwives were provided by the District Health Directorate. Text messages were sent to each midwife by the first author to inform them about the study. Each midwife was then called and asked whether they would like to receive more information about the study. If they agreed, they were sent printed copies of detailed information about the study, and a consent form. All written material was available in both English and Twi, the local language. Seven out of nine invited midwives agreed to take part in the study.

2.4. Data Collection

A convenient date and time for the interview was agreed with each of the midwives. Data for this study were collected using a semi-structured topic guide for individual in-depth interviews, covering areas such as the midwives' views on their own profession regarding engagement in abortion services, their perceptions on the existing law, and their knowledge about the practices used for performing abortions. The interviews were conducted in Twi, a language that the participants were comfortable with and which was also spoken by the interviewer. The interviews were recorded using a voice recorder after seeking permission from the participants. The recorded audios were transcribed verbatim and translated into English for analysis, in order to include the non-Twi speaking collaborator.

2.5. Data Analysis

Content analysis, as described by Graneheim and Lundman, was used to analyze the data, in order to obtain the manifest meaning of the discussions [10]. Transcripts were read several times by the researchers, to allow them to become familiar with the text. Using Nvivo 11 (QRS International, Melbourne, Australia), the meaning units were condensed and coded. The coded groups were created into sub-categories, which were merged into categories, depending upon their associated findings. The categories and subcategories were discussed between the researchers until consensus was reached.

2.6. Ethical Reflection

This study was conducted in accordance with the Declaration of Helsinki, and the protocol was approved by the Regional Committee for Medical and Health Research Ethics (REK 2016/874) at NTNU, Norway, and the Ghana Health Service Ethical Review Committee. Consent was sanctioned from the District Directors of Health Services. All midwives gave their informed consent before they participated in the study. Participants were informed that, when the transcriptions of the recordings were made, the voice recording would be deleted, that it would not be possible to trace who said what during the individual interviews, and that results would only be provided at a group level. It was also made clear that, if they wanted to withdraw their consent, they could contact the researchers afterwards but before the analysis was completed. No monetary reimbursement was given to the participants.

3. Results

Seven practicing midwives participated, with ages ranging from 31 to 59 years. Their working experience ranged from 2 to 20 years. The individual midwives are referred to in the quotes as MW, with numbers 1–7. During the analysis, three main categories were identified, out of eight subcategories, from the individual in-depth interviews (Table 1).

Table 1. Categories and subcategories from participants' responses.

Categories	Subcategories
Motivation to be a midwife	Passion for maternal health
	Previous experiences
	Lack of professional opportunities
Unsafe abortions common and hidden	Stigmatization
	Unsafe abortion practices
The law and abortion	Knowledge and ignorance of existing law
	Views on abortion law
	Willingness to provide safe abortion care

3.1. Motivation to Be a Midwife

3.1.1. Passion for Maternal Health

Midwives described how a strong desire for improving the health of pregnant women had motivated them to choose midwifery as a profession. They used the word "passion" and expressed the need that someone who is educated should care for women to avoid preventable ill health. They described experiences that had motivated them in their choice of profession. Living in a rural area had made them see the importance of having access to a health facility, especially to antenatal services. Furthermore, they were aware of positive outcomes where pregnant women were well cared for.

My main motivation is to help improve the health of pregnant women and to help save their lives. (MW2)

I wanted to provide care for pregnant women. I have a passion for the health of pregnant women. (MW3)

The midwives were highly aware of the high level of mortality that occurs among young pregnant women in Ghana and wished to improve the situation. The knowledge of these mortalities was a strong motivating factor for becoming a midwife and an issue that they wanted to help to reduce. They appreciated that their profession as educated midwives provided them with the possibility to assist in preventing maternal mortalities in dangerous situations.

I want to help reduce maternal mortalities. (MW4)

I studied nursing before midwifery, so during my training as a nurse, I made up my mind that I needed to study midwifery so that I could help to reduce maternal mortalities. (MW1)

Midwives expressed worries that maternal mortality is high in deprived areas of the country due to the apparent low access to antenatal services. They emphasized that pregnant women in rural communities without health facilities are at a high risk of maternal death, and they showed motivation and readiness to work in rural areas to help improve access to safe motherhood.

Women in rural areas who are usually poor do not have access to quality maternal health services during pregnancy. I did midwifery so that I could add to the few numbers of midwives so that maternal health will be accessible to pregnant women irrespective of where they live. (MW5)

3.1.2. Previous Experiences

These midwives were also community members and had been raised in rural areas. They had seen and heard of the dangers during pregnancies and deliveries and of the disastrous consequences after unsafe abortions. They were influenced by what they had learned and witnessed in the areas in which they lived during their childhood and youth. Mothers had told their daughters about maternal deaths, which they remembered. The study revealed that participants had become midwives due to such previous experiences. These participants revealed that they had heard several stories of maternal deaths in their community due to a lack of access to health care. This motivated them to become midwives so that they would help to save the lives of women in their communities.

> When I was growing up I used to hear about women going into labor and dying, especially in the community I was living. My mother also told me about these issues. I also saw some myself that a woman . . . died. All [these] stories and what I heard encouraged me to study nursing and for that matter went ahead to study midwifery. (MW1)

3.1.3. Lack of Professional Opportunities

An alternative perception that was disclosed was that nothing special had motivated the participants to become midwives. Becoming a midwife was the only available opportunity and not necessarily the desired profession. They described how they wanted to get a professional job and secure their own income. They may initially have wanted to do something else and admitted that they became midwives only because they did not have the opportunity to pursue their desired career. However, as they expressed, they did not see any other possibility, and, given that they had been accepted on the midwifery education program, they had accepted this opportunity. Nothing came forward during the interviews about whether they now appreciated this choice or not.

> For me, nothing motivated me, I was interested in becoming a disease control officer. I opted for midwifery when I did not get the opportunity to study disease control. I needed to develop my career and midwifery was the only available opportunity. (MW7)

3.2. Unsafe Abortions Are Common and Hidden

3.2.1. Stigmatization

Midwives admitted that unsafe abortion practices are common in the communities, and that living and working there, and having to take care of women with related complications made them well aware of it. However, abortions are hidden procedures, as it is perceived to be a taboo and not spoken about openly, except with very close friends, and hardly ever with health care providers. The midwives explained that society frowns on abortions and stigmatizes those who seek abortion services and those who provide the service alike.

> It is something that goes on in the communities and because of the stigma attached to abortion, women who do abortions always do it under the cover of darkness. (MW7)

> . . . relating to unsafe abortions, it is unknown because of the way society perceives abortion. People hide to do it. (MW3)

Another opinion expressed was that the extent of unsafe abortion was unknown, because victims only seek their help when there are complications. They said that they were not aware of the magnitude of illegal and unsafe abortions in society; however, they were regularly contacted when complications arose.

> People do in the blindside of society, so it is something that goes on, but because of how society perceives it, it only comes to us when the victim suffers complications. When unsafe abortion is done and the victim does not suffer any complication, we do not hear about it. (MW5)

3.2.2. Unsafe Abortion Practices

The participants expressed worries about how pregnancies are terminated outside health facility settings. They emphasized that the methods used were dangerous and were the cause of complications of unsafe abortions. The midwives were aware of many crude ways in which women attempted to terminate pregnancies, such as the use of herbal mixtures to drink or as an enema, administering un-prescribed drugs, ground-up bottles mixed with Guinness beer, or the insertion of cassava sticks or herbs in the vagina. They described how the use of misoprostol (Cytotec®), normally used in postpartum hemorrhages, was known and used illegally for the termination of a pregnancy.

> *Some prepare herbal concoction and get it into the body through enema. The herbal concoction then forces the fetus to fall out. Some also use grinded bottles mixed with Guinness for enema. This is very dangerous! (MW5)*

> *Some use enema or drink all kinds of herbal concoctions, some insert Cytotec into the vagina; yes, they know about Cytotec! Some also drink un-prescribed drugs which they buy from the local drug stores. (MW7)*

> *Some insert herbs in the vagina. Some also use sticks; cassava stick, they insert it into the vagina. (MW6)*

3.3. The Law and Abortion

3.3.1. Knowledge and Ignorance of Existing Law

As described above, abortion is a crime under the laws of Ghana, and only permitted under certain circumstances. A common misunderstanding revealed in the interviews was concerning the legality of performing an induced abortion. Participating midwives could not demonstrate a good understanding of the abortion laws and some misinterpreted the nature of Ghana's abortion laws, while others described that they understood all abortions to be legal in Ghana. This interpretation was apparent in both old and young midwives.

> *I know that abortion is legal under the law, so if someone walks in and you are trained, you can do it for the woman. Also, if a pregnant woman attempts an unsafe abortion, you can complete it for her. (MW5)*

> *Abortion is legal in Ghana. If you get pregnant and you feel you do not want it, the law allows you to terminate the pregnancy. (MW1)*

3.3.2. Views on the Current Abortion Law

There was a general perception that legalizing abortion and making it accessible would increase the number of abortions that occur in the country. The participants who had the correct knowledge and perceptions of Ghana's abortion law thought that the law was satisfactory in its current state. They described how they thought that abortions should not be wholly legalized.

> *I do not support the termination of any pregnancy outside what the law allows. I feel that the law is good. (MW7)*

> *Providing safe abortion services should be done within the remit of the law. It should not like abortions to be allowed for every unwanted pregnancy. But if it affects the health of the pregnant women, then why not! Such a pregnancy can be terminated and that is what the law allows. (MW4)*

3.3.3. Willingness to Provide Safe Abortion Care

The participants expressed mixed views about whether safe abortion care should be offered, assuming it was legalized and could be provided on maternal request. Despite their concerns about maternal mortalities and the habit of performing unsafe, hidden abortions, expressions came forward that they felt abortion was against their religious beliefs—that it was sinful and they did not want to be involved. Those who shared this view were, however, ready to help in situations of incomplete abortions and miscarriages.

> *I am not ready and I am not willing to provide comprehensive abortion services where a woman can just walk to me and ask for an unwanted pregnancy to be terminated. The best I may offer is when the woman comes with an incomplete abortion, in that case, I will help complete the abortion for her ... I would rather refer a woman who needs comprehensive abortion care to the nearest health facility where the service is provided. (MW1)*

> *Seriously for me, it is against my religious belief and that does not allow me to provide abortion services. I can provide clients with pre-abortion counselling, but not to do the actual abortion. (MW4)*

Others felt that, although abortion was against their religious beliefs, they were ready to provide abortion care within the remit of the law, in order to save lives. They were of the opinion that it is always better to save lives than to allow the women to perish from preventable causes.

> *Providing safe abortion services and making it readily available and accessible is one way of preventing maternal deaths. For me, I am ready and willing to provide the service ... though my religion frowns on abortion, but I see this profession as a duty call, devoid of religious and moral judgement. It's more important that our women do not die from these kinds of avoidable deaths. (MW2)*

4. Discussion

It is an undeniable fact that unsafe abortions are one of the main causes of maternal mortality and morbidity [2,4]. In order to save women's lives, there is an urgent need to address the setbacks that hinder the progress of improving maternal health in the developing world. In this study, we focus on midwives' views of their potential role in the prevention of unsafe abortions and its consequences. Our results relating to the perceptions of a willingness to diminish inequality are seen from the perspective of the socio-ecologic theoretical framework, initially described by Bronfenbrenner and developed by others into four different levels: individual, relationship, community, and policy levels [11,12].

At an individual level, the midwives are concerned about the consequences of unsafe abortions. They have experiences of maternal deaths and were motivated to save lives, but simultaneously they have mixed feelings about personally engaging in abortion services. They are well aware of the illegal methods and procedures that are used, as they have a duty to deal with any complications that arise. Despite their awareness and concerns, they expressed a reluctance to participate in actual comprehensive abortion services; however, they did not object to providing post-abortion care when this was needed. They were more willing to help by referring women to the nearest health facility where abortion services were available and related this to their personal religious beliefs. This finding is also revealed in another study, where various health care professionals were interviewed and expressed conflicting dilemmas between their religious and moral beliefs about the sanctity of life and their duty to provide safe abortion care [7]. This attitude is likely to hinder midwives from providing safe abortion services. However, abortion is a sensitive topic worldwide; it raises ethical, cultural, moral, and religious questions wherever it is debated, and strong personal beliefs contribute to opposing the procedure, as revealed in research from South Africa [13]. Religious beliefs did not prevent some of the interviewed midwives from providing abortion care; however, as they perceived their profession as a duty and need to help prevent deaths from unsafe abortions, this overruled their personal feelings.

The American College of Nurse-Midwives conducted a survey among their members to determine their attitudes towards abortions, and the results showed that 79% supported unlimited access to abortion and that 52% supported abortion practice by nurse-midwives [14]. However, in another study, abortion procedures have been known to be hindered due to a lack of nurses who are willing to assist physicians with the procedure [15].

Regarding the relationship level, couples need to be able to plan the size of their families and to decide whether and when to have a child, as well as the age gap between children. Having access to modern contraceptives is important, as it will decrease the amount of unwanted pregnancies and, consequently, unsafe abortions [4]. This will further reduce the burden of the ethical dilemma that the midwives expressed. Smaller family sizes will reduce poverty, increase financial capital within the family, and may give children the possibility of participating in higher levels of education than their parents did. However, in many developing countries, fertile women are less likely to use modern contraceptives [16]. Three out of every 10 women of reproductive age in Ghana had an unmet need for contraception in 2014 [17]. A Greek study shows that cultural differences significantly affect contraceptive behavior. Nevertheless, interventions that promote contraception can still be successful in other populations [18]. Thus, contraceptives should be made readily accessible, affordable, and acceptable for use by people in relationships.

In relation to the community level, midwives in this study chose the profession because they wanted to care for pregnant women in their communities. They have much concern for reducing maternal deaths, a finding that is similar to those of a study in Papua New Guinea, in which midwifery students expressed the same motivation for choosing their profession [19]. As a result, they experience frustration about the number of unsafe abortions in their communities, which contribute to maternal losses. However, abortions do evoke religious, moral, ethical, and medical concerns. Abortion can be highly stigmatizing and poses challenges; both to the pregnant women, and health care providers and researchers. The midwives expressed that pregnant women were stigmatized in the community, whether they just talked about it or had an abortion [6]. Another study has reported similar negative attitudes among health providers towards women seeking abortions, and these are frequently driven by socio-cultural and religious norms, and contribute further to the stigmatization [7]. Midwives in this study felt that they were also frowned upon if they engaged in this service. However, where health care providers were exposed to higher levels of education, including training overseas, this seemed to result in more positive, less stigmatizing views towards the need for safe abortion services [7].

On a policy level, the health system has the responsibility to provide policies and legislation with the aim to improve and ensure the health and well-being of the people of Ghana. The legalization of the safe abortion care service is a human rights imperative, and making abortions accessible and affordable, together with improved access to contraceptives, will be an important step towards reducing the high maternal mortality ratio in Ghana. Studies report that health professionals who do not support safe abortion often lack sufficient knowledge of current legislation in their countries [20]. Health centers are the first level of primary care in rural areas, and these are usually managed by a midwife or a trained community health nurse. This study showed that midwives had limited understanding of the abortion law in Ghana, and could not clearly state the position of the law regarding safe abortion care. Contrary to this law, some midwives believe that abortion is fully legalized and hence, any person who does not want a pregnancy can request abortion at any health facility and be provided a safe service. This finding contradicts the high level of knowledge found among doctors in a similar study in Ghana [1]. Although some participants showed strong feelings about unsafe abortions and its consequences, any modification of the abortion law to make it legal was, for some, not appreciated. The successful implementation of any health sector reform is dependent on the acceptance and willingness of health professionals to implement the desired change, and midwives can play a key role in this.

There was a fear among the midwives in this study that the numbers of unsafe abortions would increase if the laws were less restrictive; however, legalization in other countries has not confirmed this concern [21]. Haddad and Nour, in their review of unsafe abortion globally, demonstrated that liberalizing abortion laws is correlated with a reduction in the rate of abortion-related morbidity and mortality [21]. However, these studies are mainly from high-income countries, as similar studies are scarce from low-income countries. When abortions are performed by skilled providers using appropriate medical techniques and drugs, and under hygienic conditions, induced abortion is a safe medical procedure. A remarkable decline in the abortion rate has been seen in developed countries where abortion is available on request and contraception readily accessible [21–23].

However, less restrictive abortion laws do not guarantee safe abortions for all in need. In India, despite abortions being legal, women with low levels of education still turn to unqualified local providers for abortion, if access is limited [24]. Complications arising from unsafe abortions are common, which the midwives in this study were very much aware of. Estimates from 2012 indicate that 6.9 million women in developing regions were treated for complications from unsafe abortions [4]. The treatment of medical complications places a considerable financial burden on women and on the public health care systems, which have limited resources and funds to devote to health services [4].

4.1. Trustworthiness

Measures were taken to promote the trustworthiness of this study [25]. Credibility was ensured as the study was undertaken by two Ghanaian researchers, both of whom work within the public health sector, are fluent in the Twi language, and are familiar with the study settings. The international researcher, an obstetrician, has experience of conducting reproductive health research in Africa and other developing regions, and is knowledgeable in qualitative research methods. Using a semi-structured interview guide, audio recording the interviews, providing verbatim transcription, and employing a systematic process of data analysis enhanced the confirmability of the results. Transferability was achieved by providing a detailed description of the methodology and setting. In addition to the detailed description of the methods, the same researcher conducted all seven individual in-depth interviews within a period of one month to increase the consistency of data and to achieve dependability.

4.2. Strengths and Limitations of the Study

The strength of this study is the qualitative approach, as, to our knowledge, no such study has previously been performed among midwives in Ghana. In order to structure the findings we used the socio-ecological model, which was suitable as it argues that individual behavior is shaped by factors at multiple levels, including individual, community, and policy levels in addition to intrapersonal and interpersonal levels [9]. A strength of this study was that interviews were performed individually, as using FGDs was anticipated as having the potential to deter the participants from disclosing their personal views on this sensitive matter.

A limitation could be that only nine midwives were available in the chosen district. More information may have been achieved if more midwives were available, or if a second district was included. However, the researcher felt that the midwives spoke freely and openly about their feeling and perceptions regarding abortions, and no more information came up after the sixth interview. One more interview was made to ensure the saturation of the material. More information may have surfaced if doctors and community members had been included in this study, but this was not the aim of this first study.

5. Conclusions

By interviewing practicing midwives in primary health care, we found that a change in the current Ghanaian abortion law to make abortion legal and to make the service available and safe, would need clarification across the health system and the provision of training and leadership support to the providers in the health facilities. As there is a shortage of physicians in the country, midwives will be the potential future providers of comprehensive abortion care, in order to reduce the tragic and preventable deaths among pregnant women who choose a dangerous, unsafe method to terminate an unwanted pregnancy. Midwives will need support, guidelines, supervision, orientation on the behavior necessary to boost confidence in providing safe abortion care, further repeated training, and the necessary equipment.

The community should be made aware of the knowledge that health providers already have: that the high numbers of maternal deaths in Ghana are partly because of unsafe abortions. Awareness of the possibility of saving lives if abortions were legal and discussion with stakeholders are necessary steps towards making a change. Further, the Ghanaian government needs to promote and make known the declarations that have already been signed and the responsibility that has been guaranteed in order to follow the international standards and the United Nations Sustainable Development Goals.

Guidelines must be disseminated and support given to the primary health providers for giving Ghanaian women access to safe health care, including abortions. Simultaneously, it is important that policy-makers not only make abortion legal but also make family planning methods accessible, as this has been proven to be one of the successes that contributes to reducing the amount of abortions in other countries.

Acknowledgments: The authors wish to express their sincere appreciation to the participating midwives, who willingly shared their views on unsafe abortions occurring in the country. Furthermore, we thank Marion Okoh-Owusu, District Director of Health Services, and the members of the District Health Management Team for their support and contribution during the data collection process. Funding for this study was received from the Norwegian University of Science and Technology, NTNU.

Author Contributions: P.O.-D. and E.D. conceived and designed the study. P.O.-D. conducted all interviews and data collection. P.O.-D. and E.D. analyzed and interpreted the data. P.O.-D. wrote the first draft of the manuscript. E.D. and K.A.-A. read and made substantial revisions to the manuscript and references. All authors have approved the submitted version.

Conflicts of Interest: The authors declare no conflicts of interest.

References

1. Morhe, E.S.K.; Morhe, R.A.S.; Danso, K.A. Attitudes of doctors toward establishing safe abortion units in Ghana. *Int. J. Gynecol. Obstet.* **2007**, *98*, 70–74. [CrossRef] [PubMed]
2. Ahman, E.; Shah, I. *Unsafe Abortion: Global and Regional Estimates of the Incidence of Unsafe Abortion and Associated Mortalities in 2008*, 6th ed.; WHO: Geneva, Switzerland, 2008; Volume 6, pp. 1–55. Available online: http://apps.who.int/iris/bitstream/10665/44529/1/9789241501118_eng.pdf (accessed on 2 November 2017).
3. World Health Organization. Safe Abortion: Technical and Policy Guidance for Health Systems. 2012. Available online: http://www.ncbi.nlm.nih.gov/pubmed/23700650 (accessed on 6 November 2017).
4. Singh, S.; Maddow-Zimet, I. Facility-Based Treatment for Medical Complications Resulting from Unsafe Pregnancy Termination in the Developing World, 2012: A Review of Evidence from 26 Countries. *BJOG Int. J. Obstet. Gynaecol.* **2016**, *123*, 1489–1498. [CrossRef] [PubMed]
5. World Health Organization (WHO). Achieving the Health-Related MDGs. It Takes a Workforce! WHO, 2014. Available online: http://www.who.int/hrh/workforce_mdgs/en/ (accessed on 20 May 2017).
6. Hord, C.E.; Delano, G.E. The Midwife's Role in Abortion Care. *Midwifery* **1994**, *10*, 136–141. [CrossRef]
7. Aniteye, P.; Mayhew, S.H. Shaping legal abortion provision in Ghana: Using policy theory to understand provider-related obstacles to policy implementation. *Health Res. Policy Syst.* **2013**, *11*, 23. [CrossRef] [PubMed]
8. Bronfenbrenner, U. Ecology of the family as a context for human development: Research perspectives. *Dev. Psychol.* **1986**, *22*, 723–742. [CrossRef]
9. Kumar, S.; Quinn, S.C.; Kim, K.H.; Musa, D.; Hilyard, K.M.; Freimuth, V.S. The social ecological model as a framework for determinants of 2009 H1N1 influenza vaccine uptake in the United States. *Health Educ. Behav.* **2012**, *39*, 229–243. [CrossRef] [PubMed]

10. Graneheim, U.H.; Lundman, B. Qualitative content analysis in nursing research: Concepts, procedures and measures to achieve trustworthiness. *Nurse Educ. Today* **2004**, *24*, 105–112. [CrossRef] [PubMed]

11. HEISE, L.L. Violence Against Women: An integrated, ecological framework. *Violence Against Women* **1998**, *4*, 262–290. [CrossRef] [PubMed]

12. Pun, K.D.; Infanti, J.J.; Koju, R.; Schei, B.; Darj, E. Advance Study Group on behalf of the AS. Community perceptions on domestic violence against pregnant women in Nepal: A qualitative study. *Glob. Health Action* **2016**, *9*, 31964. [CrossRef] [PubMed]

13. Harries, J.; Stinson, K.; Orner, P. Health care providers' attitudes towards termination of pregnancy: A qualitative study in South Africa. *BMC Public Health* **2009**, *9*, 296. [CrossRef] [PubMed]

14. Position Statement Midwives' Provision of Abortion-Related Services. Available online: http://www.internationalmidwives.org/assets/uploads/documents/PositionStatements-English/PS2008_011ENGMidwivesProvisionofAbortionRelatedServices.pdf (accessed on 14 March 2017).

15. Kade, K.; Kumar, D.; Polis, C.; Schaffer, K. Effect of nurses' attitudes on hospital-based abortion procedures in Massachusetts. *Contraception* **2004**, *69*, 59–62. [CrossRef] [PubMed]

16. Osei Kuffuor, E.; Esantsi, S.F.; Tapsoba, P.; Quansah-Asare, G.; Askew, I. Introduction of Medical Abortion in Ghana. Available online: http://www.popcouncil.org/uploads/pdfs/2011RH_IntroMedAbortionGhana.pdf (accessed on 24 Februrary 2017).

17. Service, G.S. Ghana Demographic and Health Survey. *Stud. Fam. Plan.* **2014**, *21*, 1–5.

18. Tsikouras, P.; Koukouli, Z.; Psarros, N.; Manav, B.; Tsagias, N.; Galazios, G. Contraceptive behaviour of Christian and Muslim teenagers at the time of abortion and post-abortion in Thrace, Greece. *Eur. J. Contracept. Reprod. Health Care* **2016**, *21*, 462–466. [CrossRef] [PubMed]

19. Moores, A.; Catling, C.; West, F.; Neill, A.; Rumsey, M.; Samor, M.K.; Homer, C.S. What Motivates Midwifery Students to Study Midwifery in Papua New Guinea? *Pac. J. Reprod. Health* **2016**, *1*, 60–67.

20. Abdi, J.; Gebremariam, M.B. Health providers' perception towards safe abortion service at selected health facilities in Addis Ababa. *Afr. J. Reprod. Health* **2011**, *15*, 31–36. [PubMed]

21. Haddad, L.B.; Nour, N.M. Unsafe abortion: Unnecessary maternal mortality. *Rev. Obstet. Gynecol.* **2009**, *2*, 122–126. [PubMed]

22. WHO. *Abortion Rates Drop in More Developed Regions but Fail to Improve in Developing Regions*; WHO: Geneva, Switzerland, 2016. Available online: http://www.who.int/reproductivehealth/news/abortion-rates/en/ (accessed on 6 November 2017).

23. Bardin, C.W.; Robbins, A.; O'Connor, B.M.; Spitz, I. Medical Abortion. *Curr. Ther. Endocrinol. Metab.* **1997**, *6*, 305–311. [PubMed]

24. Mundle, S.; Elul, B.; Anand, A.; Kalyanwala, S.; Ughade, S. Increasing Access to Safe Abortion Services in Rural India: Experiences with Medical Abortion in a Primary Health Center. *Contraception* **2007**, *76*, 66–70. [CrossRef] [PubMed]

25. Shenton, A.K. Strategies for ensuring trustworthiness in qualitative research projects. *Educ. Inf.* **2004**, *22*, 63–75. [CrossRef]

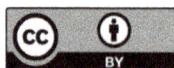

© 2017 by the authors. Licensee MDPI, Basel, Switzerland. This article is an open access article distributed under the terms and conditions of the Creative Commons Attribution (CC BY) license (http://creativecommons.org/licenses/by/4.0/).

MDPI
St. Alban-Anlage 66
4052 Basel
Switzerland
Tel. +41 61 683 77 34
Fax +41 61 302 89 18
www.mdpi.com

International Journal of Environmental Research and Public Health Editorial Office
E-mail: ijerph@mdpi.com
www.mdpi.com/journal/ijerph

www.ingramcontent.com/pod-product-compliance
Lightning Source LLC
Chambersburg PA
CBHW051852210326
41597CB00033B/5864